MULTICULTURAL NEUROREHABILITATION

Jay M. Uomoto, PhD, is a rehabilitation psychologist and neuropsychologist and the Training Director for the Clinical Neuropsychology Postdoctoral Residency Program at the Veterans Affairs Northern California Health Care System. He is a Fellow of the National Academy of Neuropsychology and a Fellow of the American Psychological Association, Division 22—Rehabilitation Psychology, and he is Certified in Health Care Ethics. Prior to his current position, Dr. Uomoto served in the Department of Veterans Affairs Central Office as the National Mental Health Director for Veterans Affairs/Department of Defense Collaboration and was a Deputy Director for the Defense Centers of Excellence for Psychological Health and Traumatic Brain Injury. He also served on the faculty of the Department of Rehabilitation Medicine at the University of Washington and Emory University, in the Department of Clinical Psychology at Seattle Pacific University, and in the Department of Neuropsychology at the Barrow Neurological Institute.

MULTICULTURAL NEUROREHABILITATION

CLINICAL PRINCIPLES FOR REHABILITATION PROFESSIONALS

Jay M. Uomoto, PhD

EDITOR

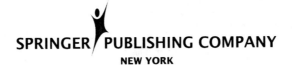

SPRINGER PUBLISHING COMPANY

NEW YORK

Springer Publishing Company, LLC
11 West 42nd Street
New York, NY 10036
www.springerpub.com

Acquisitions Editor: Nancy S. Hale
Production Editor: Michael O'Connor
Composition: Westchester Publishing Services

ISBN: 978-0-8261-1515-7
e-book ISBN: 978-0-8261-1528-7

15 16 17 18 19 / 5 4 3 2 1

Unless otherwise stated, the opinions expressed in this book are those of the individual authors and do not represent the official position of the Department of Veterans Affairs, Department of Defense, U.S. government, or any specific VA facility or program.

Library of Congress Cataloging-in-Publication Data
Multicultural neurorehabilitation : clinical principles for rehabilitation professionals / edited by Jay M. Uomoto.
  p. ; cm.
Includes bibliographical references.
ISBN 978-0-8261-1515-7 (hardcopy : alk. paper)—ISBN 978-0-8261-1528-7 (ebook)
I. Uomoto, Jay M. (Jay Matthew), 1956–, editor.
[DNLM: 1. Brain Injuries—rehabilitation. 2. Cultural Diversity. 3. Culturally Competent Care—ethnology. 4. Disabled Persons—rehabilitation. 5. Healthcare Disparities—ethnology. WL 354]
RC387.5
617.4'810443—dc23

2015019043

CONTENTS

CONTRIBUTORS

Julie Alberty, PhD, Department of Clinical Neuropsychology, Barrow Neurological Institute, St. Joseph's Hospital and Medical Center, Phoenix, Arizona

Juan Carlos Arango-Lasprilla, PhD, Department of Psychology, University of Deusto, IKERBASQUE, Basque Foundation for Science, Bilbao, Spain

Heather G. Belanger, PhD, ABPP (CN), James A. Haley Veteran's Hospital, Department of Mental Health and Behavioral Sciences, University of South Florida, Department of Psychiatry and Neurosciences, Tampa, Florida

William L. Brim, PsyD, Center for Deployment Psychology, Uniformed Services University of the Health Sciences, Bethesda, Maryland

Alison N. Cernich, PhD, ABPP (CN), Defense Centers of Excellence for Psychological Health and Traumatic Brain Injury, Silver Spring, Maryland; Veteran's Affairs/Department of Defense Mental Health Integration, Office of Mental Health Services, Department of Veterans Affairs, Washington, DC

Nicole Ditchman, PhD, CRC, LCPC, Department of Psychology, Illinois Institute of Technology, Chicago, Illinois

Fernando Gonzalez, PhD, ABPP (RP), Ranchos Los Amigos National Rehabilitation Center, Downey, California

Stephanie L. Hanson, PhD, ABPP (RP), College of Public Health and Health Professions, University of Florida, Gainesville, Florida

Brick Johnstone, PhD, ABPP (CN), School of Health Professions, University of Missouri, Columbia, Missouri

Joseph Keawe'aimoku Kaholokula, PhD, Department of Native Hawaiian Health, John A. Burns School of Medicine, University of Hawai'i—Manoa, Honolulu, Hawaii

Thomas R. Kerkhoff, PhD, ABPP (RP), Department of Clinical and Health Psychology, University of Florida (Retired), Gainesville, Florida

Pamela S. Klonoff, PhD ABPP (CN), Center for Transitional NeuroRehabilitation, Barrow Neurological Institute, St. Joseph's Hospital and Medical Center, Phoenix, Arizona

Eun-Jeong Lee, PhD, CRC, Department of Psychology, Illinois Institute of Technology, Chicago, Illinois

Anthony H. Lequerica, PhD, Kessler Foundation, West Orange, New Jersey; Department of Physical Medicine and Rehabilitation, Rutgers, New Jersey Medical School, Newark, New Jersey

Vicky T. Lomay, PhD, Tsinajini Psychology Services, Mesa, Arizona

Jennifer Loughlin, PhD, Center for Transitional NeuroRehabilitation, Barrow Neurological Institute, St. Joseph's Hospital and Medical Center, Phoenix, Arizona

Fred Loya, PhD, VA Northern California Health Care System, Martinez, California; Helen Willis Neuroscience Institute, University of California, Berkeley; Department of Neurology, University of California, San Francisco

Janet P. Niemeier, PhD, ABPP (RP), Department of Physical Medicine and Rehabilitation, Carolinas Rehabilitation, Carolinas Healthcare System, Charlotte, North Carolina

Ivan Panyavin, MS, Department of Psychology and Education, University of Deusto, Bilbao, Spain

Kavitha R. Perumparaichallai, PhD, Center for Transitional NeuroRehabilitation, Barrow Neurological Institute, St. Joseph's Hospital and Medical Center, Phoenix, Arizona

Michael Pramuka, PhD, James A. Haley Veteran's Hospital, Psychology Service, Tampa, Florida

Aida Saldivar, PhD, ABPP (RP), Ranchos Los Amigos National Rehabilitation Center, Downey, California

Charlotte Sykora, PhD, Ranchos Los Amigos National Rehabilitation Center, Downey, California

Jay M. Uomoto, PhD, VA Northern California Health Care System, VA Martinez Outpatient Clinic, Martinez, California

Shawn O. Utsey, PhD, Department of African American Studies, Virginia Commonwealth University, Richmond, Virginia

Marlene Vega, PsyD, Pate Rehabilitation, Dallas, Texas

Foreword

Multicultural Neurorehabilitation: Clinical Principles for Rehabilitation Professionals provides a much-needed view of how culture is implicated and intertwined with our attempts to serve the mental and neurological health of human beings. By "culture," I am loosely referring to the rules, norms, patterns of behavior, values, and attitudes that characterize particular groups. In three major analyses of mental health services over many decades, we have learned about the importance of culture, as well as about problems that occur when culture is not appreciated. In 1978, President Jimmy Carter's Commission on Mental Health noted that mental health services are often poorly delivered because they are not consistent with the cultural traditions of clients. In 2001, the U.S. Surgeon General's Report called for culturally competent services because ethnic minorities often have poorer access to services and lower quality of care. Finally, in 2003, President George W. Bush's Freedom Commission on Mental Health lamented the fact that the needs of culturally diverse groups are often underserved or inappropriately served and that the histories, traditions, beliefs, and value systems of clients should be incorporated into treatment.

Multicultural Neurorehabilitation: Clinical Principles for Rehabilitation Professionals reminds us that despite the greater attention on cultural factors in health and service delivery, we have been remiss in dealing with cultural issues involving persons with neurological disorders or diseases. The book proceeds to illustrate the dilemmas and issues facing service providers and researchers who work with ethnic and culturally diverse clients who experience disability because of central nervous system disorders, diseases, and traumas. It is all the more important because it is one of the few contributions that provides a comprehensive look at these issues and offers recommendations to remedy problems. The contributions made by the authors are pioneering, challenging, and substantive.

Human beings come from cultural backgrounds that may involve ethnicity, sexual orientation, gender, social class, and religious affiliation.

These backgrounds are important to understand in neurorehabilitation. They raise important questions. For example, in trying to determine the neurological disability of a client who has suffered a cerebral hemorrhage, are assessment procedures valid across different cultural groups? How can one provide effective rehabilitation services to an immigrant who has limited English proficiency? Questions such as these are difficult to address because of the lack of research and theory on disability within the context of culture. Nevertheless, they are critically important, especially because, as noted by contributors to this book, disparities exist. Members of ethnic minorities who suffer from neurological disabilities are often receiving inadequate and lower quality services than mainstream Americans.

Interestingly, because "culture" loosely refers to the rules, norms, patterns of behavior, values, and attitudes that characterize particular groups, disability itself may be the basis for a cultural group. Disability culture can evolve and develop. Human beings are a part of many different cultures, some by birth (e.g., one's culture as a man or woman) and others by choice or upbringing (e.g., religious affiliation). In the case of the neurological disability culture, I am reminded of the observation that many elderly persons who suffer from neurological problems join support groups concerned with health, medications, and aging. We see many military service members who experienced neurological injuries in combat joining the "wounded warrior" movement. Both in the cases of the elderly and the wounded warriors, we see the formation of cultures—group identification, similar attitudes, and behavioral patterns. Even those with disabilities who do not specifically identify with a disability cultural group are often forced into a disability culture because of reactions from others, limitations caused by the disability, and social stereotypes and stigmas.

How those with neurological disability or how disability culture is accepted by one's other cultures is important to ascertain. For example, are Mexican Americans more tolerant of disability than other ethnic groups? What family or community resources are available to Chinese who have disabilities? How can service providers utilize existing resources in the client's ethnic culture to achieve more effective outcomes? What are the best ways to reduce stigmas and misunderstandings over neurological disability that may exist within one's ethnic culture? In the United States, the mainstream cultural orientation toward disability rights has been relatively strong and has resulted in important legislation such as the Americans with Disabilities Act.

Finally, there is growing realization that multicultural rehabilitation issues are pertinent to all human beings. No one is immune to neurological impairment and disability. They can affect, and probably have affected, everyone at some point in their lives. Brain traumas or neurological disorders can develop slowly or occur suddenly and immediately impact one's functioning, social relationships, and socioeconomic standing. When they occur, rehabilitation is certainly more effective when cultural factors are utilized, as revealed in this book.

Stanley Sue, PhD
Palo Alto University

PREFACE

The basic categories of human mental life can be understood as products of social history—they are subject to change when the basic forms of social practice are altered and thus are social in nature.

—A. R. Luria[1]

This is just the start of a conversation, and in this context a conversation regarding how we best develop and deliver effective neurorehabilitation services to *all* who walk through our rehabilitation doors. As Luria so eloquently stated, our mental life, which is our cognitive experience, is shaped by social history and practice. We are social creatures, and as such we cannot extract ourselves from the cultural influences and environments in which we live. The neurorehabilitation setting is a special and unique culture in and of itself. It is a microcosm of intersecting cultures, and we must understand that as such, neurorehabilitation service delivery requires thoughtful and intentional acknowledgment of cultural dimensions in all facets of care. Such acknowledgment should lead to actionable practices that ultimately maximize the effectiveness of neurorehabilitation processes (e.g., team functioning, culturally shaped rehabilitation therapies) and improve the quality of life for all of those engaged in rehabilitation care.

Much has been written in the areas of multicultural and diversity issues in many areas of health care provision, and studies exist that demonstrate health care disparities in ethnic minority populations, lower socioeconomic groups of individuals, and many groups who have experienced discrimination and stigma by group membership alone. Much less has been written about issues of multicultural diversity in neurorehabilitation settings. Here, we are referring to those who are engaged in rehabilitation

---

[1]Luria, A. R. (1976). *Cognitive development: Its cultural and social foundations* (p. 164). Cambridge, MA: Harvard University Press.

of primarily central nervous system disorders, across many different stages and levels of care. To this end, this book is a collection of chapters written by expert scientist–practitioners in neurorehabilitation whose work has been in settings and populations that represent a diverse population of individuals seeking improved quality of life after acquired central nervous system injury and dysfunction.

Through a dialectic among a diverse group of clinicians, researchers, survivors of central nervous system injury, and their loved ones, we can move our knowledge forward toward more effective delivery of neurorehabilitation services. I hope this book can be a catalyst to such a dialectic. In this book, considerations of race and ethnicity, disability culture, military and veteran culture, and cultural aspects of religiousness and spirituality are all considered. The authors in this book wrote from their own perspectives as clinicians and researchers, representing diverse cultural backgrounds and neurorehabilitation contexts and roles. Hopefully, this book will generate more discussion, research, and literature on multicultural neurorehabilitation.

This project began several years ago, and it was originally meant to be a coauthored book with my good friend and colleague in rehabilitation neuropsychology, Dr. Tony Wong (Department of Physical Medicine and Rehabilitation at the University of Rochester Medical Center and Director of Neuropsychology at the Unity Health System in Rochester, New York), who tragically passed away suddenly in April 2011. His passing was a substantial loss to the field of cross-cultural neuropsychology and to neurorehabilitation.

Dr. Wong deeply appreciated within-culture variation in neuropsychology and balancing this with cross-cultural considerations. Once, at a national neuropsychology conference, an audience member questioned some assertions about testing individuals from a nonmajority culture that had been made during a symposium on cross-cultural neuropsychology. Dr. Wong's response was thoughtful and respectful. He provided information on the available science in cross-cultural neuropsychology and admitted that the science was insufficient (and still is) to provide a definitive answer as to how one can interpret certain test findings in a patient from a different culture. He, however, infused the discussion with significant wisdom by stating that neuropsychology is always a clinical endeavor, requiring the clinician to not only be aware of potential cultural considerations but to proceed forward with the best one can do under those circumstances, knowing that doing informed and educated clinical work is better than doing nothing at all. He added that we cannot ignore or always have the luxury of specifically selecting those whom we evaluate and treat, many of whom will represent a wide diversity of cultures.

Dr. Wong and I had many conversations about the vision for this book, and we agreed that it should be a scholarly yet practically oriented book—something that clinicians, researchers, administrators, and policy makers could embrace. This book is therefore dedicated to Dr. Wong and his much too short career of scholarly inquiry. Sadly, we do not have any of Dr. Wong's written thoughts that were to be a part of this book, but I truly hope that we embody his spirit of empathic clinical concern and innovative academic inquiry and, in doing so, honor his legacy in the area of multicultural neurorehabilitation.

Jay M. Uomoto

PART ONE

DIVERSITY AND THE WIDER CONTEXT OF MULTICULTURAL NEUROREHABILITATION

CHAPTER ONE

NEUROEPIDEMIOLOGY AND RACIAL DISPARITIES IN NEUROREHABILITATION CARE

Jay M. Uomoto and Jennifer Loughlin

*I*t is important to have a thorough understanding of the neuroepidemi-ology of central nervous system disorders to incorporate cultural diversity into the neurorehabilitation care of patients with these dis-orders. An awareness of the incidence and prevalence rates of neurologi-cal disorders and syndromes, and the potential disparities that exist in delivering such neurorehabilitation care, is vital to tailoring culturally competent care to each individual. It can be difficult to obtain representa-tive data from large epidemiological studies that reflect the rates of these disorders among the array of cultural groups beyond ethnicity, age, and socioeconomic status. This chapter emphasizes traumatic brain injury and stroke—two of the most common neurological disorders seen in neurorehabilitation facilities and services—to narrow the scope of our discussion.

To address the preceding issues, we begin by reviewing existing neuroepidemiological studies that include representative samples of indi-viduals from different cultures. Because many of these studies were not conducted to explicitly examine cultural differences in the incidence and prevalence rates of neurological disorders, the data compiled are not terribly helpful to our discussion. Only more recently have efforts been made to specifically define the population to better determine cultural differences.

Figure 1.1 shows how many articles appeared in PubMed on the sub-jects *epidemiology* and *traumatic brain injury* between 1964 and 2014. As with many areas of study, the number of articles about these topics increased

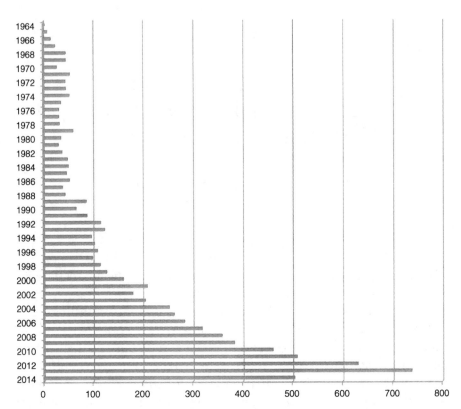

Figure 1.1 *Articles on epidemiology and traumatic brain injury published from 1964 to 2014.*
Source: PubMed.

considerably over the past 5 to 10 years. The earliest article about traumatic brain injury epidemiology was published in approximately 1963.

Figure 1.2 shows the number of articles on *epidemiology* and *stroke* that appeared in PubMed during the same years. Again, much more literature on stroke epidemiology has been written over the past few years, and it is very likely that these studies include data about racial and ethnic minorities.

Many of the earlier articles were generally categorized under *epidemiology*. What we know today as a neuroepidemiological study did not truly appear in the scientific literature until the early 1970s. The study of traumatic brain injury has seen a clear evolution in the sophistication, breadth, and depth of findings concerning neuroepidemiology as it affects racial and ethnic minorities.

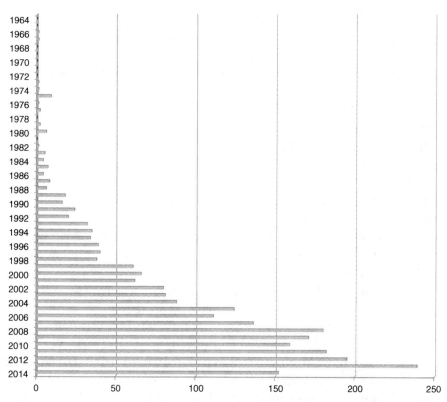

Figure 1.2 *Articles on epidemiology and stroke published from 1964 to 2014.*
Source: PubMed.

EARLY NEUROEPIDEMIOLOGICAL STUDIES
OF TRAUMATIC BRAIN INJURY

London (1967) conducted one of the earliest studies on the incidence of traumatic brain injury, in which he examined the clinical outcomes of patients with severe head injuries who had been admitted to Birmingham Accident Hospital in the United Kingdom between 1957 and 1961. The study examined the relationship between the duration of loss of consciousness and the level of disability based on the ability to return to work, which was categorized as "normal," "easier," "home care," and "special care." Based on the admission rates at the hospital, London was also able to estimate the national disability rate. The study found that every year approximately 1,000 individuals suffered a severe head injury, and about 50% of them would "never work again" (p. 473). London also reported on the problems these individuals had finding appropriate rehabilitation services. He found that a certain stigma was associated with receiving services with other categories of patients, noting that they may be "understandably reluctant to seem to be classed with, say, spastic or mentally defective persons" (p. 476). He also found that some rehabilitation centers were reluctant to admit patients who had a poor prognosis.

These results suggest a cultural bias against patients with severe head injuries in obtaining rehabilitation services. In addition, the patients feel they are being discriminated against because they are treated the same as individuals with mental disabilities. It is interesting to note that neurorehabilitation facilities and programs have faced very similar dilemmas in attempting to deliver culturally relevant services.

Cultural variables other than gender have not been widely addressed in the early neuroepidemiological literature in the United States. The earliest epidemiological study of traumatic brain injury in the United States was conducted in Olmsted County, Minnesota, by the Mayo Clinic. It involved 3,587 cases of injury that occurred between 1935 and 1974 (Annegers, Grabow, Kurland, & Laws, 1980). This was likely the first report involving the well-known high rate of incidence in the age 15 to 24 cohort in males. No studies involving race or other common cultural categories (e.g., socioeconomic status) were conducted.

In 1974, the National Institute of Neurological and Communication Disorders and Stroke (NINCDS) initiated the National Head and Spinal Cord Injury Survey, which sampled those who were hospitalized for head injury (excluding those with mild traumatic brain injury) between 1970 and 1974. The survey used a sophisticated sampling strategy that included a stratified random sampling of U.S. counties with a review of hospital discharge records for making final determinations of case inclusion based on discharge diagnoses (see Levin, Benton, & Grossman, 1982, for the data generated by the survey). No mention of incidence rates broken down by race appears in summary articles of the major findings of this survey (e.g., see Anderson, Miller, & Kalsbeek, 1983), but rates of injuries, age at injury, gender, and day of the week the injury most commonly occurred were all examined. Kraus and Nourjah (1989) also did not include race and ethnicity variables in their chapter on the epidemiology of mild traumatic brain injury. Levin, Benton, and Grossman (1982) found a high occurrence of traumatic brain injury in lower socioeconomic groups. In these groups, the injuries were most often the result of assaults, whereas in higher socioeconomic groups, the injuries were usually sports related. These findings clearly demonstrate the complex interactions between demographic and injury-related variables when examining cultural differences in neuroepidemiology.

Klauber, Barrett-Connor, Marshall, and Bowers (1981) conducted a large epidemiological study of traumatic brain injury in San Diego County, California, which is very ethnically diversified. It is not surprising, however, that neither racial nor ethnic variables were included in their study. Although they examined all deaths due to head injury and all individuals admitted to San Diego County hospitals with a diagnosis of head injury in 1978, it was not common to include race in such studies. Indeed, in 1970, U.S. Census data (U.S. Census Bureau, 1973) defined "race" only as "all persons" versus "Negro and other races."

Kraus et al. (1984) conducted a follow-up study in which they examined new cases of traumatic brain injury in San Diego County in 1981. They pointed out shortcomings in the previous study's case identification protocols, and they included a comprehensive profile of injury mechanisms, age distribution, and disposition after acute hospitalization. Unlike Klauber et al.'s study, they presented data on race and ethnicity. Hospital records showed that the vast majority of individuals who had sustained a traumatic brain injury were White, 12% were Hispanic, 6% were Black, and 2% were Asian. Because 1,198 of the 3,358 cases of traumatic brain injury did not indicate the race of the patient, no further analyses of race were conducted. Today, this information is always included in a patient's records.

RECENT INVESTIGATIONS OF TRAUMATIC BRAIN INJURY EPIDEMIOLOGY

Today, racial breakdowns on all medical and health care topics are readily available on the Internet. For example, one can easily look up statistics on motor vehicle and motorcycle accident injury and death rates by race/ethnicity in San Diego County during a certain time period. The Health and Human Services Agency's 2010 report (County of San Diego, Health and Human Services Agency, Emergency Medical Services, 2012) shows that motor vehicle accident injury and death rates were highest among

Blacks, followed by Hispanics, Whites, and Asians/Other, in that order. The highest injury rate from motorcycle accidents, however, was among Whites, followed, in order, by Blacks, Asians/Other, and Hispanics (rates for death were not calculated due to fewer than five occurrences in the non-White population). These data can help brain injury prevention campaigns to target information to certain sectors of the population. National surveillance data and statistics on traumatic brain injury, categorized by race and ethnicity, can be found on the Centers for Disease Control and Prevention (CDC) website (www.cdc.gov) in its *Morbidity and Mortality Weekly Report* (CDC, 2015).

More recent epidemiological evidence routinely includes race as a key categorical variable in understanding incidence rates of traumatic brain injury in a given population. Fletcher, Khalid, and Mallonee (2007) studied brain injuries sustained by Oklahoma individuals age 65 and older from 1992 to 2003. Race was parsed into White, African American, and Native American categories, appropriately reflecting some of the racial demographics of that state. Overall, incidence rates among Whites exceeded those of African Americans and Native Americans, as did the rates of intentionality, except in cases of assaults, where the rate among African Americans was three times greater than both Whites and Native Americans. The mean length of stay for hospitalizations due to traumatic brain injury was greater for African Americans than for Whites and Native Americans. These findings offer valuable information for determining why these rates vary so widely among races. It is also important to explore the different methodologies, measurement approaches, source data, and calculations of incidence and prevalence rates. According to Corrigan, Selassie, and Orman (2010), "Surveillance comes in many shapes and sizes, and the informed user must know the differences" (p. 78).

Statistics about disabilities that result from traumatic brain injury can facilitate the implementation of needed and appropriate neurorehabilitation services in general. Detailed analyses of the interactions among race, age, gender, and other socioeconomic variables can help the development of culturally relevant and effective services. The U.S. Department of Education's National Institute on Disability and Rehabilitation Research (NIDRR) Traumatic Brain Injury Model Systems (TBIMS) research program provides a rich database (TBIMS-NDB) from which to examine such interactions on a large scale. As discussed by Corrigan et al. (2014), although a race/ethnic breakdown is included, as with many large-scale studies of this type, representing and recruiting non-Whites can be challenging. Their database from 2001 to 2007 included 78.5% White, 9.3% African American, 7.0% Hispanic, and 5.1% Other. Since 2014, with continued enrollment in the TBIMS-NDB, however, the database consists of 19% African American, 9% Hispanic Origin, 3% Asian, 0.5% Native American, and 1% other ethnic groups (TBIMS, National Data and Statistical Center, 2014). Researchers with the TBIMS have cited some racial/ethnic disparities in outcomes, which we discuss later in this chapter.

In addition to data on incidence and prevalence rates of traumatic brain injury, information on functional outcomes based on race and ethnicity can prove important in developing strategies for resolving racial/ethnic disparities in health care. Staudenmayer, Diaz-Arrastia, de Oliveira, Gentilello, and Shafi (2007) found significant deficits in long-term functional outcomes after traumatic brain injury in minority (non-White) patients. This multicenter study through the Traumatic Brain Injury (TBI) Clinical Trials Network tracked 211 patients on the Functional Status Examination (FSE) for 6 months after they were discharged from the hospital. Grouped into categories of ethnic minority and non-Hispanic Whites, these investigators found poorer functional outcomes in the minority group in terms of being dependent on others for care across the FSE domains of standard of living, leisure, and work or school. The data gathered did not allow for a more in-depth understanding of the reasons for poorer social reintegration and lower standard of living compared to the non-Hispanic White group, and they concluded that further study was needed to "determine causes of these disparities, and to identify potential remedies to minimize this ethnic divide" (p. 1369). Also, it is important to consider that variables such as insurance coverage, local access to services, and availability of family and community supports can influence these outcomes. This has been found to be the case in examining racial disparities in health outcomes in those with spinal cord injury (Krause, Broderick, Saladin, & Broyles, 2006), where education (in years) and household income mediated the relationship between race and health. Rath (2014) summed up this point well when he stated that disparities in health care outcomes in those with cognitive disabilities occur also within the context of "patients and families from low SES [socioeconomic status] backgrounds [who are] already less likely to have insurance, stable housing, and transportation, and are at risk for poor outcomes following cognitive disability."

NEUROEPIDEMIOLOGY OF STROKE

According to the American Heart Association, stroke was the fifth leading cause of death in the United States in 2009 (Kochaneck, Murphy, Xu, & Arias, 2011) and a leading cause of long-term disability (Go et al., 2014). In 2010, the total cost of treatment for cardiovascular disease and stroke was estimated to be around $315.4 billion in the United States alone (Go et al., 2014). Potential risk factors for stroke identified in the literature include those related to lifestyle, medical history, and social factors, such as older age, hypertension, diabetes, hypercholesterolemia, atrial fibrillation, diet, obesity, smoking, amount of physical activity, region of residence in the United States, and lower socioeconomic status (Addo et al., 2012; Go et al., 2014; Obisesan, Vargas, & Gillum, 2000). Additionally, membership of certain ethnic groups has also been associated with greater risk for stroke, which we discuss later in this chapter.

Much like early studies of traumatic brain injury, race was seldom included or only categorized participants as African American/non-White or White. In a Nationwide Cerebrovascular Disease Mortality Study of stroke incidence, mortality, and clinical data, only White male and White female subjects were included (Kuller et al., 1970). As the stroke epidemiology literature grew, it became more apparent that there were stark differences in stroke incidence by race. Wylie (1970) described differences in age-adjusted incidence for Whites and non-Whites from 1949 to 1967 in his review of mortality statistics from cerebrovascular disease. He found that the rate of death was higher for non-Whites and speculated that this was due to higher hypertension rates and other factors, such as lower socioeconomic status, limited access to medical care, and "life stresses."

Ahmed et al. (1988) examined stroke mortality between 1971 and 1980 in two hospitals in Allegheny County, Pennsylvania. This included incidence data by race, which was grouped by White, Black, or "unknown" membership. They found that after adjusting for age, African American patients had a higher rate of mortality from stroke compared to White patients. Sacco (1995) and Sacco et al. (1998) also found greater prevalence of stroke in minority groups compared to Whites for those living in New York City. African Americans and Hispanics were found to have 2.4 and 2 times greater risk, respectively, compared to Whites (Sacco et al., 1998). In their review of the literature on stroke incidence published between 1995 and 2003, Stansbury, Jia, Williams, Vogel, and Duncan (2005) found higher rates of mortality, severity of stroke, and disease burden for African Americans compared to Whites. Japanese Americans, Chinese Americans, and Filipino Americans were all found to have higher rates of hemorrhagic stroke compared to Whites (Palaniappan et al., 2010).

More recent studies have also found a higher incidence of stroke among certain minority groups. For example, the CDC (2012) reported that the age-adjusted prevalence from strokes between 2006 and 2010 was 5.5% for American Indian/Alaska Natives, 3.7% for African Americans, 2.5% for Hispanics, 2.4% for Whites, and 2.3% for Asians/Pacific Islanders.

In addition to the rates of stroke in White versus minority populations, rates among ethnic minority subgroups have also been examined. For example, Daviglus et al. (2012) found that among the more than 15,000 individuals studied in the *Hispanic Community Health Study/Study of Latinos* (e.g., Cuban, Dominican, Mexican, Puerto Rican, Central American, and South American), those from a Puerto Rican heritage had a higher rate of cardiovascular disease risk factors. Additionally, lower income groups and individuals who had been living in the United States for a long time also had more risk factors. This study is significant in that data on ethnic subgroups were included, which is rarely the case in larger neuroepidemiological studies.

Moderators of Ethnic Disparities in Stroke

As a result of this new information about the differences in the rates of cardiovascular disease and stroke between ethnic minority groups and Whites, research is now focusing on identifying factors that may moderate this relationship to inform the development of public health interventions. This is an important step, given the potential for erroneous assumptions that might arise if ethnicity is used as an epidemiological variable to the exclusion of other, potentially more salient factors. Fustinoni and Biller (2000) reported on the rates of coronary heart disease and stroke among Japanese males and Japanese American males. Although all of these men were of the same ethnic background, a significantly higher stroke rate was found among the Japanese men. The rate of coronary heart disease, however, was higher among the Japanese American men. It was believed that this was due to differences in lifestyle between Japan and the United States, such as diet (Takeya et al., 1984). Other authors, however, have argued that using ethnicity as a variable in public health research serves a practical role. Although acknowledging the presence of confounding factors, Saposnik (2000) argues that ethnicity should be included as a variable in studies and in fact may provide important information in finding ways to reduce disease incidence in specific populations.

Potential moderating factors that have been identified in the literature include both common health conditions that may contribute to stroke (e.g., diabetes mellitus, hypertension, atrial fibrillation) and nonmedical influences. Among minority groups, these include lack of education about strokes (e.g., signs of stroke, benefit of urgent care as soon as possible), lack of participation in research, cultural differences (e.g., acculturation, attitudes or beliefs), and access to health care (Cruz-Flores et al., 2011). Chong and Sacco (2005) also discuss "novel risk factors" that may contribute to stroke in young minority group members, such as illicit drug use.

Disparities in Access to Health Care in Stroke

In addition to disparities in the rate of stroke, differences in access to health care following a stroke have also been identified in minority groups versus Whites, although these findings are less robust (Stansbury et al., 2005). This is especially true of African American stroke survivors. Zweifler, Lyden, Taft, Kelly, and Rothrock (1995) found that while most Whites and Mexican Americans got medical care within 24 hours of stroke onset, only about half of African Americans did. In addition, African Americans had significantly longer emergency department wait times compared to White and Hispanic patients (Karve, Balkrishnan, Mohammad, & Levine, 2011).

The results of research on acute length of stay, use of diagnostic imaging procedures, and use of postacute rehabilitation have been variable (Stansbury et al., 2005). For example, in an analysis of 10 large studies, Ellis, Breland, and Egede (2008) found that minority group members were more likely to participate in rehabilitation and to stay longer in rehabilitation facilities. The results were more variable, however, when the use of specific rehabilitation therapies was examined, with some studies demonstrating less outpatient services for minority group members and others greater use of these postacute services (Cruz-Flores et al., 2011). Additionally, Ng, Brotmas, Lau, and Young (2012) found that ethnicity was not related to increased mortality from a myocardial infarction and coronary artery event. Instead, insurance status (privately insured versus underinsured) and socioeconomic status were significant factors in their prospective cohort study of patients who suffered a cardiovascular event in the Maryland hospitals included in their database.

Disparities in Functional Outcomes in Stroke

Studies examining disparities in functional outcomes after stroke have also been variable. Roth et al. (2011) interviewed and evaluated stroke patients and their family caregivers for 1 year after the stroke. They found that even after controlling for age, education, and whether the patient resided with the caregiver, African American patients had greater deficits in activities of daily living and in instrumental activities of daily living, including mobility, hand functioning, social participation, memory, and Mini Mental State Examination scores compared to Whites. However, with regard to return to work after the stroke, a study that covered the years 1968 to 1973 found that Whites returned to work sooner than African Americans, but more recent studies found no significant difference (Stansbury et al., 2005). In their examination of the influence of stroke location on return to work following ischemic stroke, Wozniak et al. (1999) did not find that race, among other factors, predicted return to work within 1 year for those who were working full time at the time of their stroke. It should be noted, however, that in this study, race consisted of only White and non-White, with the latter group mostly African Americans.

Overall, the neuroepidemiologies of traumatic brain injury and stroke are quite similar, and the scientific literature has reported similar findings in terms of racial and ethnic disparities. Of particular concern is the variability in mortality rates by race/ethnicity after stroke, which highlights the need for addressing disparities in neurorehabilitation care.

RACIAL DISPARITIES IN NEUROREHABILITATION CARE

Racial disparities exist across the health care spectrum and are not unique to the delivery of neurorehabilitation services. This is a serious problem in the U.S. health care system, and it has gained significant attention over the past decade. The number of studies devoted to this issue has risen dramatically, and there is widespread debate on ways to reduce such disparities in health care delivery and outcomes. To better understand health risks in minority populations, the CDC initiated a large-scale annual survey called the Racial and Ethnic Approaches to Community Health Across the U.S. (REACH U.S.; Liao et al., 2011). In this survey, 28 racial/ethnic communities across 17 states used multiple evaluation methodologies (telephone calls, questionnaires, in-person interviews) to interview residents of different ethnicities about their experiences with the health care system. While the conclusions of the survey are beyond the scope of this book, it is worth noting that barriers to adequate health care, lower socioeconomic status, and greater health risks and disease burden, compared to the general population, were reported.

Racial and Ethnic Disparities in U.S. Health Care

As noted earlier, race or ethnicity variables alone do not explain racial/ ethnic disparities in health care or neurorehabilitation care. However, a report by the Institute of Medicine (IOM; 2002) stated that even controlling for variables such as insurance coverage and ability to pay, disparities continue in health care for ethnic minorities. According to the report, "social stereotypes" (p. 4) regarding race and ethnicity (e.g., the quiet and compliant Japanese American) can not only influence the patient–provider interpersonal relationship (thus affecting clinical outcomes) but also can reinforce stereotypes that may persist across clinical encounters. This is an example of how epidemiological or research study information about cultural differences relating to a particular medical condition is not enough to guide clinical practice. For example, just because a certain group of Hispanics is found to have a higher risk of cerebrovascular disease, that may not be a sufficient reason to guide clinical practice based on this one group. Stereotypes can have the effect of erroneously simplifying one variable out of the vast array of complex demographic and economic variables that may play equal or significant roles in the genesis and treatment of a cerebrovascular condition. The IOM report also mentions "health care provider prejudice and bias" (p. 4), where medical personnel may have personal prejudices against certain ethnic groups. While this may not always be openly expressed, microaggressions (see Chapter 10) may arise during the patient–provider relationship. The IOM report goes on to state:

> While there is no direct evidence that provider biases affect the quality of care for minority patients, research suggests that health care providers' diagnostic and treatment decisions, as well as their feelings about patients, are influenced by patients' race or ethnicity. (p. 4)

Of further concern is the issue of "patient response" (p. 5), where a provider finds it difficult to offer care to a patient who expresses distrust and is uncooperative about treatment. If a patient had a bad experience with medical treatment in the past, it can influence his or her feelings about the current situation. The issue of prior racial discrimination resulting in distrust of the health care system was highlighted in a study by Armstrong et al. (2013). In their survey, African American and White adults were administered a questionnaire that measures health system distrust and prior experiences of discrimination where the two variables were strongly correlated, despite adjusting for sociodemographic and residential segregation. Using a mediational model, Armstrong et al. found that distrust of the health care system was lower in the African American group than in the White group. This underscores the importance of considering preformed attitudes toward the health care system when developing care for ethnic minorities.

The neuroepidemiological literature cannot address all such problems in patient–provider clinical encounters, although such information is clearly relevant when identifying particular health risk groups and planning interventions. It may be that at the intervention level, more work is needed to identify mechanisms in which racial and ethnic disparities impact the delivery and receipt of health care and, in this context, neurorehabilitation care at the patient–provider or patient–interdisciplinary team level.

Emic and Etic Sources of Disparities in the Neurorehabilitation Setting

Recent literature has underscored racial and ethnic disparities in neurorehabilitation services for those with neurological disorders. Simpson, Mohr, and Redman (2000) conducted a study in which qualitative information was gathered through semistructured interviews of Italian,

Arabic, and Vietnamese patients and family members in a brain injury rehabilitation unit. Common themes among respondents included a variety of conceptualizations of the characteristics of brain injuries and praise for the health care staff. Common complaints included frequent staff turnover, limited access to doctors, and staff not being available during scheduled appointments. These responses are representative of *etic* (i.e., more universal experiences across cultures) elements of experiences with brain injury rehabilitation participation and do not represent unique cultural perceptions. These findings, however, also underscore more *emic* (i.e., the perspective of the individual within a specific cultural or social group) elements of their cultural experiences with rehabilitation. Many considered the social worker's questions to be intrusive. Some cultures consider family or lifestyle information to be private and not open to public scrutiny. Although the stigma and social isolation an individual with a brain injury may feel are not emic aspects of neurorehabilitation care, some participants expressed discomfort with being labeled. In this study, one Arabic respondent objected to the term *brain injury*. A Vietnamese respondent felt that having a brain injury brought shame to his family, which is consistent with what many Asian cultures believe. Therefore, it is important to include both etic and emic aspects of neurorehabilitation care when it involves individuals of minority cultures.

These concerns also apply to cases where the brain injury causes other disabilities, such as physical disfigurement, amputation, dysarthria, or decreased social cognition. Such disabilities can also make both an individual and his or her family feel stigmatized. The following case study illustrates some emic and etic aspects of neurorehabilitation.

Case Vignette: Eric is a 19-year-old Chinese male who was born and raised in Hong Kong. He and his brother have been attending a U.S. university. One night, after Eric had been drinking during a party at his dorm, he and his brother were driving on the freeway when their car struck another vehicle. Eric sustained a severe traumatic brain injury and was in a coma for 3 days. He was eventually transferred to the neurological ICU, where he was placed on a ventilator. Eric's brother sustained upper extremity fractures, but he was released after 2 days in the hospital. The boys' parents flew to the United States and visited Eric in the ICU every day. Neither parent spoke English, but Eric's father was highly involved in making decisions about Eric's care. After emerging from the coma and being weaned off the ventilator, Eric was transferred to the acute neurorehabilitation unit. A telephone translation service was offered, but Eric's parents refused, preferring and expecting Eric to translate despite his severe brain injury. The rehabilitation staff expressed frustration with this situation, as well as with what they perceived as Eric's mother's "passive" attitude toward the rehabilitation. His mother often showed little interest in Eric's physical therapy, and his father only seemed to be interested in how soon Eric would be able to go back to school to complete his studies.

This case highlights the many difficulties that can arise as a result of cultural attitudes. Having to use a translator meant that personal information would have to be revealed to a "stranger," which may be an emic preference by the parents. Eric's father's reaction could be interpreted as one of a "typical" traditional Asian parent who had high expectations for his firstborn son. This could be considered emic as well. However, it is just as possible that Eric's father was finding it difficult to accept that his son had sustained a serious cognitive disability. He may have found it too difficult to admit that Eric would possibly never be able to achieve his goal of getting a college degree. This would be an understandable etic (i.e., toward a more universal) perspective taken by a grieving and suffering father. Therefore, it is a mistake to look at this case strictly in terms of Asian emic aspects and/or etic elements of the experience of neurorehabilitation. Social stereotypes of Asians could make the rehabilitation staff misjudge the parents' participation in the rehabilitation process and could lead to ongoing health care provider bias in the future. The patient's or family's response to these interactions might be a result of overgeneralizing what "mainstream" American rehabilitation is all about. The neuroepidemiological literature on racial and ethnic disparities in neurorehabilitation is still emerging, but some key findings should inform specific case conceptualizations.

Disparities in Outcomes

The question of racial and ethnic disparities in outcomes after traumatic brain injury has recently been well documented. Much of this information comes from the aforementioned NIDRR TBI Model Systems research (Arango-Lasprilla et al., 2007). Ethnic minorities (classified as self-identified African American and Hispanic) sustained traumatic brain injury from acts of violence four times as often as Whites. Minority rating of functional status as measured by the Disability Rating Scale and the Functional Independence Measure was lower than Whites at discharge from inpatient rehabilitation, and this difference was sustained after 1 year. In another TBI Model Systems study, Perrin et al. (2014) found African Americans who sustained traumatic brain injury had elevated scores for depression at 1 and 2 year follow-ups compared to Whites. Depression among Asian/Pacific Islanders was also found to be elevated over the same time span whereas it decreased among Hispanics even more than among Whites. One year after the injury, it was found that African Americans had lower self-reported life satisfaction compared to Whites and Asian/Pacific Islanders (Arango-Lasprilla et al., 2009). In a review of the literature on racial and ethnic differences in traumatic brain injury outcomes, Gary, Arango-Lasprilla, and Stevens (2009) concluded that "after controlling for demographic and injury characteristics, discrepant postinjury outcomes are prevalent among African Americans and Hispanics with [traumatic brain injury] compared to Whites" (p. 787).

In examining differential rates of discharge after traumatic brain injury care in an Oregon group, Kane, Wright, Fu, and Carlson (2014) found that Hispanics were sent to posthospital care at a significantly lower rate than African Americans, non-Hispanic others, and Whites, after controlling for a set of demographic, injury, and insurance variables. As might be expected, those without insurance were less likely to be discharged to posthospital care. Similarly, African American and Hispanic individuals with traumatic brain injury were shown (through examination of the National Trauma Data Bank) to be less likely to receive acute neurorehabilitation services compare to Whites (Meagher, Beadles, Doorey, & Charles, 2014). In summarizing the literature on racial and ethnic disparities in outcomes after brain injury, Arango-Lasprilla and Kreutzer (2010) find the preponderance of evidence quite sobering. Their review suggests poorer treatment outcomes of ethnic minorities compared to Whites, poorer neuropsychological outcomes, poorer employment outcomes, poorer everyday functioning outcomes, poorer community reintegration outcomes, more marital instability, more psychological and neurobehavioral problems, and poorer overall quality of life experienced by ethnic minorities compared to Whites. They point out that "researchers and clinicians need to understand the linguistic, economic, and social barriers that individuals from different cultures face, preventing their access to health care and rehabilitation services" (p. 134).

CONCLUSIONS

The neuroepidemiological evidence continues to mount with generally consistent findings regarding the racial and ethnic disparities that exist in accessing neurorehabilitation care and functional outcomes for those who have sustained neurological disorders such as traumatic brain injury and stroke. As large-scale epidemiological studies increasingly include and distinguish individuals of color and linguistic minorities together with religion, sexual orientation, physical disabilities, place of residence, and key socioeconomic variables that interact with race/ethnicity, more information will be available to make changes in policy, training, and clinical service delivery. As the field advances, more specific clinical practice guidelines will be developed. The following are some recommendations for what we can do now:

1. Awareness of racial and ethnic disparities in the context of neurorehabilitation care should alert researchers, health care organizations, policy makers, and clinicians that disparities in other cultural groups may be suspected. As noted earlier, many other cultural groups may also experience disparities in their attempts to get neurorehabilitation care and the quality of the care they receive.
2. Studies of racial/ethnic disparities in neurorehabilitation should delineate key interactive variables that may account for cultural disparities. Current research has come a long way in breaking down racial and ethnic variables, but these are clearly difficult studies to carry out, especially on a larger scale. Thus, a continued call for funding priorities that are inclusive of an array of cultural experiences would be beneficial to advance the science in this area.
3. Research has resulted in actionable health care administration policies and clinical guidelines. Caregivers must be aware that different racial/ethnic groups can have different risks (e.g., increased rate of depression after discharge from the hospital in African Americans) and that other dynamics may also impact a patient's recovery (e.g., access to social support, additional medical conditions that may increase depression). There must be a balance between considering emic contributors and overgeneralizing research findings that may not be relevant to a cultural group, thus running the risk of a stereotyping.

4. Clinical researchers should be encouraged to use comparative effective research designs, as suggested by the Agency for Healthcare Research and Quality (2015). A more rapid deployment of tested clinical interventions to key stakeholders is a critical element in comparative effectiveness research. This also includes dissemination of findings and reaching out to stakeholders (an active outreach approach) to effect the implementation of findings.

5. According to Arango-Lasprilla and Kreutzer (2010), rehabilitation providers should seek out input and perspectives from diverse cultural groups. Listening to patient's perspectives and their personal experiences with having a neurological disorder or caring for someone with a neurological disorder can help design individualized care. Surveys may not always provide this information, so it is important to give different cultural groups the opportunity to talk about their experiences.

REFERENCES

Addo, J., Ayerbe, L., Mohan, K. M., Crichton, S., Sheldenkar, A., Chen, R., . . . McKevitt, C. (2012). Socioeconomic status and stroke: An updated review. *Stroke, 43,* 1186–1191.

Agency for Healthcare Research and Quality. (2015). What is comparative effectiveness research? Retrieved from http://effectivehealthcare.ahrq.gov/index.cfm/what-is-comparative-effectiveness-research1

Ahmed, O. I., Orchard, T. J., Sharma, R., Mitchell, H., & Talbot, E. (1988). Declining mortality from stroke in Allegheny County, Pennsylvania: Trends in case fatality and severity of disease, 1971–1980. *Stroke, 19,* 181–184.

Anderson, D. W., Miller, J. D., & Kalsbeek, W. D. (1983). Findings from a major U.S. survey of persons hospitalized with head injuries. *Public Health Reports, 98,* 475–478.

Annegers, J. F., Grabow, J. D., Kurland, L. T., & Laws, E. R. (1980). The incidence, causes, and secular trends of head trauma in Olmsted County, Minnesota, 1935–1974. *Neurology, 30,* 912–919.

Arango-Lasprilla, J. C., Ketchum, J. M., Gary, K., Hart, T., Corrigan, J., Foster, L., & Mascialino, G. (2009). Race/ethnic differences in satisfaction with life among persons with traumatic brain injury. *NeuroRehabilitation, 24,* 5–14.

Arango-Lasprilla, J. C., & Kreutzer, J. S. (2010). Racial and ethnic disparities in functional, psychosocial, and neurobehavioral outcomes after brain injury. *Journal of Head Trauma Rehabilitation, 25,* 128–136.

Arango-Lasprilla, J. C., Rosenthal, M., Deluca, J., Komaroff, E., Sherer, M., Cifu, D., & Hanks, R. (2007). Traumatic brain injury and functional outcomes: Does minority status matter? *Brain Injury, 21,* 701–708.

Armstrong, K., Putt, M., Halbert, C. H., Grande, D., Schwartz, J. S., Kiao, K., . . . Shea, J. A. (2013). Prior experiences of racial discrimination and racial differences in health care system distrust. *Medical Care, 51,* 144–150.

Centers for Disease Control and Prevention. (2012). Prevalence of stroke—United States, 2006–2010. *MMWR: Morbidity and Mortality Weekly Report, 61,* 379–382.

Centers for Disease Control and Prevention. (2015). *Morbidity and Mortality Weekly Report.* Retrieved from www.cdc.gov/MMWR

Chong, J. Y., & Sacco, R. L. (2005). Epidemiology of stroke in young adults: Race/ethnic differences. *Journal of Thrombosis and Thrombolysis, 20,* 77–83.

Corrigan, J. D., Cuthbert, J. P., Harrison-Felix, D., Whiteneck, G. G., Bell, J. M., Miller, A. C., . . . Pretz, C. R. (2014). U.S. population estimates of health and social outcomes 5 years after rehabilitation for traumatic brain injury. *Journal of Head Trauma Rehabilitation, 29,* E1–E9.

Corrigan, J. D., Selassie, A. W., & Orman, J. A. (2010). The epidemiology of traumatic brain injury. *Journal of Head Trauma Rehabilitation, 25,* 72–80.

County of San Diego, Health and Human Services Agency, Emergency Medical Services (2012, September). *San Diego County trauma system report: 2010.* Retrieved from http://www.sandiegocounty.gov/hhsa/programs/phs/documents

Cruz-Flores, S., Rabinstein, A., Biller, J., Elkind, M. S. V., Griffith, P., Gorelick, P. B., . . . Valderrama, A. L. (2011). Racial–ethnic disparities in stroke care: The American Experience—a statement for health-care professionals from the American Heart Association/American Stroke Association. *Stroke, 42,* 2091–2116.

Daviglus, M. I., Talavera, G. A., Avilés-Santa, M. L., Allison, M., Cai, J., & Criqui, M. H. (2012). Prevalence of major cardiovascular risk factors and cardiovascular diseases among Hispanic/Latino Individuals of diverse backgrounds in the United States. *Journal of the American Medical Association, 308,* 1775–1784.

Ellis, C., Breland, H. L., & Egede, L. E. (2008). Racial/ethnic differences in utilization of post-stroke rehabilitation services: A systematic review. *Ethnicity and Disease, 18,* 365–372.

Fletcher, A. E., Khalid, S., & Mallonee, S. (2007). The epidemiology of severe traumatic brain injury among persons 65 years of age and older in Oklahoma, 1992–2003. *Brain Injury, 21,* 691–699.

Fustinoni, O., & Biller, J. (2000). Ethnicity and stroke: Beware the fallacies. *Stroke, 31,* 1013–1015.

Gary, K. W., Arango-Lasprilla, J. C., & Stevens, L. F. (2009). Do racial/ethnic differences exist in post-injury outcomes after TBI? A comprehensive review of the literature. *Brain Injury, 23,* 775–789.

Go, A. S., Mozaffarian, D., Roger, V. L., Benjamin, E. J., Berry, J. D., Blaha, M. J., . . . American Heart Association Statistics Committee and Stroke Statistics

Subcommittee. (2014). Heart disease and stroke statistics—2014 update: A report from the American Heart Association. *Circulation, 129,* 399–410.

Institute of Medicine. (2002). *Unequal treatment: Confronting racial and ethnic disparities in health care.* Washington, DC: National Academies Press.

Kane, W. G., Wright, D. A., Fu, R., & Carlson, K. F. (2014). Racial/ethnic and insurance status disparities in discharge to posthospitalization care for patients with traumatic brain injury. *Journal of Head Trauma Rehabilitation, 6,* E10–E17.

Karve, S. J., Balkrishnan, R., Mohammad, Y. M., & Levine, D. A. (2011). Racial/ethnic disparities in emergency department waiting time for stroke patients in the United States. *Journal of Stroke and Cerebrovascular Disease, 20,* 30–40.

Klauber, M. R., Barrett-Connor, E., Marshall, L. F., & Bowers, S. A. (1981). The epidemiology of head injury: A prospective study of an entire community—San Diego County, California, 1978. *American Journal of Epidemiology, 113,* 500–509.

Kochanek, K. D., Murphy, S. L., Xu, J., & Arias, E. (2014). Mortality in the United States, 2013. *NCHS Data Brief, 178,* 1–8.

Kraus, J. F., Black, M. A., Hessol, N., Ley, P., Rokaw, W., Sullivan, C., . . . Marshall, L. (1984). The incidence of acute brain injury and serious impairment in a defined population. *American Journal of Epidemiology, 119,* 186–201.

Kraus, J. F., & Nourjah, P. (1989). The epidemiology of mild head injury. In H. S. Levin, H. M. Eisenberg, & A. L. Benton (Eds.), *Mild head injury* (pp. 8–22). New York, NY: Oxford University Press.

Krause, J. S., Broderick, L. E., Saladin, L. K., & Broyles, J. (2006). Racial disparities in health outcomes after spinal cord injury: Mediating effects of education and income. *Journal of Spinal Cord Medicine, 29,* 17–25.

Kuller, L., Anderson, H., Peterson, D., Cassel, J., Spiers, P., Curry, H., . . . Seltster, R. (1970). Nationwide cerebrovascular disease morbidity study. *Stroke, 1,* 86–99.

Levin, H. S., Benton, A. L., & Grossman, R. G. (1982). *Neurobehavioral consequences of closed head injury.* New York, NY: Oxford University Press.

Liao, Y., Bang, D., Cosgrove, S., Dulin, R., Harris, Z., Stewart, A., . . . Giles, W. (2011). Surveillance of health status in minority communities—Racial and Ethnic Approaches to Community Health across the U.S. (REACH U.S.) risk factor survey, United States, 2009. *Morbidity and Mortality Weekly Report Surveillance Summaries, 60,* 1–41.

London, P. S., (1967). Some observations on the course of events after severe injury of the head. Hunterian Lecture delivered at the Royal College of Surgeons of England on January 12, 1967. *Annals of the Royal College of Surgeons of England, 41,* 460–479.

Meagher, A. D., Beadles, C. A., Doorey, J., & Charles, A. G. (2014). Racial and ethnic disparities in discharge to rehabilitation following traumatic brain injury. *Journal of Neurosurgery, 21,* 1–7.

Ng, D. K., Brotmas, D. J., Lau, B., & Young, J. H. (2012). Insurance status, not race, is associated with mortality after an acute cardiovascular event in Maryland. *Journal of General Internal Medicine, 27,* 1368–1276.

Obisesan, T. O., Vargas, C. M., & Gillum, R. F. (2000). Geographic variation in stroke risk in the United States: Region, urbanization, and hypertension in the Third National Health and Nutrition Examination Survey. *Stroke, 31,* 19–25.

Palaniappan, L. P., Araneta, M. R. G., Assimes, T. L., Barrett-Connor, E. L., Carnethon, M. R., Criqui, M. H., . . . Wong, N. D. (2010). Call to action: Cardiovascular disease in Asian Americans—a science advisory from the American Heart Association. *Circulation, 122,* 1242–1252.

Perrin, P. B., Krch, D., Sutter, M., Snipes, D. J., Arango-Lasprilla, J. C., Kolakowsky-Hayner, S. A., . . . Lequerica, A. (2014). Racial/ethnic disparities in mental health over the first 2 years after traumatic brain injury: A model systems study. *Archives of Physical Medicine and Rehabilitation, 95,* 2288–2295.

Rath, J., (2014, July). Reducing disparities in access to health care. *Spotlight on Disability Newsletter, 6*(1). Retrieved from http://www.apa.org/pi/disability/resources/publications/newsletter/2014/07/healthcare-disparities.aspx

Roth, D. L., Haley, W. E., Clay, O. J., Perkins, M., Grant, J. S., Rhodes, D., . . . Howard, G. (2011). Race and gender differences in 1-year outcomes for community-dwelling stroke survivors with family caregivers. *Stroke, 42,* 626–631.

Sacco, R. L. (1995). Race-ethnicity and determinants of intracranial atherosclerotic cerebral infarction: The Northern Manhattan Stroke Study. *Stroke, 26,* 14–20.

Sacco, R. L., Boden-Albala, B., Gan, R., Chen, X., Kargman, D. E., Shea, S., . . . Hauser, W. A. (1998). Stroke incidence among White, Black, and Hispanic residents of an urban community: The Northern Manhattan Stroke Study. *American Journal of Epidemiology, 147,* 259–268.

Saposnik, G., (2000). Ethnicity in stroke: Practical implications. *Stroke, 31,* 2732–2733.

Simpson, G., Mohr, R., & Redman, A. (2000). Cultural variations in the understanding of traumatic brain injury and brain injury rehabilitation. *Brain Injury, 14,* 125–140.

Stansbury, J. P., Jia, H., Williams, L. S., Vogel, W. B., & Duncan, P. W. (2005). Ethnic disparities in stroke: Epidemiology, acute care, and post-acute outcomes. *Stroke, 36,* 374–386.

Staudenmayer, K. L., Diaz-Arrastia, R., de Oliveira, A., Gentilello, L. M., & Shafi, S. (2007). Ethnic disparities in long-term functional outcomes after traumatic brain injury. *Journal of Trauma, 63,* 1364–1369.

Takeya, Y., Popper, J. S., Shimizu, Y., Kato, H., Rhoads, G. G., & Kagan, A. (1984). Epidemiologic studies of coronary heart disease and stroke in Japanese men living in Japan, Hawaii, and California: Incidence of stroke in Japan and Hawaii. *Stroke, 15,* 15–23.

Traumatic Brain Injury Model Systems, National Data and Statistical Center. (2014). National database: 2014 profile of people within the Traumatic Brain Injury Model Systems. Retrieved from http://www.tbindsc.org

U.S. Bureau of the Census. (1973). *Census of the population: 1970, Vol. 1, Characteristics of the population, Part 6, California—Section 1.* Washington, DC: U.S. Government Printing Office.

U.S. National Library of Medicine, National Institutes of Health. (2015). Retrieved from http://www.ncbi.nlm.nih.gov/pubmed

Wozniak, M. A., Kittner, S. J., Price, T. R., Hebel, J. R., Sloan, M. A., & Gardner, J. F. (1999). Stroke location is not associated with return to work after first ischemic stroke. *Stroke*, *30*, 2568–2573.

Wylie, C. M., (1970). Death statistics for cerebrovascular disease: A review of recent findings. *Stroke*, *1*, 184–193.

Zweifler, R. M., Lyden, P. D., Taft, B., Kelly, N., & Rothrock, J. F. (1995). Impact of race and ethnicity on ischemic stroke: The University of California at San Diego Stroke Data Bank. *Stroke*, *26*, 245–248.

CHAPTER TWO

WORKING WITH PEOPLE WITH DISABILITIES WITHIN A MULTICULTURALISM FRAMEWORK

Eun-Jeong Lee and Nicole Ditchman

The diversity of the United States' population has been increasing more rapidly over the past couple of decades. Currently, 30% of the U.S. population consists of ethnic minorities. It is also estimated that people of color will make up about half of the population by the year 2050 (Taylor-Ritzler, Balcazar, Dimpfl, & Suarez-Balcazar, 2008). As the number of people from ethnic minority backgrounds continues to increase, so will the number of people with disabilities (PWDs) within these groups. In fact, recent findings indicate that African Americans and American Indians have the highest rates of disability (American Cancer Society, 2010; Brault, 2012; Humes, Jones, & Ramirez, 2011; World Health Organization, 2005). Individuals from all minority groups, including PWDs, are likely to share common negative experiences, including, but not limited to, stereotyping and marginalization, higher unemployment and underemployment rates, discrimination, social stigma, disempowerment in the workplace, and financial and educational barriers (Chronister & Johnson, 2009). Moreover, those individuals who belong to more than one minority group are at risk for experiencing multiple negative experiences or "double" discrimination and stigmatization (Brodwin, 1995).

The multicultural movement in counseling and psychology has begun to provide scholars and practitioners with contextually relevant, systems-based ecological approaches to counseling as alternatives to the traditional theoretical models of human behavior and intervention that are based on Western dominant culture (Chronister & Johnson, 2009). With its emphasis on historically underrepresented populations, multiculturalism calls for shifting the focus from White, middle-class clients and research participants to include people from ethnic and sexual minority groups, as well as people who hold various spiritual/religious views (Gilson & DePoy, 2000). Multiculturalism has indeed become a powerful force within psychology, yet PWDs are not well represented among psychologists. For example, less than 2% of American Psychological Association (APA) members identify as a PWD (Olkin & Pledger, 2003).

In fact, PWDs represent the largest minority group in the United States, comprising 15% of the total population (Cornish et al., 2008; Longmore, 2009; Mpofu & Conyers, 2004; Olkin, 2002). However, many psychologists experience challenges working with PWDs due to lack of knowledge about disability. In addition, if the client holds more than two minority statuses, the situation may be even more difficult for psychologists to develop a strong therapeutic relationship with the client. Therefore, the purpose of this chapter is to increase awareness of the complexity of multicultural issues among individuals with disabilities and to discuss culturally sensitive strategies to work with PWDs. The objectives of the chapter are (a) to review legislative mandates related to diversity and multiculturalism in rehabilitation, (b) to address the relationship between disability and culture in the scope of rehabilitation practice, (c) to introduce multiculturalism and multicultural counseling models as a therapeutic framework, (d) to provide guidelines to help psychologists increase their cultural sensitivity, and (e) to provide strategies to work with individuals with disabilities from minority backgrounds.

LEGISLATIVE MANDATES

In the field of rehabilitation, federal initiatives, legislative mandates, and training accreditation bodies have explicitly acknowledged the cultural diversity of PWDs (Chronister & Johnson, 2009). For example, the reauthorization of the Rehabilitation Act of 1992 added new language that specifically identified the inequitable treatment of minorities in the vocational rehabilitation process. Subsequently, the Rehabilitation Services Administration set forth the Rehabilitation Cultural Diversity Initiative (RCDI) to realize the objectives of cultural diversity (Atkins, 1995). The Rehabilitation Act amendments (1992) emphasize the significance of diversity issues in rehabilitation services, stating:

Patterns of inequitable treatment of minorities have been documented in all major junctures of the vocational rehabilitation process. As compared to White Americans, a larger percentage of African American applicants to the vocational rehabilitation system [are] denied acceptance. Of applicants for service, a larger percentage of African American cases [are] closed without being rehabilitated. Minorities are provided less training than their White counterparts. Consistently, less money is spent on minorities than their White counterparts. (p. 4364)

Although diversity and multicultural issues have been discussed extensively in the rehabilitation field, individuals with disabilities who also hold another minority status experience inadequate access to health services and have lower education and income levels, compared with their peers with disabilities who are not from minority backgrounds (Niemeier, Burnett, & Whitaker, 2003; Zea, Belgrave, Townsend, Jarama, & Banks, 1996). In public rehabilitation service programs, individuals from racial/ethnic minority groups are less likely to be accepted for rehabilitation services, have fewer successful case closures, and receive less training and case expenditures (Chronister & Johnson, 2009; Donnell, 2008; Wilson, 2000; Wilson, Harley, & Alston, 2001). As a result of the growing evidence of poor outcomes for PWDs with minority backgrounds, awareness about the importance of multiculturalism and the need for cultural competency in providing services to diverse populations in the United States has been increasing at the federal, state, and local levels.

DISABILITY, CULTURE, AND REHABILITATION

The disability experience *is* a multicultural experience. To understand disability within a multicultural context, it is important to consider the different philosophical perspectives regarding how disability is perceived in cultural groups (Chronister & Johnson, 2009). According to Barnes and Mercer (2001), people believe that individuals with disabilities share a "disability culture"—that is, that they share common experiences related to disability and have a shared social identity across age, gender, ethnic, and disability lines. Disability culture supports the idea that disability is positive and should not be the object of pity. It stresses solidarity and positive identity (Leung, 2003), which reinforces member status within a cultural group.

Although disability and other minority statuses may have features in common, there are distinct differences between the experiences of persons from ethnic/racial minority backgrounds and those of PWDs. For instance, Davis (2001) pointed out that a person with a disability may be "cured," and, therefore, can enter or leave the disability community at any time. For that reason, disability culture may not be as permanent as other minority cultures. On the other hand, disability, like other minority labels, is at risk for stigma, discrimination, and prejudice (Olkin, 1999). Moreover, the cultural context where disability occurs impacts the extent to which individuals may recognize or identify with a disability label. For example, Asian cultures often link mental illnesses or congenital disabilities to supernatural causes, such as a punishment by God or ancestors for past bad behavior, "karma," the effects of inappropriately locating an ancestor's tomb, or possession by evil spirits (Wynaden et al., 2005). As a result of these beliefs, Asians often rely on themselves and family members to manage the symptoms first or turn to spiritual healers for help (Yeung & Kung, 2004).

It is critical to identify the ways individuals, their family members, and their communities define culture and disability. The perspective of PWDs constituting a minority culture seems to have gained ground from a policy standpoint, as reflected in the broader civil rights–based legislative initiatives and policies (e.g., Americans with Disabilities Act [ADA] and subsequent amendments) to increase access and equal opportunity (Chronister & Johnson, 2009). At the same time, the notion of a disability culture, which implies specific norms and expectations that are different from the mainstream culture, should be recognized and has application to both research and clinical models of intervention.

Many PWDs are members of other minority groups. Thus, it is imperative to consider not only the individual's perception of his or her disability status but also the impact that other characteristics (e.g., race, ethnicity, gender, age, sexual orientation, socioeconomic status [SES]) may have on the client's self-concept and on the disability adjustment process. For some individuals, an existing minority status may influence a person's daily life much more than his or her disability, yet for other PWDs, disability may be the most prominent experience. It can be hypothesized that for some individuals, one minority status can lead to others. For example, there is a significantly higher rate of disability among people coming from a lower SES, given the limited access to health care. Thus, much of the work in this area should be preempted with prevention and health care policy. Regardless, the interaction among all cultural roles, expectations, and experiences in an individual's life is critical to exploring and understanding the individual's adjustment process.

The intersection of disability and multicultural competencies is complex and often difficult to negotiate. The application of multicultural competencies in practice with PWDs must be intertwined with disability awareness, sensitivity, and an ongoing recognition of the complex interactions between an individual's view of disability and cultural identities. It is important to respect the personal and contextual differences of each individual, keeping in mind how he or she identifies culturally and how this is an ongoing process (Leung, 2003). In addition to a focus on the individual, it is important that the cultural views of the family also be recognized, particularly when the family becomes involved in the rehabilitation process.

MULTICULTURALISM

The terms *multiculturalism* and *diversity* are often used interchangeably. According to Liu and Pope-Davis (2003), *diversity* is typically defined via quantity of differences represented, but it does not reflect the deeper contextual change that involves intercultural dialogue, sensitivity, and awareness. *Multiculturalism* can be defined as a philosophical framework that encompasses the experiences of various people and groups—and is not just limited to racial and ethnic minorities (Pope-Davis, Liu, Toporek, & Brittan-Powell, 2001).

Many researchers indicate that multicultural sensitivity is an essential element of an effective helping professional. Multicultural intervention can be defined as infusing within one's therapeutic or helping techniques sensitivity to the client's cultural identity, considering how this impacts the way the client views and interacts with the world (Bryan, 2007). As just mentioned, it is helpful to conceptualize PWDs within a minority group model. To adequately provide services and generate better rehabilitation outcomes, the cultural identity of the individuals, the cultural characteristics of the environment in which they function, the rehabilitation service culture, and the interaction of these variables should all be taken into account. The rehabilitation field must have a broader framework that considers the salience of each cultural role, the interaction of these roles within a given context, and the impact on adjustment (Chronister & Johnson, 2009). Rehabilitation professionals need to strengthen their focus and commitment in understanding multidimensional aspects of disability and the adjustment process among PWDs from minority backgrounds.

Multicultural Competency

To be effective at engaging in multiculturally competent intervention, it is important for rehabilitation professionals to have an understanding of culture and worldview. *Culture* involves the beliefs, customs, practices, social behaviors, and attitudes of a particular group of people (National Center for Cultural Competence, 2011). *Worldview* is the framework of ideas and beliefs through which an individual perceives the world and interacts with it based on his or her philosophy, values, emotions, and ethics (Ivey & Ivey, 2003). A person's culture and worldview are critical factors to consider in the response to disability. Culture and worldview inform how disability is defined and experienced and contribute to how PWDs seek out and access rehabilitation services and develop salient goals. For example, in contrast to the medical approach to explain disability, many cultures perceived the origin of disability from a metaphysical or spiritual realm. For other cultures, disability is a condition predetermined by an individual's fate (Sotnick & Jezewski, 2005).

Culture-centered clinical practice emphasizes the integration and awareness of culture in skill-based clinical practice. Culturally competent practitioners recognize the cultural considerations that influence all levels of the client–provider working alliance, including the communication process, health care practices, values and beliefs, treatment efficacy, and service utilization. Based on a series of studies, the field of counseling psychology has developed multicultural counseling models that recognize that individuals hold multiple cultural identities, including age, disability, gender, language, race, sexual orientation, social class and educational background, geographic location, relationship status, spirituality or religion, work experience, and hobbies/recreational interests (Arredondo & Toporek, 2004). According to these models, helping professionals who are culturally competent try to understand the different experiences of people within a particular group, have an understanding of potential barriers to communication that exist as a result of cultural differences, and possess a set of skills that increase the professionals' cultural awareness and allow them to work more effectively with their clients (Pope-Davis et al., 2001).

The contributions of Sue et al. (1982) and Sue, Arredondo, and McDavis (1992) in multicultural counseling competence (MCC) have had a profound impact on the multicultural movement, providing the conceptual foundation for competencies and standards with which practitioners can skillfully and competently serve culturally diverse populations. Sue and colleagues originally conceptualized the model to encompass three broad characteristics, including (a) practitioner's awareness of his or her own assumptions, values, and biases; (b) understanding the worldview of the culturally different client; and (c) developing appropriate and culturally sensitive intervention strategies and techniques. Each of these characteristics is conceptualized to include three components: beliefs and attitudes, knowledge, and skills (Sue et al., 1992; Exhibit 2.1).

Several MCC models have extended Sue et al.'s work. These MCC models have enhanced the conceptualization and understanding of multicultural competency and have provided other allied health specialties with ways to systematically apply a multicultural approach in training,

Exhibit 2.1 *Characteristics of the Multiculturally Competent Practitioner*

Beliefs and attitudes	A practitioner's mental framework about ethnic and racial minorities, their biases and stereotypes about specific groups, the development of a positive outlook toward multicultural perspectives, and the recognition of how his or her own biases and values may affect working with individuals from different cultures.
Knowledge	A practitioner's understanding of his or her worldview, knowledge of cultural groups, and the sociopolitical factors that may affect the cross-cultural therapeutic relationship.
Skills	Specific abilities are needed to work effectively with different cultural minority groups (Ridley & Kleiner, 2003). Skills to assess the level of acculturation, family structure, and worldview to which the client ascribes are critical elements in multicultural interventions.

Source: Sue et al. (1992).

research, and practice. However, there remain a few challenges that psychologists still face and need to overcome. Major limitations of these frameworks include: (a) the inabilities to provide specific and concrete guidance in the achievement of specific competency areas; (b) limited research supporting the empirical validation of these models (Atkinson & Israel, 2003; Weinarch & Thomas, 2002); (c) lack of training and supervision opportunities to develop the level of competency and cultural sensitivity required; and (d) lack of attention given to the client perspective related to multicultural competencies (Pope-Davis et al., 2001). Despite these limitations, these models underscore the importance of recognizing the complexity of the professional–client interaction, highlighting the myriad cultural and contextual factors involved.

The Multicultural Counseling Approach for PWDs

PWDs from racial/ethnic and sexual minority groups often present situations that challenge psychologists and do not adhere to the rehabilitation treatment process. Therefore, psychologists in rehabilitation settings require not only multicultural competence but also disability competence. An awareness and understanding of disability may be quite different from what most rehabilitation practitioners have been previously confronted with (Leung, 2003).

Another issue is the complexity of the individual's personal experience when demographic characteristics (e.g., ethnicity, gender, SES, sexual minority status) intersect with disability. For example, racial discrimination can influence access to appropriate health care, work, and assistive technology among PWDs. People from lower SES backgrounds may have substantial trouble affording health care, health insurance, transit, and necessary assistive technology as well. Gender issues can interact with disability for both men and women, especially if a person's disability affects her or his ability to maintain a culturally accepted gender role. People who identify as lesbian, gay, bisexual, or transsexual also face additional challenges, because there are even fewer legislative protections for these individuals and additional social stigma (Balcazar, Suarez-Balcazar, & Taylor-Ritzler, 2009; Cornish et al, 2008).

According to Suarez-Balcazar and Rodakowski (2007), "Becoming culturally competent is an ongoing contextual, developmental, and experiential process of personal growth that results in professional understanding and ability to adequately serve individuals who look, think, and behave differently from us" (p. 15). Researchers have applied MCC models to the context of rehabilitation (e.g., Balcazar et al., 2009; Middleton et al., 2000), developed new models of multicultural counseling for clients with disabilities, and conducted studies investigating the level of MCC among rehabilitation professionals and the relationship between MCC and rehabilitation–client outcomes (e.g., Bellini, 2002; Cumming-McCann & Accordino, 2005; Donnell, 2008). Although the field of rehabilitation has explicitly acknowledged the diversity of individuals seeking services and the inequities in service delivery, the field still remains in the early stages of developing multicultural models of training, research, and practice. Balcazar et al. (2009) pointed out that a major shortcoming in the current cultural competence literature is the lack of available validated conceptual frameworks and measures. Rehabilitation researchers and practitioners share the struggles experienced by those who are advocating for the multicultural movement, such as the ever-present challenges of balancing between-group differences with within-group heterogeneity, applying mainstream theories and treatments to those from minority cultures, and developing empirically supported, theory-driven therapeutic frameworks that are relevant and meaningful to PWDs and their families (Chronister & Johnson, 2009).

Among the many MCC models, Lewis (2006) presented a three-factor model of multicultural counseling for PWDs that applies the work of multicultural scholars regarding the process of adjustment to disability. This model was designed to assist rehabilitation professionals in gaining awareness of their readiness to engage in multicultural interventions and to guide professionals in focusing on the three primary client characteristics: adjustment to disability, stage of development, and cultural identity. According to this model, the practitioner should explore the client's stage of adjustment, meaning of adjustment, and commitment to the adjustment process. Identifying the stage of development is critical to understanding where the PWD is in terms of developmental functioning. This area is particularly important to adjustment because the age of onset of a disability can significantly influence the adjustment process (Lewis, 2006). Finally, cultural identity involves exploration and understanding of the individual's physical, mental, emotional, spiritual, social, and volitional functioning from the client's cultural perspective.

HELPING REHABILITATION PROFESSIONALS
TO INCREASE CULTURAL SENSITIVITY

PWDs are similar to other minority groups in many ways, given their history of subjugation, intolerance, and discrimination. In addition, they have been defined through the lens of the mainstream cultural group and therefore historically denied self-definition. They have been underrepresented in positions of power and have been forced to emulate and adopt the values of the majority group. Like other social movements, the disability rights and independent living movements are evidence that PWDs have fought these circumstances. Although conceptualizing PWDs within a multicultural framework is useful, it is also important for psychologists to realize both the similarities and the differences this group has with other cultural groups (Artman & Daniels, 2010). To this end, practitioners must ask themselves: What is a culturally sensitive helping professional? How can a helping professional be culturally competent?

First, the professional needs to assess his or her comfort level with regard to being around and interacting with persons who appear to be different from him or herself based on race, ethnicity, religion, sexual orientation, or disability status. Cultural sensitivity skills are required for the professional to be considered professionally competent. The success or failure of the helping relationship with a culturally different client will, to a major extent, depend on this competency (Artman & Daniels, 2010). At the same time, in situations where the practitioner and client may appear to share a common cultural identity (such as being from the same race/ethnicity or having a disability), it is important that the practitioner recognize the potential for countertransference to occur and maintain an openness to understanding the perspective and unique identity of the client.

Sue and Sue (2008) provide a broad summary of a culturally sensitive helping professional. In making their case, they refer to psychologists, but the points apply to any type of helping professional:

1. Culturally skilled helping professionals have moved from being culturally unaware to being aware and are sensitive to their own cultural heritage and to valuing and respecting differences.
2. Culturally skilled helping professionals are aware of their own values and biases and how these may affect clients from minority backgrounds.

3. Culturally skilled helping professionals are comfortable with differences that exist between themselves and their clients in terms of race and beliefs.
4. Culturally skilled helping professionals are sensitive to circumstances that may dictate referral of minority clients to another practitioner of their own race/culture or to another professional in general.
5. Culturally skilled helping professionals acknowledge and are aware of their own potentially racist or culturally biased attitudes, beliefs, and feelings.

In rehabilitation psychology, Balcazar et al. (2009) developed a cultural competence model based on an extensive review of the literature. According to this model, critical awareness, knowledge, and skill development are fundamental elements for developing cultural competence. First, *critical awareness* consists of being aware of personal biases, lack of knowledge/training, and an understanding of what privilege status one may have. Second, *knowledge* is the interest and investigation into other cultures and gaining an understanding of their core values, shared history, and customs. Third, *skills development* describes increasing critical awareness and knowledge, as well as the importance of interacting with clients in an empathic manner and being able to weave clients' cultural values and personal contexts into therapeutic interventions. Fourth, *practice/application* refers to the process of applying all three components in a specific context. Implementing individual and organizational practices is the most challenging part of addressing cultural competence. Because the application of cultural competence involves organizational and systemic changes, Balcazar et al. pointed out that organizational support is a critical factor in determining the capacity of individual practitioners to deliver culturally competent services.

Critical Awareness and Knowledge

Helping professionals must be aware of their personal language, attributions, and attitudes in working with PWDs. Most perceptions of disabilities are negatively reflected in the language that is used. Therefore, a simple, basic approach would be to use person-first language (e.g., "a person *with* a disability" as opposed to "a disabled person"). Using person-first language reminds others of PWDs' basic humanity (Mpofu & Conyers, 2004;

Olkin, 2002). PWDs have combated other terminology that appears harmless but is actually an expression of negativity toward PWDs because the use of negative language serves to perpetuate stigmatizing attitudes and assumptions that PWDs are inherently miserable or victims who should be pitied (Mpofu & Conyers, 2004). On the other hand, some groups of individuals with disabilities, such as many members of the Deaf community, have a strong tie with their disability network and often advocate language reflective of this by placing emphasis on their disability (Leung, 2003). A professional working from a multiculturalism framework would take into account the particular labels and style of language preferred by the client.

Exposure to and building relationships with PWDs are also invaluable learning tools. According to Artman and Daniels (2010), local Centers for Independent Living are community resources that can assist in a fuller understanding of PWDs as a cultural group. Longmore (2009) provides other resources for learning about the history of disability, such as books and journals that have devoted substantial attention to the topic and an encyclopedic series that provides a detailed disability history in the United States.

Skills Development

Olkin and Taliaferro (2006) point out common mistakes that professionals make when working with PWDs. In addition to assuming the disability is central to the presenting concerns (or ignoring the disability completely), practitioners sometimes fall victim to the spread effect—that is, allowing the disability to completely define the individual and subsume other aspects of the person, such as personality, gender, race, sexuality, religion, age, ethnicity, interests, and employment status, among others. Another error involves misinterpreting affect. For example, just because a PWD is depressed does not mean it is a normal part of adjustment or is inevitable. Similarly, anger over lack of accommodations and discrimination may be justified rather than labeled as maladjustment. In addition, many professionals may hold PWDs to lower standards and expectations related to personal achievement, such as in the areas of academics, employment, intimate relationships, or leadership in the community because of their own negative attributions about the abilities of PWDs (Middleton et al., 2000; Wheaton & Granello, 1998). To help avoid these mistakes, conceptualizing clients within social contexts helps remove the effects of these pathological labels, viewing some of the difficulties they face in terms of the physical and social barriers inherent in being a cultural minority rather than being a "damaged" individual (Olkin, 1999).

Olkin (1999) notes that many psychologists are reluctant to ask questions directly of PWDs regarding their disability and adjustment when they come in for psychotherapy. Similarly, psychologists often hesitate to ask about racial or ethnic issues when the client is culturally different from the psychologist. It is generally acceptable to ask about the nature of the disability or condition. If the client does not broach the subject during the discussion of presenting issues in therapy, the psychologist can open a dialogue by asking if the client feels her or his disability plays a role in the presenting issues. The main message is that it is important to remember that disability may or may not be central to the client's concerns, but it should not be completely ignored (Olkin, 1999).

Accessibility/Accommodation

As rehabilitation professionals, it is often the first step to think about accommodation and accessibility issues for PWDs to provide more inclusive and culturally sensitive practice. In addition, professionals should be able to provide simple action steps to help the clients advocate for themselves and direct them to additional resources and options to promote informed choice (Artman & Daniels, 2010). Professionals must consider several factors when they provide services. First, to what extent is the building physically accessible? If the clinic is considered a nonprofit or public rehabilitation facility, it will be covered by Title II of the ADA, and if the setting is in a federally owned facility, it is covered by Section 504 of the Rehabilitation Act of 1973 (Artman & Daniels, 2010). Therefore, the building needs to be accessible and adhere to the accessibility guidelines. As rehabilitation professionals, separate entrances, elevators, and accessible restrooms are important to culturally sensitive work with PWDs. Second, public transportation or paratransit should also be considered with regard to scheduling appointments. Depending on the client's disability condition, appointments should be made considering sleep/wake cycles and levels of fatigue. Third, it is important to consider the psychotherapy and assessment milieu, including the accessibility of the actual room, the frequency of breaks given, seating arrangements, lighting, and room temperature. In addition, professionals should take into consideration the language and verbal communication abilities of the client and may use written handouts, visual aids, voice amplifiers, or recordings. Alternative formats of consent forms and handouts such as large print, font color, and Braille should be considered as well (Artman & Daniels, 2010).

Strategies for Working With PWDs From Different Cultural Backgrounds

Psychologists may be concerned with how they can implement their knowledge and create a more accessible practice as well as improve advocacy skills for their clients with disabilities. The following strategies are presented to help psychologists start thinking about a more inclusive practice, provide simple steps, and direct them to additional resources for further learning. In general, it may be helpful for psychologists to let all clients know that they wish to make psychotherapy as accessible and successful as possible and to empower clients to advocate for any considerations or modifications to improve their service experience. Overall, the most important skill for psychologists to possess is the ability to listen to their clients with disabilities, while taking their feedback and concerns seriously (Artman & Daniels, 2010).

Cultural and Racial Identity

Most PWDs who receive rehabilitation services have multiple identities that are connected to beliefs, attitudes, values, and goals that shape their unique worldviews and how they choose to interpret and respond to disability and the adjustment process (Atkins, 1988). It is important to consider the interrelationship between racial and other cultural identity processes and adjustment to disability. Cultural identity development is a critical aspect of psychosocial adjustment and is fundamental to the psychological health of all individuals. In fact, several studies show a relationship between racial identity and various psychological outcomes salient in the adjustment to disability literature, including self-esteem, depression, anxiety, stress, hope, and internal locus of control (Alston, 2003; Alston & Turner, 1994; Jarama & Belgrave, 2002; Zea et al., 1996). Among the many unique cultural identities an individual has, racial identity includes the psychological, cultural, physical, and sociopolitical dimensions of belonging to a particular group (Alston, 2003). Racial identity reflects the lens through which people position themselves in relation to others who may be racially different (McCowen & Alston, 1998; Sue, 2003). Racial identity (Mpofu & Harley, 2006; Sellers & Shelton, 2003) has also been defined by the following:

- *Degree of identity salience:* significance of race to an individual's self-concept
- *Centrality:* the extent to which an individual regards racial membership as primary to his or her self-definition
- *Ideology:* the individual's set of beliefs about how members of his or her own racial group should behave
- *Regard:* the individual's feelings and evaluative judgments regarding one's racial group

These definitions are useful not only for considering racial identity, but they also provide a framework for working with clients to understand their perceptions regarding other identities of importance to their lives (e.g., sexual orientation, religious group, disability).

Cultural Characteristics

A relatively robust body of literature is available on the unique characteristics, values, and norms of particular cultural minority groups. An individual's culture is not a diagnostic category, and no cultural heritage will explain the way any given individual will think and act. However, it can help rehabilitation professionals anticipate and understand how and why individuals and their families make certain decisions. Understanding cultural characteristics and differences is a new task for rehabilitation professionals. For example, the culturally perceived cause of a chronic illness or disability is significant in all culture studies to date. The reason why an illness or disability is believed to have occurred will play a significant role in determining family and community attitudes toward the individual. Often, disability is viewed as a form of punishment by many cultures. In many African and Caribbean societies, as well as in many Native American tribes, witchcraft is often linked to chronic illness and disability (Chronister & Johnson, 2009). It is imperative that the professional work with the client to understand the salience and significance of disability in the individual's life, taking into account the culture or cultures that have shaped the client's identity.

Acculturation

Assessing the individual's level of acculturation regarding the client's racial/ethnic background is important. Because many helping professionals often concentrate on only one dimension (either race or ethnic culture), in many cases, disability becomes an extra dimension that must be considered in assessing acculturation level. The assessment of an individual's and/or family's level of disability acculturation will primarily revolve around attitudes. Attitudinal barriers often become the major hindrance for most individuals with disabilities. The societal attitudes toward PWDs significantly influence the community integration and quality of life among individuals with disabilities (Chan, Livneh, Pruett, Wang, & Zheng, 2009). Therefore, it is important to assess the multidimensional aspect of acculturation by including not only racial acculturation but also disability acculturation. Bryan (2007) suggested the process of assessing the disability culture of a person with a disability:

- The professional must have knowledge of societal attitudes toward individuals with disabilities.
- The professional must have an awareness of the subtle and sometimes not-so-subtle ways society expresses attitudes toward persons with disabilities.
- The professional must be knowledgeable about the client's "environment attitudes (the client's local surroundings, such as neighborhood, city, state, etc.)" toward disabilities and the ways in which these attitudes are manifested.
- The professional must determine the client's attitudes toward his or her disability.
- The professional must determine the attitudes of the client's family regarding disability in general and also for the individual's life situation. (p. 123)

Family Structure

It is critical to understand the family structure when a helping professional works with a PWD (e.g., Who is the authority figure in the family? Who makes decisions? How are decisions made?). An individual with a disability within a family unit, regardless of whether the onset of the disability was sudden, gradual, or congenital, does not necessarily mean that a family will be thrust into a state of crisis (Bryan, 2007). The professional needs to observe carefully each family member's reaction to the disability situation, which will reveal strengths and weaknesses within the family unit. Identifying a family's strengths and weaknesses will help the professional to work with the family. The family can be the strongest emotional and practical support system for the individual. Both PWDs and their families face a variety of needs, including service information, advocacy, a system of care, emotional and social support, and financial support (Bryan, 2007; Rosenthal, Kosciulek, Lee, Frain, & Ditchman, 2009).

For example, in Asian and Latino cultures, families often play a key role in deciding on appropriate treatments due to a strong familial connection. For that reason, family members typically assume that it is their responsibility to be with the clients when the client communicates with the practitioner. Research findings support this assertion and highlight the importance of the family in treatment among culturally different clients (Bao & Lam, 2008). It is imperative that the professional recognize and assess the extent to which these needs are being met and provide resources and intervention strategies to address those that are not being met adequately.

CONCLUSIONS

In the field of rehabilitation, little attention has been given to the uniqueness of PWDs from a multicultural context. Given the increased diversification of American society, more attention should be given to how PWDs identify due to the different worldviews held by minority individuals. In addition, more rehabilitation professionals are experiencing challenges working with PWDs and have become increasingly concerned with understanding racial/ethnic minority individuals with disabilities. Moreover, cultural sensitivity is important for enhancing the therapeutic working relationship between the practitioner and the client.

In this chapter, we addressed the challenges and issues facing rehabilitation professionals when working with PWDs and provided an overview of multiculturalism, related conceptual models, and strategies to work with PWDs from a culturally sensitive approach. It is necessary for rehabilitation professionals to engage in ongoing education, supervision, and training related to how to most effectively work with various minority populations. It is imperative that practitioners recognize the complexity of the client identity and the intersection of culture and disability.

REFERENCES

Alston, R., & Turner, W. L. (1994). A family strengths model of adjustment to disability for African American clients. *Journal of Counseling & Development, 72,* 378–383.

Alston, R. J. (2003). Racial identity and cultural mistrust among African American recipients of rehabilitation services: An exploratory study. *International Journal of Rehabilitation Research, 26,* 289–295.

American Cancer Society. (2010). *Cancer facts & figures 2010.* Atlanta, GA: American Cancer Society.

Arredondo, P., & Toporek, R. (2004). Multicultural counseling competencies-ethical practice. *Journal of Mental Health Counseling, 26,* 44–55.

Artman, K. J., & Daniels, J. A. (2010). Disability and psychotherapy practice: Cultural competence and practical tips. *Professional Psychology: Research and Practice, 41*(5), 442–448.

Atkins, B. J. (1995). "Diversity: A continuing rehabilitation challenge and opportunity." In S. Walker, K. A. Turner, M. Haile-Michael, A. Vincent, & M. D. Miles (Eds.), *Disability and diversity: New leadership for a new era* (pp. 34–38). Washington, DC: President's Committee on Employment of People with Disabilities and Howard University Research and Training Center. Retrieved from http://files.eric.ed.gov/fulltext/ED394233.pdf

Atkinson, D. R., & Israel, T. (2003). The future of multicultural counseling competency. In D. B. Pope-Davis, H. L. K. Coleman, W. M. Liu, & R. Toporeks (Eds.), *Handbook of multicultural competencies in counseling and psychology* (pp. 591–606). Thousand Oaks, CA: Sage.

Balcazar, F. E., Suarez-Balcazar, Y., & Taylor-Ritzler, T. (2009). Cultural competence: Development of a conceptual framework. *Disability and Rehabilitation, 31,* 1153–1160.

Bao, X. H., & Lam, S. F. (2008). Who makes the choice? Rethinking the role of autonomy and relatedness in Chinese children's motivation. *Child Development, 79,* 269–283. doi:10.1111/j.1467-8624.2007.01125.x

Barnes, C., & Mercer, G. (2001). Disability culture: Assimilation or inclusion. In G. Albrecht, K. D. Seelman, & M. Bury (Eds.), *Handbook of disability studies.* (pp. 515–534). Thousand Oaks, CA: Sage.

Bellini, J. (2002). Correlates of multicultural counseling competencies of vocational rehabilitation counselors. *Rehabilitation Counseling Bulletin, 45,* 66–75.

Brault, M. W. (2012). *Americans with disabilities: 2010* (Current Population Report No. P70–131). Washington, DC: U.S. Census Bureau.

Brodwin, M. G. (1995). Barriers to multicultural understanding: Improving university rehabilitation counselor education programs. In S. Walker, K. A. Turner, M. Haile-Michael, A. Vincent, & M. D. Miles (Eds.), *Disability and diversity: New leadership for a new era* (pp. 39–45). Washington, DC: President's Committee on Employment of People with Disabilities and Howard University Research and Training Center. Retrieved from http://files.eric.ed.gov/full text/ED394233.pdf

Bryan, W. V. (2007). *Multicultural aspects of disabilities: A guide to understanding and assisting minorities in the rehabilitation process.* Springfield, IL: Charles C. Thomas.

Chan, F., Livneh, H., Pruett, S., Wang, C-C., & Zheng, L. X. (2009). Societal attitudes toward disability: Concepts, measurements, and interventions. In F. Chan, E. D. S. Cardoso, and J. A. Chronister (Eds.), *Understanding psychosocial adjustment to chronic illness and disability: A handbook for evidence-based practitioners in rehabilitation* (pp. 333–370). New York, NY: Springer Publishing Company.

Chronister, J., & Johnson, E. (2009). Multiculturalism and adjustment to disability. In F. Chan, E. D. S. Cardoso, and J. A. Chronister (Eds.), *Understanding psychosocial adjustment to chronic illness and disability: A handbook for evidence-based practitioners in rehabilitation* (pp. 479–520). New York, NY: Springer Publishing Company.

Cornish, J. A. E., Gorgens, K. A., Monson, S. P., Olkin, R., Palombi, B. J., & Abels, A. V. (2008). Perspectives on ethical practice with people who have disabilities. *Professional Psychology: Research and Practice, 39,* 488–497. doi:10.1037/a0013092

Cumming-McCann, A., & Accordino, M. P. (2005). An investigation of rehabilitation counselor characteristics, white racial attitudes, and self-reported multicultural counseling competencies. *Rehabilitation Counseling Bulletin, 48,* 167–176.

Davis, L. (2001). Identity politics, disability, and culture. In G. L. Albrecht, K. D. Seelman, & M. Bury (Eds.), *Handbook of disability studies* (pp. 535–545). Thousand Oaks, CA: Sage.

Donnell, C. M. (2008). Examining multicultural counseling competencies of rehabilitation counseling graduate students. *Rehabilitation Education, 22,* 47–58.

Gilson, S. F., & DePoy, E. (2000). Multiculturalism and disability: A critical perspective. *Disability and Society, 15,* 207–218.

Humes, K. R., Jones, N. A., & Ramirez, R. R. (2011). *Overview of race and Hispanic origin: 2010.* Washington, DC: U.S. Department of Commerce, Economics and Statistics Administration, U.S. Census Bureau.

Ivey, A. E., & Ivey, M. B. (2003). *Intentional interviewing and counseling: Facilitating client development in a multicultural society* (5th ed.). Pacific Groove, CA: Brooks/Cole.

Jarama, S. L., & Belgrave, F. Z. (2002). A model of mental health adjustment among African Americans with disabilities. *Journal of Social and Clinical Psychology, 31,* 323–342.

Leung, P. (2003). Multicultural competencies and rehabilitation counseling/ psychology. In D. B. Pope-Davis, H. L. K. Coleman, W. M. Liu, & R. T. Toporek (Eds.), *Handbook of multicultural competencies in counseling & psychology* (pp. 493–455). Thousand Oaks, CA: Sage.

Lewis, A. M. (2006). Three-factor model of multicultural counseling for consumers with disabilities. *Journal of Vocational Rehabilitation, 24,* 151–159.

Liu, W. M., & Pope-Davis, D. B. (2003). Moving from diversity to multiculturalism: Exploring power and its implications for multicultural competence. In D. B. Pope-Davis, H. L. K. Coleman, W. M. Liu, & R. Toporek (Eds.), *Handbook of multicultural competencies in counseling and psychology* (pp. 90–102). Thousand Oaks, CA: Sage.

Longmore, P. K. (2009, July). Making disability an essential part of American history. *OAH Magazine of History,* 11–15.

McCowen, C., & Alston, R. (1998). Multicultural counseling issues among African American college students. *Journal of Multicultural Counseling and Development, 76,* 237–249.

Middleton, R. A., Rollins, C. W., Sanderson, P. L., Leung, P., Harley, D. A., Ebener, D., & Leal-Idrogo, A. (2000). Endorsement of professional multicultural rehabilitation competencies and standards: A call to action. *Rehabilitation Counseling Bulletin, 43,* 219–240.

Mpofu, E., & Conyers, L. M. (2004). A representational theory perspective of minority status and people with disabilities: Implications for rehabilitation education and practice. *Rehabilitation Counseling Bulletin, 47,* 142–151.

Mpofu, E., & Harley, D. A. (2006). Racial and disability identity: Implications for the career counseling of African Americans with disabilities. *Rehabilitation Counseling Bulletin, 50,* 14–23.

National Center for Cultural Competence. (2011). *Report of significant accomplishments. Center for child and human development.* Washington, DC: Georgetown University.

Niemeier, J. P., Burnett, D. M., & Whitaker, D. A. (2003). Cultural competence in the multidisciplinary rehabilitation setting: Are we falling short of meeting needs? *Archive of Physical Medicine and Rehabilitation, 84,* 1240–1245.

Olkin, R. (1999). *What psychotherapists should know about disability.* New York, NY: Guilford Press.

Olkin, R. (2002). Could you hold the door for me? Including disability in diversity. *Cultural Diversity and Ethnic Minority Psychology, 8,* 130–137. doi:10.1037/1099-9809.8.2.130

Olkin, R., & Pledger, C. (2003). Can disability studies and psychology join hands? *American Psychologist, 58,* 296–304. doi:101037/0003-066X.58.4.296

Olkin, R., & Taliaferro, G. (2006). Evidence-based practices have ignored people with disabilities. In J. C. Norcross, L. E. Beutler, R. F. Levant (Eds.), *Evidence-based practices in mental health: Debate and dialogue on the fundamental questions* (pp. 353–359). Washington, DC: American Psychological Association.

Pope-Davis, D. B., Liu, W. M., Toporek, R. I., & Brittan-Powell, C. S. (2001). What's missing from multicultural competency research: Review, introspection, and recommendations. *Cultural Diversity and Ethnic Minority Psychology, 7,* 121–138.

Rehabilitation Act Amendments of 1992. (1992). Public Law No. 102-569. *U.S. Statutes at Large, Vol. 106,* pp. 4344–4488.

Ridley, C. R., & Kleiner, A. J. (2003). Multicultural counseling competence: History, themes, and issues. In D. B. Pope-Davis, H. L. K. Coleman, W. M. Liu, & R. Toporek (Eds.), *Handbook of multicultural competencies in counseling and psychology* (pp. 3–20). Thousand Oaks, CA: Sage.

Rosenthal, D. A., Kosciulek, J., Lee, G. K., Frain, M., & Ditchman, N. (2009). Family and adaptation to chronic illness and disability. In F. Chan, E. D. S. Cardoso, and J. A. Chronister (Eds.), *Understanding psychosocial adjustment to chronic illness and disability: A handbook for evidence-based practitioners in rehabilitation* (pp. 185–206). New York, NY: Springer Publishing Company.

Sellers, R., & Shelton, N. J. (2003). The role of racial identity in perceived racial discrimination. *Journal of Personality and Social Psychology, 82,* 1079–1092.

Sotnick, P., & Jezewski, M. A. (2005). Culture and the disability services. In J. H. Stone (Ed.), *Culture and disability: Providing culturally competent services* (pp. 15–36). Thousand Oaks, CA: Sage.

Suarez-Balcazar, Y., & Rodakowski, J. (2007). Becoming a culturally competent occupational therapy practitioner. *Occupational Therapy Practice, 12,* 14–17.

Sue, D. W. (2003). *Overcoming racism: The journey to liberation.* San Francisco, CA: Jossey-Bass.

Sue, D. W., Arredondo, P., & McDavis, R. J. (1992). Multicultural counseling competencies and standards: A call to the profession. *Journal of Counseling and Development, 70,* 477–486.

Sue, D. W., Bernier, J. E., Durran, A., Feinburg, L., Pederson, P., Smith, E. J., . . . Vasquez-Nuttall, E. (1982). Position paper: Cross-cultural counseling competencies. *The Counseling Psychologist, 10,* 45–52.

Sue, D. W., & Sue, D. (2008). *Counseling the culturally diverse: Theory and practice.* Hoboken, NJ: Wiley.

Taylor-Ritzler, T., Balcazar, F., Dimpfl, S., & Suarez-Balcazar, Y. (2008). Cultural competence training with organizations serving people with disabilities from diverse cultural backgrounds. *Journal of Vocational Rehabilitation, 29,* 77–91.

Weinarch, S. G., & Thomas, K. R. (2002). A critical analysis of the multicultural counseling competencies: Implications for the practice of mental health counseling. *Journal of Mental Health Counseling, 24,* 20–35.

Wheaton, J. E., & Granello, D. H. (1998). The multicultural counseling competencies of state vocational rehabilitation counselors. *Rehabilitation Education, 12,* 51–64.

Wilson, K. B. (2000). Predicting vocational rehabilitation eligibility based on race, education, work status, and source of support and application. *Rehabilitation Counseling Bulletin, 43,* 97–105.

Wilson, K. B., Harley, D. A., & Alston, R. J. (2001). Race as a correlate of vocational rehabilitation acceptance—Revisited. *Journal of Rehabilitation, 67,* 35–41.

World Health Organization. (2005). *Mental Health Atlas.* Geneva: World Health Organization.

Wynaden, D., Chapman, R., Orb, A., McGowan, S., Zeeman, Z., & Yeak, S. H. (2005). Factors that influence Asian communities' access to mental health care. *International Journal of Mental Health Nursing, 14,* 88–95.

Yeung, A., & Kung, W. W. (2004). How culture impacts on the treatment of mental illnesses among Asian Americans. *Psychiatric Times, 21,* 34–36.

Zea, M. C., Belgrave, F. Z., Townsend, T. G., Jarama, S. L., & Banks, S. R. (1996). The influence of social support and active coping on depression among African Americans and Latinos with disabilities. *Rehabilitation Psychology, 41,* 225–242.

PART TWO

MULTICULTURAL ISSUES IN THE NEUROREHABILITATION SETTING

CHAPTER THREE

CULTURAL VARIABLES AND THE PROCESS OF NEUROPSYCHOLOGICAL ASSESSMENT IN THE NEUROREHABILITATION SETTING AFTER BRAIN INJURY

Anthony H. Lequerica and Ivan Panyavin

Neuropsychological assessment involves the administration of a battery of tests that assess a variety of cognitive domains to obtain a clinical picture of brain behavior relationships. Within the inpatient rehabilitation setting, neuropsychologists often perform various functions, including neuropsychological assessment, psychotherapy, and assistance with adjustment issues for patients and their families. In this setting, the goal of the neuropsychological assessment can serve several purposes beyond obtaining a diagnosis. Findings are often used to track patient progress, direct patient care, improve staff–patient interactions to be more appropriate to the patient's level of impairment, and guide discharge planning. This chapter discusses some of the common cultural issues that impact neuropsychology in an inpatient rehabilitation setting. The major focus is on potential sources of bias that can threaten the validity of neuropsychological tests. We also examine the process of the neuropsychological evaluation within the inpatient setting when working with individuals from diverse cultural backgrounds.

Although recently it has been argued that significant differences exist between races on measures of cognitive abilities due to heritable characteristics (Rushton & Jensen, 2005), the prevailing data and scientific consensus indicate that differences in human behavior and cognition are not biologically determined (Gould, 1981; Nisbett, 2005). Ethnic and racial differences have been noted in practically every sphere of neuropsychological functioning (O'Bryant, Humphreys, Bauer, McCaffrey, & Hilsabeck, 2007), and they are of particular relevance to neuropsychological test performance. However, terms like *race* and *ethnicity* are currently understood to be socially or politically determined with little basis in genetics or biology (Helms, Jernigan, & Mascher, 2005). Race and ethnicity are two aspects of culture that have appeared repeatedly in the neuropsychology research literature examining cultural differences. The term *culture* in this context refers to an integrated system of learned behavior patterns that are characteristic of the members of a society and not solely the result of biological inheritance (Hoebel, 1966). These patterns of behavior are based on an underlying set of learned traditions, living styles, beliefs, and values common to individuals within a given social milieu (Harris, 1983) that shape their view of the world. It is important to understand that when discussing *culture*, we often deal with a complex composite of sociodemographic factors that include education, socioeconomic status (SES), race, ethnicity, language, and worldview, all of which interact with one another to influence brain–behavior relationships. Even the development and organization of the human brain can be differentially affected by these components, depending on the way in which the environment interacts with personal factors to shape experience.

EDUCATION

Most neuropsychological testing utilizes normative data that are collected through standardized administration of a test to a large sample of neurologically intact individuals. When a particular patient receives a certain raw score, it is compared with scores from a matched normative cohort of healthy individuals in the community. Normative data in the field of neuropsychology are typically stratified by age and education. Previous research has demonstrated a complex interaction between education and normal aging (Ardila, Ostrosky-Solis, Rosselli, & Gómez, 2000; Lam et al., 2013). Education alone has been shown to influence performance on seemingly simple tasks such as object naming for neurologically intact individuals (Reis, Guerreiro, & Castro-Caldas, 1994). The impact of education on test performance is quite complex and has been shown to differ across various populations (Manly, Jacobs, Touradji, Small, & Stern, 2002).

Cross-cultural differences have been found in brain mechanisms underlying many academic skills learned in most educational systems, such as reading and arithmetic (Siok, Perfetti, Jin, & Tan, 2004; Tang et al., 2006), and the interaction between culture and education to impact brain plasticity is gaining attention in the research literature (Ansari, 2012). Many studies have shown the effects of culture on brain development. For example, a study examining the development of inhibitory control among children from two eastern European countries found that performance differed depending on whether the target outcome involved accuracy or efficiency (Cheie, Veraksa, Zinchenko, Gorovaya, & Visu-Petra, 2015).

Although there is little doubt that education impacts cognitive test performance, normative data stratified by years of education can lose their utility when used among individuals from diverse cultures. Education among children growing up in countries where the educational system is not well regulated can present as heterogeneous to the point where the same relationships between years of education and cognitive test performance are not universally shared. Cognitive development can be impacted by the structure of the school system, the academic content of classes, and the quality of the education.

The structure of the educational system can vary greatly in terms of the student–teacher ratio or the degree to which children are grouped according to age or aptitude. In some cultures, children of all ages attend a one-room school where they are all taught the same material. This may be more common in areas that are sparsely populated or communities that lack resources or a sufficient number of qualified individuals to teach.

The content of what is taught in school is often a reflection of what is valued in a given culture. For example, in a farming community, there may be less emphasis on computer programming and greater emphasis on the skills children will need to function as productive members of the community. Ostrosky-Solis, Ramirez, and Ardila (2004) found that indigenous peoples performed better than nonindigenous individuals on visual–spatial tests, and education was associated with performance on tests of working and verbal memory. They concluded that the educational system can be viewed as a subculture that promotes certain skills over others for the purpose of survival.

Cultural experiences exert powerful influences on behavior (Brickman, Cabo, & Manly, 2006), especially when mediated by one's educational history. As shown by Luria (1976) during his seminal field work in Central Asia during the 1930s, and subsequently by other researchers (e.g., Cole, Gay, Glick, & Sharp, 1971), individuals with no formal education use dramatically different strategies on tasks of object classification than those with even a modicum of organized schooling. Instead of the expected taxonomic or categorical classification of objects into linguistic categories (e.g., "tools," "foods"), individuals with no history of formal education approached such problems with a concrete, graphic/functional method that directly reflected their predominant worldview—that of solving practical problems in their environment that are related to everyday work and survival.

Studies have examined literacy as a key variable that may provide more useful information than duration of education (Ostrosky-Solis, Ardila, Rosselli, Lopez-Arango, & Uriel-Mendoza, 1998). Schneider and Lichtenberg (2011) found that among African American elders, reading ability, and not education, was associated with performance on tasks such as the Trail Making Test, Controlled Oral Word Association Test, animal naming, Digit Span, and the Stroop Test, but not with tests of memory. Reading ability has also been shown to act as a mediator between years of education and performance on a number of executive functioning tests (Johnson, Flicker, & Lichtenberg, 2006). Other studies have also found reading recognition to be a better predictor of premorbid functioning after brain injury because it is said to provide a better measure of educational quality than the number of years of education (Silverberg, Hanks, & Tompkins, 2013). Differences in cognitive development due to illiteracy have been studied previously, and many have advocated for using literacy over years of education because it more accurately captures educational quality (Manly, Byrd, Touradji, Sanchez, & Stern, 2004; Reis & Castro-Caldas, 1997).

It is important to obtain detailed information about education beyond number of years to become familiar with the cultural context and quality of the educational system in which the examinee has been raised. Understanding the individual's educational background can help in deciding which cognitive tests might be most appropriate to capture performance in a given domain. Whenever possible, incorporating measures of literacy can provide a more accurate means of examining educational quality to aid in the interpretation of test results when evaluating individuals from diverse cultural backgrounds.

LANGUAGE

Diversity of culture often comes along with diversity of language, which can pose challenges for communication between the professional and the rehabilitation patient. More than 55 million Americans speak a language other than English in their homes (U.S. Census Bureau, 2008). Non-English-speaking immigrants to the United States often reside in neighborhoods with higher densities of individuals of their culture and/or country of origin. For this reason, it is not uncommon for an immigrant to live in the United States for years without learning English. The effects of limited English proficiency (LEP) on daily life can be far reaching, impacting everything from health care utilization to quality of care (Timmins, 2002). A communication barrier due to LEP can make patients from diverse linguistic backgrounds feel more vulnerable and be less likely to self-advocate, ask relevant health questions, and express their basic needs (Ledger, 2002). This barrier can be especially problematic in neurorehabilitation settings due to the level of patient involvement required. This is an important consideration in neuropsychological assessment, where the patient is required to apply effort in a variety of tasks designed to measure cognitive functioning.

It is commonly assumed that using an interpreter in the administration of neuropsychological tests can bridge a gap of understanding when working with linguistically diverse populations. The assumption that the use of an interpreter can yield valid test results falsely reduces cultural differences to nothing more than differences in language. It has been shown that cultural groups can speak the same language but be quite diverse in aspects of their lives (i.e., SES, nutrition, education) that can cause disparities in neuropsychological test results (Artiola i Fortuny, Heaton, & Hermosillo, 1998). It has even been suggested that a particular culture's linguistic characteristics (e.g., Mandarin Chinese vs. English) may exert influence over cognition in unexpected ways, such as attentional and memory processes, abstract thinking, or estimating brief durations of time (Boroditsky, 2001; Casasanto et al., 2004).

The use of a translator has been shown to yield lower scores than the administration of a language-appropriate version of the tests (Casas et al., 2012). This effect was much stronger on verbal tests that relied heavily on the skills of the translator. Many problems can arise when an interpreter is used. The threat of error, which is always present to some degree when working with an interpreter, can be compounded due to the nature of the test-taking process. For example, for administration of cognitive tests in the United States, test instructions must first be translated from English into the foreign language. The examinee's responses must then be translated back into English for the evaluator. This two-way process leaves greater room for error in communication that is increased if the examinee has questions. In addition, there may be discussion between the patient and the interpreter about the testing material during that process that the examiner will not be able to understand and/or control. An ethical decision must be made whether an adequate evaluation can be conducted with the use of an interpreter. The clinician must always keep in mind that the divergence from standardized administration can call into question the validity of the results, especially if the examinee's culture is not adequately represented in the test's normative sample.

The majority of neuropsychological tests in languages other than English have been derived from tests developed in English and normed on English speakers. The existence of translated tests and their publication as a non-English version of the tests does not mean that they can be treated just like the English version. In many cases, the quality of the translations may be poor (Artiola i Fortuny et al., 2005). The problem of details getting lost in translation may be minimized by the use of back-translation, in which the translated material is translated back into the original language to examine the concordance with original information, or by consensus generation (Sumathipala & Murray, 2000). However, these practices do little to ensure construct validity that may be compromised due to cultural differences beyond language (Bender, Martin Garcia, & Barr, 2010). Translation and adaptation guidelines have been developed (Bartram, 2001; International Test Commission, 2000). This process can be viewed as having four main categories: those of cultural context, technicalities of instrument development and adaptation, test administration, and those concerned with documentation and interpretation, with direct implications for test use and users (Hambleton, 2005).

When using tests that have been formally translated and published in other languages, it is important to be aware of the translation process, as well as the steps taken to adapt the measure to the given culture through procedures such as cognitive interviewing. Even with cultural adaptation, however, one still needs to be aware of the source of normative data. If the normative sample is the original cohort of English speakers, the norms are of no use in analyzing or interpreting test findings. Anytime a standardized test is being administered, it is important to know the degree to which the characteristics of the respondent are represented in the normative sample. Becoming familiar with the technical manual can provide important information that can help in the decision whether or not to administer a given test or alert the clinician that the results must be interpreted with caution.

A common problem in using non-English tests with a heterogeneous population where the same general language is spoken is that regional dialects and variations in word usage can present a problem. Among Latin American Spanish speakers, there are certain words that can mean something different depending on the geographic location. For example, the EIWA-III is a Spanish version of the Wechsler Adult Intelligence Scale adapted for usage in Puerto Rico. The norms may not generalize to all Hispanic subgroups, and certain terms in the instructions may be problematic. On the similarities subtest, the word *china* is used for *orange* (the fruit). *China* is a slang term, and that meaning is specific to Puerto Rico. A colleague from Mexico once told the author that *china* was a slang term for drugs. In other regions, however, it refers to the country China. It is important to be aware of these subtle differences because words that are quite benign to some Hispanic subgroups may be very offensive to others. It is useful to have a multilanguage dictionary that is sensitive to multiple meanings depending on regional differences in language usage.

SOCIOECONOMIC STATUS

Accumulated empirical evidence from the past decades indicates a relationship between ethnic/racial differences in morbidity/mortality and socioeconomic resources that can potentially impact performance on cognitive tests (Hayward, Crimmins, Miles, & Yu, 2000; Williams & Collins, 1995). A number of explanations have been suggested for this observed relationship between SES and health outcomes, including differential access to health care, differential exposure to environmental hazards, health behaviors (behavior and lifestyle choices such as smoking, poor diet, lack of exercise, etc.), and differential exposure to stress (Saegert et al., 2007).

SES, a measure of one's position and status in society, is one of the most widely studied constructs in the social sciences (Bradley & Corwyn, 2002). It is generally conceptualized as including income, education, and occupation (White, 1982). The effect of SES on neuropsychological functioning has been of increased interest in recent years. It appears to exert its influence primarily in an indirect way—that is, via its effect on other variables such as education (Strauss, Sherman, & Spreen, 2006). Mehta et al. (2004) proposed that individuals from higher SES experience more (and more enriched) educational experiences and opportunities, resulting in protective influence of cognitive reserve. Disparities in educational experiences and cognitive performance begin early in life (Lee & Burkam, 2002). Even at the earliest stages of education, children from different SES groups achieve at different levels. Though the age when children begin their formal education (i.e., entering kindergarten) is generally approximately five years old, their cognitive status has been shown to substantially vary: Average scores on measures of cognition of children in the highest SES group were 60% above the scores of the lowest SES group (Lee & Burkam, 2002). Compounding this difference is the reality that children from low SES are more likely to attend a kindergarten or school of substantially lower quality—that is, with fewer school resources, fewer qualified teachers, and higher student-to-teacher ratios—which further reinforces the preexisting inequalities (Lee & Burkam, 2002). Byrd et al. (2006) identified a number of potential socioenvironmental correlates of cognitive test performance, including education and occupational backgrounds of the parents, access to health care, and availability of reading and other educationally oriented materials in the home.

Limited education or education of lower quality can lead to a restricted range of employment opportunities (e.g., menial or unskilled work, repetitive and monotonous factory jobs), which can actually increase the risk of brain injury due to unsafe working conditions, such as exposure to toxic substances or dangerous equipment (Llorente, 2000). Undocumented immigrants often have jobs "off the books," where the employers get away with failing to provide proper protective gear or safety education.

With a limited income, the place of residence is often restricted to certain affordable neighborhoods that may have high levels of noise, crime, overcrowding, and greater exposure to violence, conflict, drugs, and stress (Evans & Kantrowitz, 2002; Saegert et al., 2007). The fact that these elements are more common in lower SES environments has been referred to as "residential segregation" (a form of institutional racism), which is said to affect health outcomes of minorities (compared to Whites) by patterning residence in impoverished neighborhoods and thus limiting their potential lifetime socioeconomic advancement (Acevedo-Garcia & Osypuk, 2008;

Williams & Collins, 2001). Moreover, low SES, poverty, and income inequality are all associated with violent crime (Hsieh & Pugh, 1993), drug and alcohol abuse, inadequate health care, poor nutrition (Gurland et al., 1997), and higher likelihood of being a pedestrian fatality (National Complete Streets Coalition, 2014).

Indirect effects of SES on cognitive functioning have been described primarily via effects on the developing nervous system, especially in children. Poor nutrition affects brain growth both pre- and postnatally (Pollitt et al., 1996) and is a key pathway to poor health. Inadequate dietary intake produces defective nutrient absorption and utilization and leads to poor defenses against infection, contributing to a variety of morbidities (Mortorell, 1980) that can potentially impact the developing brain. Oria, Costa, Lima, Patrick, and Guerrant (2009) observed that children from Brazilian shantytowns who suffered from malnutrition-related diarrhea at ages 1 to 3 years exhibited not only physical and growth deficits but also impairments on tasks of executive functioning and semantic fluency at 6 to 12 years of age.

Additional risks to child development in low SES environments may be seen in the adverse effects on parenting styles, leading to early-onset conduct and attention problems in childhood, as well as higher rates of anxiety and depression (Dodge, Pettit, & Bates, 1994; Goodman, Slap, & Huang, 2003; Merikangas et al., 2010; Shanahan, Copeland, Costello, & Angold, 2008; Tracy, Zimmerman, Galea, McCauley, & Vander Stoep, 2008), low academic performance, underachievement, and lack of school readiness via multiple pathways (Bornstein & Bradley, 2003; Hochschild, 2003; McLoyd, 1998).

In low SES adults, a pattern of problems with mental health functioning has been documented, with disproportionately higher rates of depression among low-income individuals (particularly in households headed by women of color; Cutrona et al., 2005; Hobfoll, Johnson, Ennis, & Jackson, 2003) and greater lifetime exposure to chronic stress (Schwartz et al., 2004). Higher SES is consistently associated with better health compared to both low and middle SES (Saegert et al., 2007), implicating lifetime exposure to stress as a possible mediating factor (Sapolsky, 2005).

Because SES often underlies certain cultural differences, it is important to consider as an issue in the rehabilitation setting. A recent study showed that difference in income was a significant predictor of rate of progress for individuals with brain injury in an inpatient rehabilitation setting even after controlling for age, education, and injury severity (Lequerica, Krch,

Lavrador, & Chiaravalloti, 2012). Every individual in this sample was treated at the same location, so differences in care should not be a factor. It was hypothesized that those with a lower income may have had a history of lack of access to health care resources or limited knowledge of the importance of preventive medicine over the long term such that their premorbid state of health made them less resilient after injury. SES has been shown to impact the rates of incidence, mortality, and subsequent impairments in neurological disorders such as stroke (Kapral, Wang, Mamdani, & Tu, 2002; Li et al., 2008; McFadden, Luben, Wareham, Bingham, & Khaw, 2009) and the rate of recovery after stroke. Patients with less education had substantially lower rates of good functional outcome 3 months after their stroke that were not fully explained by variations in their clinical and demographic characteristics (Grube et al., 2012). A large-scale epidemiological study of over 300,000 young men identified low education and SES as independent strong risk factors for at least one mild traumatic brain injury (Nordström, Edin, Lindstrom, & Nordström, 2013).

ACCULTURATION

One of the most time-tested and frequently used conceptualizations of acculturation defines it as "those phenomena which result when groups of individuals having different cultures come into continuous firsthand contact, with subsequent changes in the original culture patterns of either or both groups. . . . This is to be distinguished from . . . assimilation, which is at times a phase of acculturation" (Redfield, Linton, & Herskovits, 1936, pp. 149–152). There is strong evidence that level of acculturation can influence performance on cognitive tests. Complex effects have been shown in performance on tests of attention, information processing, and executive functioning, among others (Coffey, Marmol, Schock, & Adams, 2005; Razani, Burciaga, Madore, & Wong, 2007). Among Latinos, U.S. acculturation has been associated with verbal fluency and processing speed, whereas Latina/Latino acculturation was associated with tests of motor and executive functions (Arentoft et al., 2012). Differences in acculturation also have been shown to affect performance on the subscales from the Wechsler Adult Intelligence Scale (Kennepohl, Shore, Nabors, & Hanks, 2004; Manly et al., 1998). With education being such an important predictor of performance, this finding is not surprising, given the lack of stratification by education in the normative data on these subscales.

Many of the measures of acculturation focus on language usage and are very specific to particular dyads of cultures. Many factors commonly associated with acculturation can be used as estimates in the absence of formal measures. For example, correlations have been found among neuropsychological test scores, the amount of time educated outside of the United States, and the amount of English spoken when growing up (Razani et al., 2007). Other studies have found the age of entry to the United States and the length of time spent living in the United States to be associated with cognitive test performance. It is important to realize that these acculturation variables need to be considered together with other demographic characteristics due to the complex interactions involved. For example, using time spent living in the United States as a proxy for acculturation without any other information can lead to error. Immigrants to the United States tend to find places of residence in neighborhoods where their culture of origin predominates (Zhou, 1997). Because all of their needs can often be met without leaving their neighborhood, it is not uncommon for individuals to live in the United States for decades without learning how to speak English. There may be no need to speak English in their neighborhood because store proprietors, supermarket cashiers, bank tellers, and hairdressers communicate with their clientele in the predominant native language within the limits of that geographic region. When an appropriate measure of acculturation is not available for a given individual, obtaining information such as country of origin, age of immigration to the United States, years (and indicators of quality) of education both outside and in the United States, and number of years of residency can help in estimating level of acculturation and should be taken into account (Chun, Balls Organista, & Marín, 2003; Manly et al., 2002).

CULTURE AND WORLDVIEW

The effects of worldview and culture have been noted on a number of processes potentially related to the outcome of neuropsychological evaluation, ranging from visual perception to interpersonal relations with strangers (i.e., the evaluators). Nonverbal tests, once believed to be "culture-free," are likely to rely on stimuli that may not be culturally appropriate for diverse populations. Social practices, customs, and environment may exert meaningful influences even on low-level perceptual processes.

Once held as the prime example of a universal human trait in sensory perception, susceptibility to optical illusions is a phenomenon that varies as a function of culture. As early as the turn of the 20th century, and multiple times since then, it was demonstrated that members of indigenous populations (who generally lack formal schooling, engaged in simple farming or hunter–gatherer activities for sustenance and survival) are not only less susceptible to, but are at times completely unaffected by, for instance, the Muller-Lyer illusion (Luria, 1976; Rivers, 1901). It appears that the individual's worldview—that is, experiences with the surrounding environment—mediates this phenomenon. In Western societies the very structure of cities, houses, rooms, and furniture consists mainly of vertical and horizontal lines that converge in a variety of angles (e.g., the carpentered environment hypothesis; Segall, Campbell, & Herskovits, 1966). Due to visual experiences and ontological familiarity with such environments, Westerners tend to form the perception and consequent belief that lines ending in inward-facing arrows are longer than they appear (which is the basis for the Muller-Lyer illusion). Although other hypotheses have been suggested to account for this apparent cross-cultural difference (e.g., density of retinal pigmentation; Jahoda, 1971), Segall et al.'s work highlights the importance of environmental differences on visual perception. Basic abilities, when fostered in particular environments, are subject to modification as a culturally evolved by-product (Kotik-Friedgut & Ardila, 2014).

Other recent studies have identified cross-cultural differences in scene perception and pattern of eye movements. Chua, Boland, and Nisbett (2005) found that Westerners (Americans) and Easterners (Japanese) demonstrated different patterns in allocation of attentional resources when presented with static scenes. The former tended to focus more on the objects in the foreground, whereas the latter exhibited a marked tendency to focus on the background objects, consistent with other reports of focal versus holistic processing of visual scenes as a function of culture (Kitayama, Duffy, Kawamura, & Larsen, 2003; Masuda, 2009; Masuda & Nisbett, 2001). Performance on tasks such as Picture Completion on the Wechsler Adult Intelligence Scale in which the examinee must identify which important part of the depicted object is missing can potentially be impacted by such cultural differences in perception.

As mentioned earlier, educational practices and content often reflect the worldview of the respective culture. Agranovich and Puente (2007) demonstrated a significant difference in performance on timed tasks between Russian and American participants, whereas no difference in performance was found on measures of tests that did not require timed performance (e.g., digit span, verbal memory). They attributed the observed difference to lack of emphasis on speedy, timed completion of tasks in the Russian education system. Whereas the American system of schooling uses assessments that consist of multiple-choice tests that are timed, the Russian education system tends to emphasize essay-type or oral examinations, where extra time for test completion is often granted. American culture is very focused on speed and efficiency, whereas other cultures see speed as a detriment to quality of performance. It is not uncommon for a patient from another culture to respond to instructions on timed tests with questions like "Do you want me to do it fast, or do you want me to do it well?" Accuracy and speed are seen as having a negative relationship, and it is not uncommon for other cultures to value accuracy over speed (Ardila, 2007).

THERAPEUTIC ENGAGEMENT IN THE REHABILITATION SETTING

Patients from culturally diverse backgrounds may exhibit greater difficulty in engaging with rehabilitation activities due to a variety of factors. The stress of being away from their family may be compounded by difficulty communicating, aversion to the hospital food, and difficulty understanding the purpose of the neuropsychological assessment, ultimately leading to an underestimation of their cognitive functioning (Uomoto & Wong, 2000). In addition, because the acute rehabilitation setting often mimics the acute care hospital setting from which patients often come, it is common for culturally diverse patients to view the rehabilitation team according to their traditional view of organized medicine. For example, doctors may be seen as highly respected individuals who prescribe medications and administer treatments, whereas the patients typically play a more passive role. However, such "background authority," which implicitly belongs to medical (or neuropsychology) professionals, is not necessarily shared by all cultures (Ardila, 2005).

Individuals from diverse cultures should be fully informed that the rehabilitation setting requires their involvement with the understanding that forming a partnership with health care providers may be an unfamiliar concept to many. The importance of giving their best effort in therapies and on neuropsychological measures should be emphasized. Here again exists a potential for a clash or incompatibility of cultural values. "Best effort" or "best performance" may not necessarily mean the same thing to the evaluator and the patient, as when timed tests scored for speed of completion are administered (Ardila, 2005).

The patient's predominant worldview, shaped by both his or her learned values as well as beliefs and patterns of behavior, is likely to manifest itself in the interpersonal interaction that is the neuropsychological evaluation. It is important to consider how diverse individuals may perceive the interaction because it can impact their performance. There are also a variety of factors about the testing situation that need to be considered by the neuropsychologist and possibly explained fully to the patient to minimize the chance of misunderstanding.

It is important to remember that even the U.S. health care system and its approaches to serving individuals with an illness or disability are not culture-free but are a distinctive by-product of the history and the very fabric of the United States (Groce & Zola, 1993). The neuropsychology professionals themselves also bring their potential cultural biases and idiosyncrasies into the interpersonal interaction that is the assessment/evaluation. During graduate and postgraduate training, after much instruction, practice, and supervision, the neuropsychologists likely internalize many of the aspects of the assessment process that may be foreign to individuals who are not from the same culture. Ardila (2005, 2007) addresses these aspects of the assessment process. For example, neuropsychological evaluation presupposes that two individuals who are virtual strangers to each other (and who may not meet again in the future once the evaluation is over) will find themselves in relative privacy (e.g., behind closed doors to reduce distracting stimuli). Patients are expected to answer questions about their internal states, such as emotional or mental functioning. Evaluators, in the process of administering standardized instruments, read the instructions in a specific (ideally unvarying) way and use particular testing materials or strategies that may not be familiar to patients. Another way to construe such process of neuropsychological evaluation from a cross-cultural perspective is that patients may find themselves in an isolated environment (away from possible or expected sources of advice or social support) and being forced to answer potentially private or intrusive questions and engage in tasks that may have little sense or meaning to them, all in the context of a social interaction that bears little resemblance to their normal or typical interactions (Ardila, 2005, 2007). It is conceivable that any or all of these factors may influence an individual's performance on the assessment battery, and the potential complexity of the situation must be appreciated by the clinician. Additionally, this area is ripe for investigation and clinical research into how such cultural values, beliefs, and interpersonal interactions come to bear on evaluation and rehabilitation outcomes.

Although it is recommended that practitioners conduct background research (e.g., via the Internet, literature, or professional or personal contacts) on their patients' linguistic and cultural practices and customs (Judd & DeBoard, 2010), it is most important to spend time with patients and ask questions about their particular cultural backgrounds. Getting the patients' perspective on their culture, life, and current situation provides more relevant information that can be useful in terms of choosing measures and interpreting results. In addition, showing an interest in the person as an individual can convey a sense of respect and improve rapport. In addition to gathering information, the clinician should be careful to provide information about the purpose of testing and how the information obtained from the neuropsychological assessment will be used to inform their treatment or discharge planning. Patients should be encouraged to ask questions.

RELIGION AND SPIRITUALITY

Due to prevailing attitudes and worldviews in the country/environment of origin, ideas of what causes disease/pathogenesis can be drastically different from the predominant Western conceptualization. Certain neurological conditions (e.g., epilepsy), seen as debilitating and obviously undesirable in the Western culture, can be interpreted as something akin to a divine gift of communication with the spirit realm in some indigenous cultures (Fadiman, 2012). In the Hmong (an Asian ethnic group) culture, for example, the traditional worldview and religion are characterized by shamanistic animism. The shamans serve as health care providers who attempt to restore health and balance to body and soul through ritual practices, which may involve animal sacrifice and other seemingly eso-teric ceremonies (Plotnikoff, Numrich, Wu, Yang, & Xiong, 2002). Other cultures may view illnesses or neurological conditions as a form of pun-ishment (i.e., something the patient may have brought upon himself or herself by violating a societal taboo, angering or displeasing God or gods), the consequences of being bewitched (as in some Native American tribes and African and Caribbean societies), or the result of "bad blood" or the "evil eye" (Groce & Zola, 1993). Health care providers must there-fore exercise culturally conscious practices when engaging in therapeutic relationships—whether via assessment, rehabilitation/treatment, or fol-low-up—with members of minority cultures that are drastically different from their own, and they should attempt to understand the culture and worldview of such patients and their families to avoid alienation and instead forge therapeutic alliances to achieve successful outcomes.

Certain cultures have very strict gender roles. What may be thought of as a universal skill in Western cultures may be gender specific in others. Prescribed gender roles or behaviors may be associated with religious beliefs. In certain religions, the husband is the only male permitted to touch a woman or view certain body parts such as face, hair, or legs. Although neuropsychologists are not typically in physical contact with patients, one must be aware of how seemingly common gestures or customary greetings in Western culture may be perceived by individuals from diverse reli-gious backgrounds. For example, it is often best for a male not to extend a hand upon greeting a woman from certain diverse religious backgrounds unless she initiates the handshake.

INTERACTIONS AMONG MULTIPLE DIVERSITY FACTORS

It should be mentioned that cultural differences can interact with one another in complex ways. For example, gender identity and sexual orien-tation can vary greatly from culture to culture. Among many Native Amer-ican tribes, a homosexual or transgendered individual may be seen as possessing both male and female spirits. Such individuals may have spe-cific roles within their community. Whether these individuals are feared, respected, accepted, or ostracized could vary, depending on tribal beliefs or the influence of acculturation that often carries with it homophobia. Within certain cultures with strong disparities in gender roles, a male who exhibits typically feminine behaviors may be ostracized or shunned. The experience of discrimination throughout one's life can manifest as internalized homophobia and cause a patient to blame himself for his injury, which can impact motivation and participation with treatment. This issue of attribution and other existential issues often arise based on religious background. These interactions among elements of culture can create challenges when working with families (see Lequerica & Krch, 2014, for an example).

CONCLUSIONS

Living in a society that is rich in cultural diversity requires us to diversify our clinical approaches in order to provide services that are culturally appropriate and patient-centered. Improving one's cultural awareness can seem like a daunting task given the potential variations and interactions. However, cultural competence does not necessarily mean that one must know all there is to know about all cultures. It can be viewed as a process by which one increases the awareness of his or her own worldview and recognition of potential cultural biases (Niemeier, Burnett, & Whitaker, 2003). This can lead to consideration of alternative hypotheses when interpreting a patient's behavior in the rehabilitation setting and a decreased chance of making assumptions. Cultural competence begins with greater cultural sensitivity.

In addition to greater multicultural awareness and knowledge, Monica Rivera-Mindt, Byrd, Saez, and Manly (2010) advocate for steps to be taken at multiple levels of the health care system, starting with the education and training of neuropsychology students who have yet to enter into their careers. There is also much work to be done in terms of neuropsychology research and cognitive test development so that more valid measures of cognition can be available for use in serving the diverse population within the United States. In the meantime, neuropsychologists working with culturally diverse patients should follow the ethical guidelines set forth by the American Psychological Association (2003) regarding multicultural education, training, research, practice, and organizational change. As awareness of these issues increases among clinicians, and as the research progresses in the investigation of multicultural assessment, the challenges currently faced by neuropsychologists working in multicultural environments could eventually be overcome in our continuing efforts to improve the quality of care we provide to patients in the rehabilitation setting.

REFERENCES

Acevedo-Garcia, D., & Osypuk, T. L. (2008). Impacts of housing and neighborhoods on health: Pathways, racial/ethnic disparities, and policy directions. In J. Carr & N. Kutty (Eds.), *Segregation: The rising costs for America* (pp. 197–235). New York, NY: Routledge.

Agranovich, A. V., & Puente, A. E. (2007). Do Russian and American normal adults perform similarly on neuropsychological tests? Preliminary findings on the relationship between culture and test performance. *Archives of Clinical Neuropsychology, 22*(3), 273–282.

American Psychological Association. (2003). American Psychological Association guidelines on multicultural education, training, research, practice, and organizational change for psychologists. *American Psychologist, 58,* 377–402.

Ansari, D. (2012). Culture and education: New frontiers in brain plasticity. *Trends in Cognitive Sciences, 16*(2), 93–95.

Ardila, A. (2005). Cultural values underlying psychometric cognitive testing. *Neuropsychology Review, 15*(4), 185–195.

Ardila, A. (2007). The impact of culture on neuropsychological test performance. In B. P. Uzzell, M. Ponton, & A. Ardila (Eds.), *International handbook of cross-cultural neuropsychology* (pp. 23–44). Mahwah, NJ: Lawrence Erlbaum Associates.

Ardila, A., Ostrosky-Solis, F., Rosselli, M., & Gómez, C. (2000). Age-related cognitive decline during normal aging: The complex effect of education. *Archives of Clinical Neuropsychology, 15*(6), 495–513.

Arentoft, A., Byrd, D., Robbins, R. N., Monzones, J., Miranda, C., Rosario, A., . . . Rivera Mindt, M. (2012). Multidimensional effects of acculturation on English-language neuropsychological test performance among HIV+ Caribbean Latinas/os. *Journal of Clinical and Experimental Neuropsychology, 34*(8), 814–825.

Artiola i Fortuny, L., Garolera, M., Romo, D. H., Feldman, E., Barillas, H. F., Keefe, R., . . . Maestre, K. V. (2005). Research with Spanish-speaking populations in the United States: Lost in the translation. A commentary and a plea. *Journal of Clinical and Experimental Neuropsychology, 27*(5), 555–564.

Artiola i Fortuny, L., Heaton, R., & Hermosillo, D. (1998). Neuropsychological comparison of Spanish-speaking participants from the U.S.-Mexico border region versus Spain. *Journal of the International Neuropsychological Society, 4*(4), 363–379.

Bartram, D. (2001). The development of international guidelines on test use: The International Test Commission Project. *International Journal of Testing, 1*(1), 33–53.

Bender, H. A., Martin Garcia, A., & Barr, W. B. (2010). An interdisciplinary approach to neuropsychological test construction: Perspectives from translation studies. *Journal of the International Neuropsychological Society, 16*(2), 227–232.

Bornstein, M. H., & Bradley, R. H. (Eds.). (2003). *Socioeconomic status, parenting, and child development.* New York: Routledge.

Boroditsky, L. (2001). Does language shape thought? Mandarin and English speakers' conceptions of time. *Cognitive Psychology, 43*(1), 1–22.

Bradley, R. H., & Corwyn, R. F. (2002). Socioeconomic status and child development. *Annual Review of Psychology, 53*(1), 371–399.

Brickman, A. M., Cabo, R., & Manly, J. J. (2006). Ethical issues in cross-cultural neuropsychology. *Applied Neuropsychology, 13*(2), 91–100.

Byrd, D. A., Walden Miller, S., Reilly, J., Weber, S., Wall, T. L., & Heaton, R. K. (2006). Early environmental factors, ethnicity, and adult cognitive test performance. *The Clinical Neuropsychologist, 20*(2), 243–260.

Casas, R., Guzmán-Vélez, E., Cardona-Rodriguez, J., Rodriguez, N., Quiñones, G., Izaguirre, B., & Tranel, D. (2012). Interpreter-mediated neuropsychological testing of monolingual Spanish speakers. *The Clinical Neuropsychologist, 26*(1), 88–101.

Casasanto, D., Boroditsky, L., Phillips, W., Greene, J., Goswami, S., Bocanegra-Thiel, S., . . . Gil, D. (2004). How deep are effects of language on thought? Time estimation in speakers of English, Indonesian, Greek, and Spanish. *Proceedings of the 26th Annual Conference of the Cognitive Science Society* (pp. 575–580). Hillsdale, NJ: Lawrence Erlbaum Associates.

Cheie, L., Veraksa, A., Zinchenko, Y., Gorovaya, A., & Visu-Petra, L. (2015). A cross-cultural investigation of inhibitory control, generative fluency, and anxiety symptoms in Romanian and Russian preschoolers. *Child Neuropsychology 21*(2), 121–149.

Chua, H. F., Boland, J. E., & Nisbett, R. E. (2005). Cultural variation in eye movements during scene perception. *Proceedings of the National Academy of Sciences of the United States of America, 102*(35), 12629–12633.

Chun, K. M., Balls Organista, P., & Marín, G. (Eds.). (2003). *Acculturation: Advances in theory, measurement, and applied research.* Washington, DC: American Psychological Association.

Coffey, D. M., Marmol, L., Schock, L., & Adams, W. (2005). The influence of acculturation on the Wisconsin card sorting test by Mexican Americans. *Archives of Clinical Neuropsychology, 20*(6), 795–803.

Cole, M., Gay, J., Glick, J. A., & Sharp, D. W. (1971). *The cultural context of learning and thinking: An exploration in experimental anthropology.* New York, NY: Basic Books.

Cutrona, C. E., Russell, D. W., Brown, P. A., Clark, L. A., Hessling, R. M., & Gardner, K. A. (2005). Neighborhood events, personality, and stressful life events as predictors of depression among African American women. *Journal of Abnormal Psychology, 114,* 3–15.

Dodge, K. A., Pettit, G. S., & Bates, J. E. (1994). Socialization mediators of the relation between socioeconomic status and child conduct problems. *Child Development, 65*(2), 649–665.

Evans, G. W., & Kantrowitz, E. (2002). Socioeconomic status and health: The potential role of environmental risk exposure. *Annual Review of Public Health, 23,* 303–331.

Fadiman, A. (2012). *The spirit catches you and you fall down: A Hmong child, her American doctors, and the collision of two cultures.* New York, NY: Macmillan.

Goodman, E., Slap, G. B., & Huang, B. (2003). The public health impact of socioeconomic status on adolescent depression and obesity. *American Journal of Public Health, 93,* 1844–1850.

Gould, S. J. (1981). *The mismeasure of man.* New York, NY: Norton.

Groce, N. E., & Zola, I. K. (1993). Multiculturalism, chronic illness, and disability. *Pediatrics, 91*(5), 1048–1055.

Grube, M., Koennecke, H-C., Walter, G., Thummler, J., Meisel, A., Wellwood, I., & Heuschmann, P. (2012). Association between socioeconomic status and functional impairment 3 months after ischemic stroke: The Berlin Stroke Register. *Stroke, 43,* 3325–3330.

Gurland, B., Wilder, D., Lantigua, R., Mayeux, R., Stern, Y., Chen, J., . . . Killeffer, E. (1997). Differences in rates of dementia among ethno-racial groups. In L. Martin & B. Soldo (Eds.), *Racial and ethnic differences in the health of older Americans* (pp. 233–269). Washington, DC: National Academy Press.

Hambleton, R. K. (2005). *Issues, designs and technical guidelines for adapting tests into multiple languages and cultures.* In R. K. Hambleton, P. F. Merenda, & C. D. Spielberger (Eds.), Adapting psychological and educational tests for cross-cultural assessment. Hillsdale, NJ: Lawrence Erlbaum Associates.

Harris, M. (1983). *Culture, people, nature: An introduction to general anthropology* (3rd ed.). New York, NY: Harper and Row.

Hayward, M. D., Crimmins, E. M., Miles, T. P., & Yu, Y. (2000). The significance of socioeconomic status in explaining the racial gap in chronic health conditions. *American Sociological Review, 65,* 910–930.

Helms, J. E., Jernigan, M., & Mascher, J. (2005). The meaning of race in psychology and how to change it: A methodological perspective. *American Psychologist, 60*(1), 27–36.

Hobfoll, S. E., Johnson, R. J., Ennis, N., & Jackson, A. P. (2003). Resource loss, resource gain, and emotional outcomes among inner city women. *Journal of Personality and Social Psychology, 84,* 632–643.

Hochschild, J. L. (2003). Social class in the public schools. *Journal of Social Issues, 59,* 821–840.

Hoebel, E. A. (1966). *Anthropology: The study of man.* New York, NY: McGraw-Hill.

Hsieh, C., & Pugh, M. D. (1993). Poverty, income inequality, and violent crime: A meta-analysis of recent aggregate data studies. *Criminal Justice Review, 18,* 182–202. doi:10.1177/073401689301800203

International Test Commission. (2000). *International guidelines for test use.* Retrieved from http://www.intestcom.org/page/17

Jahoda, G. (1971). Retinal pigmentation, illusion susceptibility and space perception. *International Journal of Psychology 6*(3), 199–207.

Johnson, A. S., Flicker, L. J., & Lichtenberg, P. A. (2006). Reading ability mediates the relationship between education and executive function tasks. *Journal of the International Neuropsychological Society, 12*(1), 64–71.

Judd, T., & DeBoard, R. (2010). Assessment of linguistic minorities. *NAN Bulletin, 25*(1), 6–10.

Kapral, M., Wang, H., Mamdani, M., & Tu, J. (2002). Effect of socioeconomic status on treatment and mortality after stroke. *Stroke, 33,* 268–273.

Kennepohl, S., Shore, D., Nabors, N., & Hanks, R. (2004). African American acculturation and neuropsychological test performance following traumatic brain injury. *Journal of the International Neuropsychological Society, 10,* 566–577.

Kitayama, S., Duffy, S., Kawamura, T., & Larsen, J. T. (2003). Perceiving an object and its context in different cultures: A cultural look at the New Look. *Psychological Science, 14*(3), 201–206.

Kotik-Friedgut, B., & Ardila, A. (2014). Cultural-historical theory and cultural neuropsychology today. In A. Yasnitsky, R. van der Veer, & M. Ferrari (Eds.), *The Cambridge handbook of cultural-historical psychology* (pp. 378–399). New York, NY: Cambridge University Press.

Lam, M., Eng, G. K., Rapisarda, A., Subramaniam, M., Kraus, M., Keef, R. S. E., & Collinson, S. L. (2013). Formulation of the age–education index: Measuring age and education effects in neuropsychological performance. *Psychological Assessment, 25*(1), 61–70.

Ledger, S. D. (2002). Reflections on communicating with non-English-speaking patients. *British Journal of Nursing (Mark Allen Publishing), 11*(11), 773–780.

Lee, V. E., & Burkam, D. T. (2002). *Inequality at the starting gate: Social background differences in achievement as children begin school.* Washington, DC: Economic Policy Institute.

Lequerica, A., Krch, D., Lavrador, S., & Chiaravalloti, N. (2012). Demographic factors associated with rehabilitation progress after traumatic brain injury. Poster presentation at the Annual Convention of the American Psychological Association, Orlando, Florida.

Lequerica, A., & Krch, D. (2014). Issues of cultural diversity in ABI rehabilitation. *NeuroRehabilitation, 34*(4), 645–653.

Li, C., Hedblad, B., Rosvall, M., Buchwald, F., Khan, F. A., & Engstrom, G. (2008). Stroke incidence, recurrence, and case-fatality in relation to socioeconomic position: A population-based study of middle-aged Swedish men and women. *Stroke, 39,* 2191–2196.

Llorente, A. M. (2000). Evaluation of developmental neurocognitive and neurobe-havioral changes associated with pesticide exposure: Recommendations for the U.S. Environmental Protection Agency on the assessment of health effects of pesticide exposure in infants and young children. In D. Otto, R. Calderon, P. Mendola, & E. Hilborn (Eds.), *Assessment of health effects of pesticide exposure in young children* (pp. 22–32). Research Triangle Park, NC: Environmental Protection Agency.

Luria, A. R. (1976). *Cognitive development: Its cultural and social foundations.* Cambridge, MA: Harvard University Press.

Manly, J. J., Byrd, D., Touradji, P., Sanchez, D., & Stern, Y. (2004). Literacy and cognitive change among ethnically diverse elders. *International Journal of Psychology, 39*(1), 47–60.

Manly, J. J., Jacobs, D. M., Touradji, P., Small, S. A., & Stern, Y. (2002). Reading level attenuates differences in neuropsychological test performance between African American and White elders. *Journal of the International Neuropsychological Society, 8*(3), 341–348.

Manly, J. J., Miller, S. W., Heaton, R. K., Byrd, D., Reilly, J., Velasquez, R. J., . . . Grant, I. (1998). The effect of African-American acculturation on neuropsychological test performance in normal and HIV-positive individuals. *Journal of the International Neuropsychological Society, 4*(3), 291–302.

Masuda, T. (2009). Cultural effects on visual perception. In E. B. Goldstein (Ed.), *Sage encyclopedia of perception, vol. 1* (pp. 339–343). Thousand Oaks, CA: Sage.

Masuda, T., & Nisbett, R. E. (2001). Attending holistically vs. analytically: Comparing the context sensitivity of Japanese and Americans. *Journal of Personality and Social Psychology, 81*, 922–934.

McFadden, E., Luben, R., Wareham, N., Bingham, S., & Khaw, K. T. (2009). Social class, risk factors, and stroke incidence in men and women: A prospective study in the European prospective investigation into cancer in Norfolk cohort. *Stroke, 40*, 1070–1077.

McLoyd, V. C. (1998). Socioeconomic disadvantage and child development. *American Psychologist, 53*, 185–204.

Mehta, S. E., Rooks, R., Newman, A. B., Pope, S. K., Rubin, S. M., & Yaffe, K. (2004). Black and white differences in cognitive function test scores: What explains the difference? *Journal of American Geriatric Association, 52*, 2120–2127.

Merikangas, K. R., He, J. P., Brody, D., Fisher, P. W., Bourdon, K., & Koretz, D. S. (2010). Prevalence and treatment of mental disorders among U.S. children in the 2001–2004 NHANES. *Pediatrics, 125*(1), 75–81.

Mortorell, R. (1980). Interrelationships between diet, infectious disease, and nutritional status. In H. S. Greene & F. E. Johnson (Eds.), *Social and biological predictors of nutritional status, physical growth and neurological development* (pp. 188–213). New York, NY: Academic Press.

National Complete Streets Coalition. (2014). *Dangerous by design.* Retrieved from www.smartgrowthamerica.org/dangerous-by-design

Niemeier, J. P., Burnett, D. M., & Whitaker, D. A. (2003). Cultural competence in the multidisciplinary rehabilitation setting: Are we falling short of meeting needs? *Archives of Physical Medicine and Rehabilitation, 84*(8), 1240–1245.

Nisbett, R. E. (2005). Heredity, environment, and race differences in IQ: A commentary on Rushton and Jensen. *Psychology, Public Policy, and Law, 11*(2), 302–310.

Nordström, A., Edin, B. B., Lindström, S., & Nordström, P. (2013). Cognitive function and other risk factors for mild traumatic brain injury in young men: Nationwide cohort study. *BMJ: British Medical Journal, 346*, 723f.

O'Bryant, S. E., Humphreys, J. D., Bauer, L., McCaffrey, R. J., & Hilsabeck, R. C. (2007). The influence of ethnicity on symbol digit modalities test performance: An analysis of a multi-ethnic college and hepatitis C patient sample. *Applied Neuropsychology, 14*(3), 183–188.

Oria, R. B., Costa, C. M. C., Lima, A. A., Patrick, P. D., & Guerrant, R. L. (2009). Semantic fluency: A sensitive marker for cognitive impairment in children with heavy diarrhea burdens? *Medical Hypotheses, 73*(5), 682–686.

Ostrosky-Solis, F., Ardila, A., Rosselli, M., Lopez-Arango, G., & Uriel-Mendoza, V. (1998). Neuropsychological test performance in illiterate subjects. *Archives of Clinical Neuropsychology, 13*(7), 645–660.

Ostrosky-Solis, F., Ramirez, M., & Ardila, A. (2004). Effects of culture and education on neuropsychological testing: A preliminary study with indigenous and nonindigenous population. *Applied Neuropsychology, 11*(4), 186–193.

Plotnikoff, G. A., Numrich, C., Wu, C., Yang, D., & Xiong, P. (2002). Hmong shamanism. Animist spiritual healing in Minnesota. *Minnesota Medicine, 85*(6), 29–34.

Pollitt, E., Golub, M., Gorman, K., Grantham-McGregor, S., Levitsky, D., Schurch, B., . . . Wachs, T. (1996). A reconceptualization of the effects of undernutrition on children's biological, psychosocial, and behavioral development. *Social Policy Report, 10*(5), 1–22.

Razani, J., Burciaga, J., Madore, M., & Wong, J. (2007). Effects of acculturation on tests of attention and information processing in an ethnically diverse group. *Archives of Clinical Neuropsychology, 22*(3), 333–341.

Redfield, R., Linton, R., & Herskovits, M. J. (1936). Memorandum for the study of acculturation. *American Anthropologist, 38*, 149–152.

Reis, A., & Castro-Caldas, A. (1997). Illiteracy: A cause for biased cognitive development. *Journal of the International Neuropsychological Society, 3*(5), 444–450.

Reis, A., Guerreiro, M., & Castro-Caldas, A. (1994). Influence of educational level of non brain-damaged subjects on visual naming capacities. *Journal of Clinical and Experimental Neuropsychology, 16*(6), 939–942.

Rivera-Mindt, M., Byrd, D., Saez, P., & Manly, J. (2010). Increasing culturally competent services for ethnic minority populations: A call to action. *Clinical Neuropsychologist, 24*(3), 429–453.

Rivers, W. H. R. (1901). The measurement of visual illusion. *Report of the British Association for Advancement of Science*, 818.

Rushton, J. P., & Jensen, A. R. (2005). Thirty years of research on race differences in cognitive ability. *Psychology, Public Policy, and Law, 11*(2), 235–294.

Saegert, S. C., Adler, N. E., Bullock, H. E., Cauce, A. M., Liu, W. M., & Wyche, K. F. (2007). Report of the APA Task Force on socioeconomic status. Washington, DC: American Psychological Association.

Sapolsky, R. (2005). Sick of poverty. *Scientific American, 293*(6), 92–99.

Saunders, L., Krause, J., Peters, B., & Reed, K. (2010). The relationship of pressure ulcers, race, and socioeconomic conditions after spinal cord injury. *Journal of Spinal Cord Medicine, 33*(4), 387–395.

Schneider, B. C., & Lichtenberg, P. A. (2011). Influence of reading ability on neuropsychological performance in African American elders. *Archives of Clinical Neuropsychology, 26*(7), 624–631.

Schwartz, G. T., Bolla, K. I., Stewart, W. F., Glass, G., Rasmussen, M., Bressler, J., . . . Bandeen-Roche, K. (2004). Disparities in cognitive functioning by race/ethnicity in the Baltimore Memory Study. *Environmental Health Perspectives, 112*(3), 314–320.

Segall, M. H., Campbell, D. T., & Herskovits, M. J. (1966). *The influence of culture on visual perception.* New York, NY: The Bobbs-Merrill Company.

Shanahan, L., Copeland, W., Costello, E. J., & Angold, A. (2008). Specificity of putative psychosocial risk factors for psychiatric disorders in children and adolescents. *Journal of Child Psychology and Psychiatry, 49,* 34–42.

Silverberg, N. D., Hanks, R. A., & Tompkins, S. C. (2013). Education quality, reading recognition, and racial differences in the neuropsychological outcome from traumatic brain injury. *Archives of Clinical Neuropsychology, 28*(5), 485–491.

Siok, W. T., Perfetti, C. A., Jin, Z., & Tan, L. H. (2004). Biological abnormality of impaired reading is constrained by culture. *Nature, 431,* 71–76.

Strauss, E., Sherman, E. M., & Spreen, O. (2006). *A compendium of neuropsychological tests: Administration, norms, and commentary.* New York, NY: Oxford University Press.

Sumathipala, A., & Murray, J. (2000). New approach to translating instruments for cross-cultural research: A combined qualitative and quantitative approach for translation and consensus generation. *International Journal of Methods in Psychiatric Research, 9*(2), 87–95.

Tang, Y., Zhang, W., Chen, K., Feng, S., Ji, Y., Shen, J., . . . Liu, Y. (2006). Arithmetic processing in the brain shaped by cultures. *Proceedings of the National Academy of Sciences, 103*(28), 10775–10780.

Timmins, C. L. (2002). The impact of language barriers on the health care of Latinos in the United States: A review of the literature and guidelines for practice. *Journal of Midwifery and Women's Health, 47*(2), 80–96.

Tracy, M., Zimmerman, F. J., Galea, S., McCauley, E., & Vander Stoep, A. (2008). What explains the relation between family poverty and childhood depressive symptoms? *Journal of Psychiatric Research, 42,* 1163–1175.

Uomoto, J. M., & Wong, T. M. (2000). Multicultural perspectives on the neuropsychology of brain injury assessment and rehabilitation. In E. Fletcher-Janzen,

T. Strickland, & Cecil R. Reynolds (Eds.), *Handbook of cross-cultural neuropsy-chology* (pp. 169–184). New York, NY: Springer Science+Business Media.

U.S. Census Bureau. (2008). *American community survey.* Retrieved from http://www.census.gov/acs/www/data_documentation/2008_release/

White, K. R. (1982). The relation between socioeconomic status and academic achievement. *Psychological Bulletin, 91,* 461–481.

Williams, D. R., & Collins, C. (1995). U.S. socioeconomic and racial differences in health: Patterns and explanations. *Annual Review of Sociology, 21,* 349–386.

Williams, D. R., & Collins, C. (2001). Racial residential segregation: A fundamental cause of racial disparities in health. *Public Health Reports, 116,* 404–416.

Zhou, M. (1997). Segmented assimilation: Issues, controversies, and recent research on the new second generation. *International Migration Review, 31*(4), 975–1008.

CHAPTER FOUR

LANGUAGE, ETHNICITY, CULTURE, AND THE NEUROREHABILITATION PATIENT EXPERIENCE

Aida Saldivar, Fernando Gonzalez, Marlene Vega, and Charlotte Sykora

---

Mr. N

You get a consult to evaluate Mr. N, who had a left ischemic stroke 2 weeks ago. The consult request seems relatively straight-forward; you have done it over a hundred times before. You begin to hypothesize that he may have language deficits and right-sided weakness, and, because it has been 2 weeks since the stroke, he may be experiencing, at a minimum, an adjustment disorder. You prepare your evaluation materials and review his chart. Then you discover the patient is from Nigeria. Perhaps you have worked with other patients from Nigeria, perhaps not. Now what? Should your approach to this consult be different?

This chapter explores multicultural variables to consider when pro-viding neurorehabilitation services to inpatients in an acute neuro-rehabilitation center. The cases presented involve inpatients who have recently suffered brain injuries, strokes, and other conditions that have led to acute and/or chronic disability and potential cognitive changes that are in need of physical, occupational, and speech therapy to address declines in functioning due to cognitive changes and physical disability, as well as medical treatment to manage secondary conditions. We look at several cases that involve clinicians working with patients and families from diverse backgrounds and of varying English-speaking abilities. We examine how culture, education, religion, and language may affect your clinical evaluations of patients in acute neurorehabilitation settings and at a clinician's experience in providing multicultural neurorehabilitation.

MAXIMIZING CULTURAL RESPECT AND INTEGRATING RESPECT INTO TREATMENT

All stories usually have at least two sides when it comes to appreciating how people understand and respond to unfamiliar situations, such as when they are unexpectedly thrust into a catastrophic medical situation, as is frequently seen in inpatient rehabilitation for events such as traumatic brain injury, spinal cord injury, or stroke. Many factors contribute to how patients and their families perceive and engage with the rehabilitative process: attitudes, values and beliefs, social roles, religion and spirituality, communication styles, time orientation, health practices, language, acculturation level, and socioeconomic status (Arango-Lasparilla & Niemeier, 2007; Castillo & Caver, 2009; Glover & Blankenship, 2007; Hays, 2008; Sue & Sue, 2008). These factors need to be appreciated to effectively develop the collaborative process necessary for optimal outcomes. It is clearly understood that the integration of culture and diversity into neurorehabilitation is essential, but how do we go about integrating all the relevant variables? How do we ensure that as clinicians providing Western-oriented interventions to ethnically and culturally diverse patients with acute brain dysfunction that we are practicing from a nonethnocentric—or what is described in anthropology as *culturally relativistic*—perspective?

The patient's perspective is critical to the development of a treatment plan, with the two sides (patient and provider) needing to collaboratively work toward reducing obstacles and working toward a meaningful outcome. The obstacles often come in the form of culture and the various aspects that color the individual's perceptions and expectations. The hospital culture is a unique environment that may be more familiar to individuals from the dominant culture, but it will usually require a tour or explanation of the system to be able to begin to function in the environment. A quick review of the hospital system and expectations regarding patient behavior and patient's rights can be sufficient for someone of the dominant culture to begin to function in the environment. For someone not from the dominant culture, the hospital environment and culture can appear confusing and overwhelming given the activity and behavior of staff and the required onboarding. For instance, during the admission process, the patient and/or family are expected to sign forms (e.g., Health Insurance Portability and Accountability Act [HIPAA], hospital policies, insurance, schedules, Patient Bill of Rights) that may be explained to them to varying degrees; this process can increase confusion and lead to little retention of information.

In the following sections we look at how to address and improve cultural competency, enhance communication through the use of interpreters, integrate spiritual beliefs with the Western medical model, work with collectivistic cultures, and assess acculturation. The goal is to help inform the provider's perspective, while at the same time appreciate the analogous process patients go through in developing their perspective.

CULTURAL COMPETENCY

Psychologists should strive to practice from a transcultural framework and aim to continually develop their knowledge about the cultural groups they serve (American Psychological Association, 2002). Because definitions and beliefs are often tied into culture and how we educate ourselves about culture, we need to reduce confusion by explaining or defining many of the terms we use. Culture, race, ethnicity, and nationality are not interchangeable concepts. *Race* generally refers to physical characteristics that differentiate Caucasoid, Negroid, and Mongoloid, whereas *ethnicity* refers to groups of people who share a common nationality, culture, or language. *Nationality* refers to country of origin. *Culture* is not as easily defined, but in general, it has been conceptualized as the human-made part of the environment that can have several different meanings. Typically these characteristics are learned and used by certain groups and are passed down from one generation to the next (Betancourt & Lopez, 1993; Rohner, 1984). Thus, two Americans (nationality) can be racially different, ethnically similar (e.g., second-generation Americans from Brazil), and culturally different (one from a high socioeconomic status [SES] family, college educated, with a stable job, and the other from a low SES family, dropped out of high school, and has had problems with law enforcement).

In the United States, knowledge of an individual's generational status (i.e., first-generation versus third-generation American) is also important because it can provide information about acculturation level, value system, and how self-defined the person is versus defined by his or her culture of origin. A first-generation Mexican American is more likely to hear and speak Spanish in the home, to be familiar with traditional Mexican food and music, and to have collectivistic values, whereas a third-generation Mexican American may not speak or understand Spanish, be less familiar with the more traditional Mexican dishes, prefer English-language music, and demonstrate more individualistic values. Conflicts between immigrant parents' values and those of their U.S.-born children are common in first- and second-generation American families but are not in families that have lived in the United States for extended generations. These generational cultural conflicts can be magnified when a family member becomes ill and enters the medical system. For instance, it may be challenging for second-generation adult children to make medical decisions for a parent that are consistent with the parent's values but not their own more Americanized values. It is therefore essential for clinicians working in a neurorehabilitation setting to understand the subtle differences between these concepts and their effect on a patient's worldview and perception and understanding of disability, medicine, and mental health.

Given our unique and individual upbringings, we are all, to some degree, ethnocentric, viewing the world through the lenses provided to us by our own experiences, health and disability statuses, socioeconomic statuses, sexual orientations, languages, and political and spiritual belief systems—in essence, our own culture. Therefore, if we can better understand our own cultural world viewpoint and its development, we can improve on our awareness and acknowledgment of cultural differences with our patients. Sometimes our viewpoints develop inadvertently (e.g., we or a loved one is hospitalized, and we suddenly develop a greater degree of understanding and empathy for the inpatient experience in a hospital setting), and sometimes it is deliberate (e.g., we decide to travel to a foreign country where we do not know the language and immerse ourselves as much as we can in its culture). Purposefully trying to learn about others' perspectives, others' ways of life, and others' worldviews can help us increase our awareness and provide more effective neurorehabilitation services to all of our patients.

We should be aware that as individuals we can opt to learn another language, read about other cultures, or spend time in an environment that is different from our own, but this does not ensure understanding of the fine nuances found in other languages and cultures. In other words, we may be able to read the text, but we can still miss the cultural or political references if we are not current on the history and context in which the words were written and used. We may misinterpret a section of what we read or the whole premise of the text. For instance, political humor is not funny if you are unfamiliar with the event that is being ridiculed. A dictionary may indicate that the Spanish translation for the word *discuss* is "discutir," but if you say in Spanish "Let's discuss this some more" ("Vamos a discutir esto mas"), what you are actually saying is "Let's argue about this some more," which can be offensive to a patient. Colloquialisms do not translate well either and can also be difficult to understand. What does it mean if someone says, "Don't go chasing windmills" or "You're mad as a hatter?"

As professionals we can become familiar with the research pertaining to cross-culture and seek out opportunities to increase cultural competency through continuing education and programs such as those offered by The Cross Cultural Health Care Program (www.xculture.org) and Think Cultural Health (www.ThinkCulturalHealth.hhs.gov). We can consult with colleagues or organizations that are more knowledgeable about the culture or diversity issue we are trying to better understand. For instance, the Center for International Rehabilitation Research Information and Exchange (CIRRIE; www.cirrie.buffalo.edu) facilitates the sharing of rehabilitation research in the United States and other countries and provides educational resources related to culture and disability geared toward enhancing cultural competency.

As we provide mental health services, we can ask our patients to educate us about their worldview instead of trying to pretend we understand something we do not. Asking about their beliefs about health, mental health, disability, and decision making can help us provide treatment in a manner that is consistent with and respectful of their cultural belief system. Having an accurate understanding of their belief system helps us to understand their behaviors and how best to merge their views with the treatments we are trying to provide. This type of communication helps to empower patients and develop a collaborative approach to their treatment between themselves and the clinician. Patients who are more active in treatment decisions and perceive their clinician as someone who respects them will have a greater degree of trust in the physician and will increase the likelihood of compliance with treatment.

It is also important to remember that our knowledge about culture helps us to develop hypotheses to be tested with each patient, but we must remember that these are just hypotheses. We can just as easily make the mistake of assuming that all cultural groups are the same, and our behavior can be analogous to racial profiling. Clinicians need to remember that although we are all members of a variety of groups, our experiences are unique and shape our own (and our patients') cultural identification and unique responses to psychological stressors, including health problems and our approach to neurorehabilitation.

In addressing culture and language, we should not forget that we have our own lexicon that may not be fully understood by our patients.

Mr. N, continued . . .

The rehabilitation psychologist is evaluating Mr. N, a middle-aged man from Nigeria, 2 weeks after a left ischemic stroke. Records note he speaks English. He received a college degree in Nigeria and has lived in the United States for over 30 years. His work history includes owning his own business, and recently he has been working as a security guard. The rehabilitation psychologist identifies himself as the team psychologist and reminds Mr. N that they had an appointment and asks if it is a good time to talk. Mr. N smiles and nods yes. The rehabilitation psychologist notes that Mr. N is quiet and wonders about his English language comprehension and language production. After taking a seat, the psychologist identifies himself again, explains why he is there, and reviews confidentiality limitations. Mr. N consents to the evaluation, and the psychologist proceeds with the interview. Although Mr. N was initially reserved and quiet, it becomes apparent that he can comprehend and speak English without difficulty. He discusses his current medical circumstances and provides a health history that is consistent with medical records. After about 20 minutes, when questions about his mood and mental health history come up, the psychologist asks Mr. N if he has ever seen a psychologist before or if he had ever felt the need to see a psychologist in the past. Mr. N replies, "I don't know. I have always wondered what a psychologist does. Can you tell me what a psychologist does?"

In Mr. N's case, although he is well educated and agreeable to participating in the evaluation, his understanding of who the psychologist is and a psychologist's role in his treatment was probably unclear. One solution is to ask patients—regardless of culture, ethnic, and linguistic background—at the beginning of the evaluation if they have ever met with a psychologist before, what that experience was like, and what they believe a psychologist is and does. Once this is discussed, the rehabilitation psychologist has an opportunity to clarify the psychologist's role in the patient's rehabilitation treatment plan and go from there. Other team members may want to do the same, as patients may participate without fully understanding or appreciating the purpose of the therapies being provided.

For instance, in addition to psychology, neurorehabilitation teams often include a physiatrist, occupational therapist, speech therapist, and physical therapist. It is not uncommon for people not to know what a physiatrist is or to think an occupational therapist is someone who helps you find a job or wonder what a speech and language pathologist (i.e., speech therapist) has to do with memory. Terms such as *FIM* (functional independence measure) *scores* and *capacity* (for making medical decisions, to live independently, etc.) are regularly used, and it is assumed that everyone knows what they mean. It is therefore highly recommended that clinicians in neurorehabilitation settings be conscious of the language (e.g., medical terminology, abbreviations) they are using and make an effort to assess whether their patients are fully comprehending what is being discussed or simply being agreeable for fear of being perceived as ignorant.

LANGUAGE AND EDUCATION

The number of people in the United States who speak a language other than English at home has increased in recent decades (U.S. Census Bureau, 2010). In 2007, 19.7% of adults and children older than 5 years spoke a language other than English at home, and about half of these had limited English proficiency (U.S. Census Bureau, 2010). Given the projected population growth in racial and ethnic minorities, precise communication between patients and providers is essential to provide appropriate care. According to Jacobs et al. (2001), "The physician–patient relationship is dependent on effective communication. Limited English–speaking patients need to be able to communicate adequately with their health care providers if we are to improve access to health care for this large and growing U.S. population" (p. 473).

Limited English proficiency (LEP) has been associated with adherence to treatment, accuracy of medical diagnosis, health treatment adequacy, patient satisfaction, and quality of the patient–provider relationship (Baker, Hayes, & Puebla-Fortier, 1998; Flores, 2006; Jacobs et al., 2001). Studies examining the effectiveness of professional interpreter services have demonstrated an increase in the delivery of health care, including clinical, prescription, and preventive services, in patients with LEP (Jacobs et al., 2001).

Clear communication is thus essential to providing culturally competent health services to prevent patient–clinician miscommunication and minimize any lack of trust or confidence in the clinician. Working with LEP individuals can be challenging. Language knowledge is on a spectrum. On the ends of the spectrum you have "speaks English very well" and "does not speak any English," with a broad range of language capabilities in between.

From the patients' perspective, they may feel ashamed for not speaking better English and may just smile and nod even though they do not fully understand what is being said to them. Some patients may self-identify as English speakers and may be embarrassed or ashamed to admit that unfamiliar medical concepts and terminology are difficult to understand. From the clinician's perspective, it may be difficult to gauge a patient's LEP status. Clinicians may think that because an individual has lived in the United States for over 20 years, he or she must speak and understand at least some English. Clinicians may not be aware that the person has had limited opportunities to learn English because the person has always lived in a predominantly non-English-speaking neighborhood and has always worked in an environment where coworkers speak their native language. Clinicians should be wary when patients ask few questions, rarely initiate conversation, simply nod or say "yes" in response to the clinician's questions or comments, or provide inappropriate or inconsistent responses to questions. Having patients repeat back what was discussed can help clarify the level of understanding and whether an interpreter is needed (American Medical Association [AMA], 2013).

Determining a patient's English proficiency is critical primarily to provide appropriate medical care and improve compliance but also to ensure that recipients of federal financial assistance are not violating their obligation to enforce and implement Title VI of the Civil Rights Act of 1964, which prohibits national origin discrimination. Additionally, Executive Order 13166, which went into effect on August 11, 2000, was implemented to improve access to services for LEP individuals. It requires that federal agencies provide recipient guidance to agencies that provide federal financial assistance in how to provide meaningful access to their services to LEP individuals. This applies to both written and oral information. Institutions that are not federally funded and not legally obligated to implement Title VI of the Civil Rights Act of 1964 should still strive to provide equal services to their LEP patients.

It is also important to consider that well-intentioned clinicians may overestimate their ability to communicate with LEP patients and inadvertently violate patients' civil rights and the right to be provided with language assistance services and receive health care information in their native language (Hunt, 2007). This can happen in one of two ways: overestimating the patient's ability to effectively understand and communicate in English or overestimating one's own ability to effectively understand and communicate in the patient's native language. Many clinicians may know a second language, but, again, it is one thing to know how to speak another language and another thing to know how to explain medical terms and conditions in that language.

Here is an example. A medical resident was overheard saying the following to a Spanish-speaking patient when explaining the recommendation for a surgical toe amputation versus a transmetatarsal amputation scheduled for the next day to address osteomyelitis: "Necesitamos cortar un dedo. Posiblemente todos mañana. Esta bien?" ("We need to cut a toe off, possibly all of them, tomorrow. Is that okay?"). Just imagine how the patient felt when she heard this alarming news. Fortunately, a certified bilingual staff member was nearby and was able to clarify with both the medical resident and the patient what the resident meant and help answer the patient's questions. Although knowledge of another language can be extremely helpful to clinicians, caution should be used in determining when it can be used and when bringing in a certified interpreter is warranted.

It is not uncommon for patients to state they understand English or report they are bilingual, only to later be confused by the discussions or not grasp important aspects of the discussion. In working with Spanish–English bilinguals, the authors have frequently noted that patients will "code-switch" or bounce back and forth between English and Spanish. The idea that receptive language or the ability to understand and appreciate English is better than their ability to express themselves in English is a pattern often noted in students of a new language. Other patients who have requested to speak in English are often noted to have delays and hesitations in their speech patterns that suggest the patient hears the questions in English, translates the questions into Spanish, and then translates their answers back into English, all of which can result in a variety of issues. At one level the cognitively inefficient approach of translating back and forth during discussions or during testing may lead to the patient performing more poorly than in his or her primary language and coloring the interpretations that can be made. This process may also be made worse in situations where the individual is under stress, medicated, or in pain.

An analogous concern often seen with LEP patients is limited education and literacy in their primary language. The literature has shown that limited English proficiency has a negative influence on overall health care, while functional illiteracy in patients' primary language and English further reduces the likelihood of understanding or appreciating their medical conditions and further exacerbates the overall picture of their health care. The assessment process can easily be complicated, especially if trying to establish prior levels of functioning following a stroke or brain injury. Education and literacy level can further complicate the degree, and quality of, bilingualism patients possess and complicate communication, especially if they insist on speaking in English and translating information for themselves. Additionally, the process may also increase the likelihood of errors of all kinds from the provider and patient. Patients may incorrectly state that they do or do not take medications or have specific medical conditions, or inaccurately endorse or deny medical and psychiatric symptoms. Clinicians are very likely to assume understanding when the patient says "yes" in response to every question and are less likely to ask follow-up or complicated questions. Anecdotally, when asked to continue the interviews or examinations in their primary language, many of these same individuals present as smarter, more quickwitted, more capable of using humor, and more engaged in the process.

Mr. R

Mr. R is a 65-year-old man from Russia who was stabilized and admitted to the neurorehabilitation inpatient hospital after suffering a right hemisphere stroke. He had immigrated to the United States 15 years earlier and identified himself as an English speaker. At the time of admission, he was confused and agitated, but this improved during his first week as an inpatient, and he was able to participate in his rehabilitation therapies. His English-language comprehension and production abilities appear to be grossly intact as assessed by the speech therapist. During his admission, blood was found in his stool, and the team suspected he might be bleeding internally. Two weeks after his admission, the team asked the rehabilitation psychologist to evaluate his capacity for medical decision making due to the fact that he was refusing an endoscopy to help determine the source of the bleeding.

Mr. R was evaluated by a Russian-speaking rehabilitation psychologist. Initially he insisted on using English, but as the evaluation proceeded, he switched to Russian. The evaluation revealed that he understood the team's concerns and treatment recommendations, was able to appreciate his medical circumstances, was able to reason through his situation, and was able to express a choice and thus had the capacity to make informed medical decisions. What also became clear was that Mr. R understood that the endoscopy required that a tube be put down his throat. What he did not grasp was that it was a small, thin tube that would be put in his throat temporarily for only a few minutes. He erroneously thought that it would be a large tube, like the one he required when he was initially hospitalized (a ventilation tube had been inserted to help him breathe) and that it would be left in his throat for an indefinite amount of time.

Mr. R's case shows how easily critical information can be lost in translation and how this can negatively affect patient–physician collaboration and can potentially cause harm. Mr. R's insistence on communicating only in English with staff caused him to misunderstand a key element of recommendations being made by the physician and to delay an examination that needed to be done for his own benefit. Once Mr. R understood the difference between an endoscopy tube and a ventilation tube, and that the discomfort he would experience would be minimal compared to his experience of being placed on a ventilator, he was agreeable to the procedure.

Clinicians should gather a good history about education and academic functioning to better appreciate whether what is being observed is related to true delays or lack of opportunity. Six years of education does not always equal 6 years of education. On the one hand, it may mean an individual came from a family of certain means who could afford to keep them in school rather than put them to work and that they were very good students who wanted to go further in school but could not. On the other hand, it may mean a person went to school for 6 years but repeated third grade twice or did not graduate from school until he was 20 years old and did not learn much. Or it may mean the individual is thinking, "I'm going to say I have 6 years of education because that is what I tell everybody, but I barely know how to read or write, and I do not want anyone to know I only have 1 year of formal education." Thus, patients, and sometimes their families, often misrepresent their education level for a multitude of reasons, and it is not uncommon for a team member to report a level of education that differs from what the patient has reported to the psychologist. Level of education plays such a critical role in brain injury resiliency, concrete versus abstract thinking, a person's worldview, and psychological testing norms that it is essential that the clinician have a clear picture of how to translate number of years into the patient's proxy for knowledge attained and ability to problem solve.

Clinicians can determine a more accurate level of education in various ways. For instance, when gathering patient history, clinicians typically ask how many years of education the patient completed, but it is essential that clinicians not only ask how far a person got in school but also about what kind of student the patient was. Providers might ask, "Can you tell me more about your school system? What does 6 years of education in Korea equal in U.S. education?" Providers can clarify, "Were special education classes available where you went to school? Where could a student go if he or she had difficulty learning?" Patients can be asked if they experienced difficulties in learning or if they received special education classes. It is helpful to inform them that within the hospital setting, they are going to receive a lot of important written information, so it is important to know how well they can read or if it might be better for information to be read to them to ensure they understand it. This can make a world of a difference for some patients, because they understand they can ask for help with not only health documents but with something as basic as their daily menu selections.

In an ideal situation, a brief reading comprehension test can be given to patients, but the clinician must first determine if patients will get written information in their native language or in English. If they will receive information in their native language, this would require having standardized measures in multiple languages. If patients are to receive medical information in English, then the clinician can evaluate their English reading comprehension, keeping in mind that the test will be measuring the English language comprehension of individuals with limited English proficiency. In either case, the test's usefulness will depend on whether it includes the medical language that is used in a neurorehabilitation setting.

WORKING WITH A QUALIFIED MEDICAL INTERPRETER

In today's busy medical settings where clinicians may feel pressured to provide services as quickly as possible and increase productivity, waiting for an interpreter or working with an interpreter may seem burdensome, but when working with neurorehabilitation patients who may be cognitively compromised, providing services in their native language is critical. Providing medical information and services in patients' native languages increases their knowledge and understanding, encourages their compliance with treatments, empowers them, and reduces medical errors.

Because patients have a legal right to receive medical information and services in their native language, many hospitals have interpretation services available. These include telephonic interpretation, in which the clinician calls an interpreter center and is provided with an interpreter over the phone; a video monitor interpreter (VMI) system, in which the interpreter is in a different location but can be seen on a portable screen, such as a computer tablet or video monitor on wheels (visually it functions like Skype); and onsite interpretation, in which the interpreter is in the room with the clinician and the patient. Trained onsite interpreters and trained telephonic/VMI interpreters are likely to provide a high level of interpreting quality, be professional and knowledgeable about the ethics of interpretation, and are appropriate under all circumstances. Untrained bilingual staff and bilingual family members or friends may supply poor interpretations and demonstrate low professionalism and knowledge about the ethics of interpretation. They may also be unfamiliar with terminology and confidentiality, and they may omit information when the discussion is about sensitive topics (AMA, 2013). Only if absolutely necessary should untrained staff and family members be used, and then only in low-risk circumstances (e.g., to schedule an appointment).

Providing services with an interpreter in an acute neurorehabilitation inpatient setting can be challenging. Patient schedules are often generated a week ahead, and availability may be limited due to the fact that neurorehabilitation inpatients spend 3 to 4 hours a day in therapy. Additionally, patients may have medical appointments or outings that are also scheduled around their therapy time. The challenge for rehabilitation psychologists is coordinating the patient's availability with their own schedule and that of the interpreter. If it becomes difficult to find a mutually agreeable time, the psychologist could do the evaluation with a speech therapist, who is likely already scheduled to see the patient with an interpreter or another discipline. This can be beneficial as well, because it gives the rehabilitation psychologist an opportunity to observe behaviors and determine cognitive deficits that must be taken into consideration when conducting the full psychological evaluation at a later time. It is usually easy to get an interpreter for a language such as Spanish, but in cases of a very rare language, such as Mayan or Kankanae, the clinician may have to use a telephonic interpreter and wait for that person to be available. Sometimes the language is so rare that the clinician has no choice but to rely on family members.

Ms. S

The rehabilitation psychologist has received an inpatient consult to evaluate Ms. S for depression. She is described as having a flat affect and acting apathetic, with limited initiation in her therapies. Her family has reported that she often says she wants to die. Ms. S, who is Samoan, had a left posterior cerebral artery territory stroke. She immigrated to the United States as a young child and received her education in English. Prior to her stroke, she was bilingual and

(continued)

Ms. S (*continued*)

spoke both Samoan and English. In reviewing the records, it was noted that after the stroke, Ms. S no longer used English to communicate. She spoke and responded only to her first language, Samoan. The psychologist contacted the hospital's Language and Culture Center (the department that arranges interpreters, assists with providing oral and written information to non-English-speaking patients, and provides training to increase interpreter certification and availability and cultural awareness in the hospital) and was informed that the one staff member who was certified as a Samoan interpreter no longer worked at the hospital and that they encountered difficulties finding an interpreter for other team members working with Ms. S. No one was available through the language line/VMI, and they had not been able to identify anyone in the interpreter schools that the hospital contracted with to assist with interpretation. Consequently, since Ms. S's admission, her husband has been acting as her interpreter.

In this case, the rehabilitation psychologist encountered several obstacles in attaining an interpreter to assist with the evaluation. The clinician had two choices: Use Ms. S's husband as an interpreter or decline to do the evaluation due to the potential ethical and confidentiality conflicts. Although the use of an untrained family member is discouraged, in this situation it was determined that conducting the evaluation was necessary to assess suicidal ideation, assist with her participation in rehabilitation, and determine if any behavioral interventions could help improve her participation. The staff also felt it would be beneficial to both Ms. S and her husband if they could determine if her presentation was secondary to stroke, a mood disorder, or a combination of both and address the problem as an inpatient. It was ultimately decided that it was in her best interests to do the evaluation with her husband as interpreter. Ethical principles should be paramount in guiding decisions and actions, but in some cases, the approach ends up being guided by what is the least worst option versus the best-case scenario.

Many hospitals are lucky to have interpreters for multiple languages who have experience in the medical setting. Other hospitals may have to rely on phone interpreters, who may not be familiar with medical vocabulary or concepts, particularly the relatively unusual terminology used in neurorehabilitation. Although phone interpreters are usually available up to 24 hours a day, in-person interpreters are limited, and they may not be available at the time they are needed. Additionally, translators may not be fluent in the dialect spoken by the patient, particularly for languages with multiple dialects such as Chinese and Filipino. At times, the only translator available may be a friend who speaks the patient's dialect. In one instance, a patient with an unusual rural Chinese dialect talked to his friend, who translated to Cantonese for the interpreter, who translated to English for the doctor.

Working with an interpreter can at times feel awkward, but there are things a clinician can do to make the experience more comfortable. Trained interpreters know that they should interpret everything accurately and completely and may ask clinicians to repeat themselves or slow down. Paraphrasing and answering for the patient should be avoided. Clinicians should be aware of this if they are working with someone other than a trained interpreter. The interpreter should preferably sit next to and a bit behind the patient. The interpreter should be greeted, and her role should be introduced to the patient, but after that, the clinician should speak directly to the patient, not the interpreter. The interpreter should reflect exactly what is being said by each party—for instance, "I don't understand," not "She says she doesn't understand." If the clinician notes that the interpreter is not doing this, she should be asked to do so. In the same manner, if the clinician believes that the interpreter is not interpreting everything the patient says, she should be asked to do so, and should also be reminded not to add anything to what the patient is saying. The clinician should speak at an even pace and pause often to allow time to interpret. The clinician should be aware that psychological terms, technical medical terms, slang, and complicated sentences may not translate well, so it may take the interpreter a bit longer to interpret, or she may ask for the question or information to be rephrased. Changing ideas in the middle of a sentence or asking multiple questions at once should be avoided. If the patient and the interpreter get into a conversation, the clinician should interrupt and ask that the interpreter share everything that was just said. Asking that the patient repeat back or summarize information that was just discussed can help the clinician ascertain the patient's understanding of the discussion and the information that was provided (AMA, 2013).

Psychologists who are conducting assessments may want to review the protocols to some degree with the interpreter beforehand if possible to determine the best approach and increase cultural sensitivity. For instance, when doing a memory list with the patient, it may be better for the interpreter to see the list and read it to the patient herself rather than the clinician reading the words aloud in English and having the interpreter repeat them to the patient in his native language. The interpreter can alert the clinician about any culturally inappropriate or linguistically challenging items that could be difficult to translate. Interpreters can also be rich sources of cultural and observational information; for instance, they can provide information about the individual's acculturation; their speech rate, rhythm, and prosody; and possible dysarthria and aphasia. Interpreters can inform clinicians about any potential cultural misunderstandings.

Mr. K

Mr. K is a 49-year-old man who was born in Korea. He had a right parietal lobe stroke and has a history of hypertension and hyperlipidemia. He has been referred to psychology for an evaluation of depression 3 weeks after the stroke. A trained onsite Korean interpreter was used to facilitate the evaluation. The evaluation revealed that as a teenager, Mr. K moved with his family to South America and learned to speak Spanish. At the age of 24, he moved to the United States. He worked in a factory for several years, but due to a non-work-related injury, he has not been able to work full time in over 3 years. He never married, and he has no children.

The interpreter noted to the psychologist that Mr. K's Korean language abilities lacked a higher level of understanding and language usage that is often attained in late adolescence and in higher education in Korea. The team noted that his Spanish was also poor because he had not received formal instruction in Spanish. Mr. K's unique cultural and linguistic situation had led to difficulties with cultural adaptation in the United States and limited social support.

(continued)

Mr. K (*continued*)

He has reported that since the stroke, he has had difficulties interacting with others. He often appears withdrawn.

His cognition was assessed with the use of the Montreal Cognitive Assessment (MoCA) Korean version. He demonstrated deficits in executive function, attention, immediate and delayed memory, and language. In regard to mood, he showed symptoms that were suggestive of moderate depression. Mr. K shared that he was not satisfied with his life, felt his life was empty, was afraid something bad would happen to him, and sometimes felt hopeless. Mr. K reported that he was never sad or depressed until after the stroke and acknowledged that he had experienced suicidal ideation with a vague plan immediately after but denied intention or current ideation.

The psychologist incorporated knowledge regarding right hemisphere brain function with the cultural information gathered during the evaluation. The right hemisphere is often involved in mediating nonverbal stimuli and the perception of tone quality and rhythm of speech. Additionally, the right hemisphere has been found to be involved in affective prosody (i.e., patterns of stress and intonation in a language that convey emotion; Ross, 2000). Mr. K had right hemisphere involvement in his stroke, suggesting that the emotional disconnect and language deficits observed could be stroke related. Not speaking Korean, however, it would be difficult to ascertain the degree to which the stroke had affected rhythm of speech and affective prosody. The ability to evaluate Mr. K with a trained Korean hospital interpreter and to use a cognitive measure available in Korean allowed for a richer interaction and evaluation of the patient. The interpreter provided valuable information regarding Korean culture and how Mr. K's language ability in Korean had likely affected his social interaction with others long term prior to his stroke. Post stroke these appeared to be a barrier to him connecting better with staff and other patients. Additionally, his report of time of onset of mood symptoms suggested that his presentation was not solely secondary to his stroke but that there were true clinical symptoms of depression that needed treatment. The psychologist was able to provide relevant recommendations to the team and to differentiate between culturally driven variables and true cognitive and mood problems.

Ms. H

Ms. H is a 30-year-old African American woman who was referred to inpatient psychology to evaluate her capacity to make medical decisions. She was admitted for right-foot cellulitis and was found to have osteomyelitis of the third and fourth toes. Her medical history included deafness and leukocytosis, and she had also reported a history of schizophrenia and depression, for which she was asymptomatic. She was homeless and had a history of substance use. Ms. H had been communicating with staff through writing, but her responses were inappropriate to the questions she was asked, and she was not acknowledging the team's recommendations that she have her third and fourth toes amputated. Given her current presentation, along with her mental health history and substance use history, her capacity for medical decision making was being questioned.

From a medical perspective, Ms. H's situation is clear: She has an infection/osteomyelitis in the bones and needs an amputation to eliminate the infection. From a cultural perspective, however, the situation is much more complex. What is her experience of the world from the perspective of a deaf African American woman, and what role is that playing in her medical decision making?

Ms. H, continued . . .

A trained American Sign Language (ASL) VMI was used to evaluate Ms. H. Through the VMI, a full clinical interview was conducted, and it was noted that her responses were appropriate to the questions being asked. Ms. H was open and forthcoming and had a lot to say, often needing to be redirected. Her thought process was linear, with fair to good judgment and insight.

The evaluation revealed that Ms. H had been raised in foster care since age 8 and after age 18 lived in a board and care for a while.

(continued)

Ms. H (*continued*)

It appeared that as a minor, Ms. H had also lived in two different state hospitals for reasons that she did not know. She reported going to school at the first state hospital. She shared that at the second hospital she was given psychotropic medications and that people there thought she was "dumb." Ms. H stated that although she had no symptoms, she was diagnosed with schizophrenia. She denied ever experiencing hallucinations, delusions, or related symptoms. She acknowledged using crack cocaine for 3 years and daily marijuana use and also acknowledged some run-ins with police that had led to an arrest a year earlier.

In discussing her current medical circumstances, it became clear that there was a miscommunication between her and the surgical team. She was aware of having osteomyelitis but thought the recommended treatment was an incision and debridement (i.e., I&D). When she was provided with the correct treatment recommendations along with risks and benefits of having her third and fourth toes amputated, she asked about alternatives and expressed understanding of the information provided.

Results of this evaluation indicated that Ms. H had the capacity to make informed medical decisions. The ASL VMI interpreter shared that the reason Ms. H's writing seemed odd was because she was using ASL grammatical construction; there was no indication in the interview of a cognitive or thought disorder. Psychology recommended that written communication be used for basic daily communication and an ASL interpreter be used for discussions regarding her medical care.

In both of these cases, the interpreters facilitated clearer communication with the patients and provided useful information regarding cultural variables that were potentially being misunderstood by the medical and rehabilitation teams. In the case of Mr. K, his presentation may have been attributed solely to his stroke. Given that he was familiar with Spanish, a language that is more commonly spoken by staff, the psychologist could have foregone the use of a Korean interpreter and conducted the evaluation in Spanish or referred it to a Spanish-speaking psychologist.

As it turned out, a Korean-speaking interpreter helped Mr. K to express himself to a greater and more accurate degree and to receive appropriate treatment.

In the case of Ms. H, the team initially failed to adequately communicate her medical problem and recommended treatment because they did not use an ASL interpreter. Because she declined surgery, they could have opted to move forward with a less effective treatment, such as long-term antibiotics, that could have led to further spreading of the infection and potential future necessity of a more extensive amputation, as well as development of complications secondary to the antibiotics, such as decreased kidney function. Having the ASL interpreter clarify that the sentence structure was consistent with ASL grammar also helped to support the psychologist's conclusion that Ms. H's cognition was intact and was not affected by her history of substance use or possible thought disorder.

ACCULTURATION

Acculturation is an interchangeable multistage process that occurs as an individual interacts with different cultures. Level of acculturation can have a significant impact on how patients engage with medical providers and treatment, how they comply with medical recommendations, their perceptions and beliefs about health and health care, their health practices and resulting incidences of certain health conditions (Eamranond, Wee, Legedza, Marcantonio, & Leveille, 2009; Lutsey et al., 2008; Mainous, Díaz, & Geesey, 2008; Mainous et al., 2006; Masel, Rudkin, & Peek, 2006; Suinn, 2010). Cultural concepts that summarize the spectrum of acculturation relate to descriptions of how individuals relate to one another, time orientation (e.g., future, past, or current), and locus of control (e.g., external or internal).

Interpersonal relationships across cultures are broadly classified as either individualistic or collectivistic. Individualistic relationships prioritize individuals' rights, goals, and uniqueness, whereas collectivistic relationships place the highest value on cohesiveness and integration for the community's best interest. Perhaps one of the best examples of collectivism is the Kenyan tradition of community self-help events *harambee*, literally meaning "all pull together" in Swahili. In this tradition, when a community member or family faces difficulty (e.g., illness, death, loss of home), the community comes together in an outpouring of emotional and financial support. These concepts are relevant to clinicians because they can affect patients' decision-making preferences and even the quantity and quality of social supports available to them. Among Latinos/Hispanics, *personalismo, familismo, respeto, marianismo,* and *machismo* are inherent values that prescribe social roles and interpersonal relationships (Cianelli, Ferrer, & McElmurry, 2008; Gottlieb, 1994a, 1994b). An individual's level of acculturation can enhance within-group differences, generating microdifferences even within members of the same family (Sue & Sue, 2008). This active process generates a unique constellation of multicultural values, beliefs and attitudes, a type of cultural fingerprint that is unique for each individual.

It is essential to assess level of acculturation as part of the initial clinical evaluation to inform treatment and interpretation of any neuropsychological screenings or tests. Pontón and Ardila (1999) explain, "Since tests and procedures tend to reflect what is relevant to a particular culture, acculturation assumes that the individual becomes familiar with those relevant elements in the new culture, and consequently has a higher probability of understanding and successfully completing test items developed within the new culture" (p. 573). Acculturation can be assessed with a variety of acculturation scales that may be incorporated into the interview, but generally it is relevant to inquire about primary language, languages spoken in various settings, exposure to English, length of residence in the United States and other countries, education, cultural practices, preferences and identities, and types of involvement in community activities.

Ms. J

Ms. J was an 85-year-old Japanese American woman with no significant medical, psychiatric, or substance abuse history, who suffered a fall and head injury. Records indicated that her Glasgow Coma Scale was a 6 (severe brain injury) in the emergency department and that she had to be intubated. Her head injury led to a hemicraniotomy for evacuation of a large right subdural hemorrhage. Her mental status gradually improved, and by the time of transfer to acute inpatient neurorehabilitation (15 days post traumatic brain injury),

---

(*continued*)

Ms. J (*continued*)

she was oriented to person and place. Because she had no family to assist in the decision-making process, an evaluation to assess her capacity for medical decision making was requested. The neurorehabilitation team noted that her level of alertness had increased significantly but that she presented with poor attention and comprehension. The team additionally noted that Ms. J often spoke to staff in Japanese even though they did not understand what she was saying. She was evaluated by a rehabilitation psychologist in the acute neurorehabilitation hospital 28 days and again 36 days post injury.

In the case of Ms. J, the clinician needed to consider various important variables when approaching the evaluation, such as language, elderly status, potential posttraumatic amnesia, and acculturation. The clinician also kept in mind that determining the accuracy of premorbid remote history provided by Ms. J would be difficult because there was no family to contact to corroborate the information. Initial contact was made with Ms. J to gather information regarding these variables and to determine how best to proceed.

Ms. J, continued . . .

Psychology made initial contact with Ms. J 28 days post traumatic brain injury. No interpreter was available at that time, and it was noted that Ms. J responded in both English and Japanese. Her speech was mumbled and of low volume. She was able to briefly engage in the evaluation, but it had to be discontinued due to her drowsiness and lethargy. She was oriented to person and vacillated between 2 months when asked what that day's date was. She was able to provide her month and date of birth but not the year or her age. She repeatedly said, "I'm sorry," when told she had suffered a fall and was in the hospital. She denied having any pain, and nursing denied that she was taking pain medicine. Nursing and her

---

(*continued*)

Ms. J (*continued*)

neurorehabilitation team noted fluctuations in her alertness and level of energy and felt that this was a barrier to rehabilitation. Her medical team was ruling out potential medication and/or medical variables that could be contributing to her drowsiness. Psychology decided to hold off on further evaluation of the patient until a time when she was more alert and able to engage in the evaluation process.

Thirty-six days post traumatic brain injury, Ms. J was awake and alert and seen while lying supine in bed. A Japanese phone interpreter was used to assist with the evaluation. Ms. J was noted to use both Japanese and English during the evaluation. She made good eye contact and joked with the nurses. She denied being in pain, and she was oriented to person, place, month, and year. She was aware of having had surgery to her head but was unable to explain why she required surgery, why she was in the hospital, or why she had a percutaneous endoscopic gastrostomy (PEG) tube. Although she consented to the evaluation, she appeared confused at times and expressed suspicion when asked mental status questions, stating that people might be listening. She would not elaborate on her work history, saying it was a secret, and declined to answer psychosocial questions related to family and daily activities. She was reminded of the purpose of the evaluation multiple times because on several occasions she inappropriately responded, "Japan is a beautiful country." She said the evaluator should not be asking her these questions because she was not asking the evaluator about her country of origin. When asked about hallucinations, Ms. J looked around the room and placed her index finger over her lips, gesturing to be silent. When asked why she was doing this, Ms. J replied that there might be listening devices in her room and that someone might be listening. Notably, she required redirection to the interpretation process when the interpreter reported on two occasions that the patient was initiating a separate conversation with the interpreter.

In the case of Ms. J, the clinician had to differentiate between what might be culturally and generationally appropriate and what might be an effect of her brain injury. Her level of acculturation was difficult to determine, but she appeared more comfortable communicating in Japanese, held Japan in high regard, and had been working in a primarily Japanese community, which suggested that she likely identified to a greater degree with Japanese culture and values than American. Her refusal to discuss personal matters, for instance, could be a result of cultural upbringing or long-standing personal preferences. Given her age, it was possible that she was interned during World War II or knew others who were, leading to a certain degree of suspicion of the majority culture. Her responses and behavior, however, were inappropriate for the setting, and although the purpose and nature of the evaluation were explained to her and she agreed to proceed, her ability to consistently recall that information seemed fleeting. It was determined that her presentation was more likely related to cognitive deficits to a greater degree than to cultural variables.

Her behavior also appeared to be influenced by a delusional process in which she believed that she had been employed in secret work and that she was currently being spied upon. It was unclear how the use of a phone interpreter affected her hallucinations or if it added to her confusion about her environment. Her inability to discuss her rehabilitation therapies suggested poor recall as well as poor insight regarding her environment and reason for hospitalization. LEP patients are more limited than English-speaking patients in learning about their hospital environment from overhearing conversations. They also are limited by the information provided to them by interpreters. In the case of Ms. J, a Japanese interpreter was not available 24 hours a day, which made it difficult to reinforce the information provided by the medical and rehabilitation teams. Notably, the observation that Ms. J was hallucinating was not as obvious without the use of the trained and observant interpreter. She was not able to talk about her delusions and hallucinations in English, so her inaccurate responses were often explained away by her low English proficiency.

At this point in time, Ms. J was deemed to have diminished capacity to make informed medical decisions, and designation of a health care proxy was recommended. Review of potential medication side effects and/or interactions that could affect her cognition was recommended. Strategies to assist with memory and socialization and follow-up neuropsychological testing to determine further cognitive improvements were also recommended.

CULTURE, REHABILITATION, AND PSYCHOTHERAPY: ADAPTING TREATMENT

Emotional changes after injury, including depression, anxiety, and adjustment to injury, can vary greatly according to the patient's culture of origin. For some cultures, the idea of talking to a stranger about emotions is seen as abnormal. However, family members who have adopted Western attitudes may encourage psychological contact. When providing mental health services, a clinician may find that it is necessary to work outside the box and accommodate the patient's specific cultural needs.

Ms. U

Ms. U, a 55-year-old Gujarati (Indian) woman, was referred to psychology after a traumatic brain injury as an outpatient at the request of her daughter and daughter-in-law for "fear of walking with and without a walker." The consult received indicated that Ms. U spoke English. When Ms. U arrived at the session, she was accompanied by her daughter and daughter-in-law. The psychologist realized quickly that Ms.U had limited English proficiency and indicated that she would use a phone interpreter. Ms. U, however, refused and stated she wanted her daughter and daughter-in-law to interpret for her. The psychologist explained the reasons for wanting to use a professional interpreter and suggested multiple times that a phone interpreter could be used, but Ms. U stated, "I don't want to talk to someone I don't know" and "They could be part of my (Gujarati) community, and I do not want them to know my information." Given the need to evaluate her, her refusal to use a Gujarati phone interpreter, and her statement that she was more comfortable with her family interpreting, the unconventional decision was made to go ahead and use her daughter and daughter-in-law as interpreters.

Ms. U was initially unsure of why she was talking to a stranger, due to both cognitive deficits and the limited exposure to psychology in her culture of origin. The psychologist educated her about the referral for "worry," and Ms. U stated, "I am fine."

The family members told the rehabilitation psychologist that Ms. U was reluctant to discuss her feelings with strangers, and this was reflected by Ms. U declining the use of an outside interpreter. She tended to minimize problems post injury, both cognitive and physical, even when her family talked about it during the session. For many non-Western cultures, family is a central focus of the patient. For patients from family-centered cultures, increasing the role of the family can improve rehabilitation (Scheermesser, Bachmann, Schäman, Oesch, & Kool, 2012). Although an "ideal" evaluation would involve an interpreter and individual time with the patient, the "ideal" evaluation would not respect the individual's right to obtain assessment and treatment in her preferred manner. The provider chose to respect Ms. U's preference (American Psychological Association's [APA's] Ethics General Principle E: Respect for People's Rights and Dignity) and in doing so, helped both Ms. U and her family to better cope with a difficult situation (APA Ethics General Principle A: Beneficence and Nonmaleficence).

Ms. U, continued . . .

Ms. U was born and raised in a rural location in India, completed 12 years of education, and came to the United States approximately 13 years ago. She has been working in a family business.

Ms. U initially denied difficulties with coping or anxiety after a traumatic brain injury. Her family reported that she was nervous about using the walker and doing household activities, especially when she was with her immediate family. They also stated that Ms. U had periods of sadness about her injury. After her family mentioned these difficulties, Ms. U acknowledged some sadness and "a little worry" but stated that she felt better after being around her family.

Although Ms. U admitted to sadness about changes in functioning and worries about doing activities, she did not believe she needed to talk to "anyone" because she was "fine," and she preferred to talk to her husband about any concerns. With the encouragement of her daughter and daughter-in-law, she agreed to return to psychology, and the provider arranged for a Hindi-speaking psychologist

(continued)

> **Ms. U (*continued*)**
>
> to be at the next session. Originally, the psychologist suggested that Ms. U could be followed by a Hindi-speaking psychologist, but both Ms. U and her family indicated that they would like the current provider to be present, due to their own comfort with a known provider and to ease any transition that might take place.

During the initial session, the psychologist became aware that cultural factors, such as limited exposure to psychology, language, and the role of family, affected the patient's perception of psychotherapy. The psychologist consulted with a Hindi-speaking psychologist to learn more about Indian culture and perspectives on psychology and to ask if attendance at the next session would be possible.

> **Ms. U, continued . . .**
>
> For the second session, Ms. U, her daughter, and her daughter-in-law were seen by the primary rehabilitation psychologist and a Hindi-speaking Indian rehabilitation psychologist. At Ms. U's request, her daughter-in-law translated when Ms. U did not understand Hindi. Ms. U and her family talked about an upcoming trip to India for a wedding, and this appeared to be a focus and motivation for her to "get better."
>
> Ms. U reported that she had extensive social support and that she preferred to do things with her family rather than "talk about things she can't do." She said she felt "more normal" around others.
>
> The Hindi-speaking psychologist normalized Ms. U's reaction and offered to provide ongoing support as needed to her and her family. After the second session, the Hindi-speaking psychologist told the English-speaking psychologist that she was not sure Ms. U was interested in or needed ongoing treatment. Ms. U appeared to benefit most from activities and upcoming goals (her trip to India).

(*continued*)

Ms. U (*continued*)

She stated that Indian culture focuses on achieving goals, normalizing a situation, and moving on, rather than processing feelings, which is more traditional in Western culture.

Though a third session was arranged with the Hindi-speaking psychologist, Ms. U and her family canceled the session, stating that Ms. U was "doing better" and looking forward to the upcoming trip to India.

The primary role of the rehabilitation psychologist in this case was to serve as an impetus for the family and Ms. U to discuss areas of concern and for the provider to educate the family about traumatic brain injury. Although psychotherapy can be beneficial across cultures, it was clear that Ms. U preferred a more traditional Indian approach to addressing her coping post injury.

The fact that the consult was generated by the younger generation in the family (her daughter and daughter-in-law) also illustrates the variability in acculturation and acceptance of psychotherapy from one generation to another. The daughter and daughter-in-law (and the physician who wrote the consult) thought that Western psychotherapy would be beneficial in identifying and addressing barriers to her worry about using the walker. Once it was modified to meet Ms. U's cultural needs, it was indeed better.

The provider learned about Indian culture and related generational norms and how culture might affect assessment and psychotherapy. Specifically, assessment of the individual may be a family affair, and the "identified patient" may not prefer the traditional psychological model. The younger generation was more comfortable with the idea of therapy and may have served as a bridge of information to Ms. U. They also may have learned some strategies from the provider that they could implement with Ms. U. Once the assessment and treatment were discussed as a family, Ms. U and her family appeared to better understand how to help her cope with the effects of the traumatic brain injury. In the future, the use of a translator might be discussed before the initial session, and the provider might consult with someone of Indian ancestry prior to the session to determine how to best help Ms. U and her family.

ADDRESSING CHALLENGES OF FAITH, RELIGION, AND SPIRITUALITY

It is not uncommon for issues of faith, religion, and spirituality to arise in acute care when patients have confronted real or perceived life-threatening experiences or traumas or are simply reminded of the frailty of human existence. Including these values in health care is important because they are directly related to how patients and families cope, beliefs about death and dying, beliefs about what are considered the most appropriate health practices, and attitudes toward illness and disability. Studies examining beliefs about disability suggest, for example, that some Hispanics/Latinos perceive disability as God's will and caring for people with disabilities as a virtue that will help one obtain God's favor (Glover & Blankenship, 2007). The search for meaning as a way of coping can surface during the acute recovery phase and continue thereafter when patients are confronted with news that they will potentially live with a chronic condition like cortical visual impairment following a traumatic brain injury (Coffey, Gallagher, & Desmond, 2014; Dezutter et al., 2013; Oaksford, Frude, & Cuddihy, 2005). Search for meaning may surface in questions like "Why did this happen to me?," "Why was I the only one to survive?," or "What am I supposed to do now?" At its core, searching for meaning is closely tied to issues of purpose, existence, and, ultimately, spirituality.

Faith, religion, and spirituality can become sources of great support for patients and their families, but at other times these values can become a challenging focus of attention when there is conflict between patients' values and those of the medical system. Those with primary Western cultural values may consider religion as pertaining almost exclusively to major world religions like Catholicism, Christianity, Hinduism, and Islam; however, as Chukwuneke, Ezeonu, Onyire, and Ezeonu (2012) point out, "native religions in which people believe in deities, spirits, and ancestor worship" (p. 331) may become entwined with more orthodox beliefs so that traditional religion and folk religion are incorporated into one value system. For instance, a Mexican American patient may identify as Catholic and value prayer to saints as well as indigenous practices like *curanderismo*, a form of folk healing that incorporates herbal medicine, healing rituals, and spiritualism (e.g., "I don't need insulin. I'm going to treat my diabetes with these leaves mailed from Guatemala, and I'm going to treat my neuropathy with hot water foot baths").

Attribution of illness and disability to supernatural causes has been documented in several ethnic and racial groups. One study surveying attitudes toward epilepsy of Hispanics/Latinos in the United States found that approximately 25% of respondents attributed the condition to spiritual causes (e.g., lack of spiritual faith, some kind of evil spirit, or sins) compared to non-Hispanics (Sirven, Lopez, Vazquez, & Haverbeke, 2005). Other studies comparing attitudes toward health and health care of Asian-born women found that Hmong women in particular attributed illness to spirits catching the soul (Helsel & Mochel, 2002; Johnson, 2002; Zhao, Esposito, & Wang, 2010). Thus, as clinicians trying to understand the variety of worldviews, we must realize that those who believe that health problems are essentially spiritual in nature will be more likely to seek help from spiritual healers that address both their physical ailments and the spiritual etiologies. Chukwuneke et al. (2012) offered an example involving malaria and witchcraft in a semirural Tanzanian community. In this case, community members who had been exposed to biomedicine for a long time believed that witchcraft could thwart medical treatments by placing a veil over the body so malaria parasites could not be detected in the blood. Patients who attribute their maladies to spiritual and supernatural causes may then delay pursuit of biomedicine, increasing their risk for medical complications (e.g., stroke with diabetes) because the spiritual issues are more fundamental. Not only this, but ethnic and racial minorities may prefer healers because they may be more accessible in minority communities (i.e., you do not need health insurance to get treatment from a *sobador*), and minorities may already feel alienated by Western health care systems due to language barriers, cost of care, or transportation.

While striving for multicultural competency in the realm of religion, one may become easily confused and overwhelmed by the many terms and concepts related to religion, faith, and spirituality. Pattison (2013) argues, "Those who inhabit and embrace the categories religion and spirituality on the one hand and health care on the other often fail to understand both the richness and the confusing complexity of the other. Even health care workers with personal religious affiliations may fail to comprehend the complexities and ambivalences of religion—they know the bit of their own religion that is relevant to them—while 'nonreligious' managers and clinicians may only have the most rudimentary understanding of what faith, religion, and spirituality are or might be" (p. 193). Responding to these dilemmas, he offers practical considerations for health care workers.

First of all, one must not assume that all religious groups are the same. Pattison (2013) says, "Religious traditions and groups vary enormously in their structures and organizations" (p. 202). This can make it "very difficult for health care workers and policy makers to identify who they should consult with in different religious groups and what authority and representativeness they should concede to those consulted" (p. 202). Psychologists may help reduce this burden by consulting with hospital chaplains and advocating for the health care institutions in which they are employed to support chaplaincy departments that are representative of the faith groups present in the communities in which they operate. Second, one must recognize that religious communities are internally pluriform and diverse. In the same way that individuals from any given ethnic or racial group are not all the same with respect to their values and identities (e.g., a Latino from Argentina is not the same as one from Mexico, even though they both speak Spanish), members of religious communities are also diverse in their views and opinions (e.g., an Orthodox Jew is not the same as a Seventh Day Adventist, even though they both keep the Sabbath). Finally, not all religious individuals relate to their religions in the same way. As Pattison (2013) explains, "Just because someone admits to a religious adherence, this does not necessarily mean that their commitment is keen and knowledgeable. There are degrees of belonging and believing, and this may also affect the ways in which 'religious' people react to and make demands upon health care" (p. 202).

A FRAMEWORK OF CULTURAL RELATIVISM FOR INPATIENT NEUROREHABILITATION

It is well known that attitudes, values, and beliefs impact patients' coping with illness and disability, conceptualization of their condition, and engagement in the rehabilitation process. Familiarity with different cultural groups or access to appropriate cultural consultation sources when this knowledge is absent is an asset for psychologists formulating clinical hypotheses. Although it would be unrealistic to presume competency of all the cultural groups we may encounter, it is essential to have a working knowledge of core cultural concepts to facilitate our conceptualizations of culturally diverse patients.

The Neurorehabilitation Psychologist as a Cultural Advocate

Cultural brokers can have a multilevel positive impact on the health care delivery system benefiting patients, providers, and the health care setting (National Center for Cultural Competence, 2004). They can facilitate more positive experiences when patients interface with the health care system, increase their motivation to seek treatment in the future, and help patients gain better understanding of their diagnosis and treatment. Patients motivated to seek treatment are more likely to engage in preventive health practices that can minimize health complications and the need for costly emergency care. Health care providers benefit from cultural brokerage by gaining more in-depth information about the patient that can facilitate the treatment process and improve diagnostic accuracy, treatment effectiveness, communication, and knowledge about the cultural community. In turn, health care settings benefit by reducing potential liabilities that may result from poor communication with patients and increasing cost-effectiveness associated with adherence to treatment and preventive care. Through this process, health care organizations develop trust within their service communities that may help ensure the organization's sustainability (National Center for Cultural Competence, 2004).

Ms. L

A middle-aged, Spanish-speaking Latina of Dominican and Puerto Rican descent was referred for outpatient psychotherapy after her presurgical bariatric team identified noncompliance to treatment recommendations as a primary barrier to her weight loss. During the initial visit, the psychologist identified that the patient, Ms. L, had been experiencing neuropathic symptoms resulting in frequent emergency department visits that had not been entirely disclosed to the medical team. The psychologist quickly noted that her symptoms were likely related to a history of poorly managed

---

(continued)

Ms. L (*continued*)

diabetes and that mistrust in the health care system and her conceptualization of illness were at the core of her nonadherence to treatment. Ms. L did not identify herself as diabetic and expressed doubt that diabetes was a real medical condition. She believed that insulin, among other medications, was not only unnecessary but was just a financial scheme to benefit physicians. Though Ms. L was followed somewhat regularly by her outpatient physician, interpreter services were not provided because she was considered sufficiently proficient in English to communicate with staff to schedule appointments and provide basic information. Upon reviewing her medical records, the psychologist discovered that Ms. L's most recent outpatient physician appointments were primarily focused on diabetes management; however, all communication was in English, and Ms. L had been hesitant to request an interpreter, fearing that she would be perceived as inadequate and uneducated. This initial appointment with the psychologist was the first occasion on which Ms. L interacted with a bilingual and bicultural health care provider.

The psychologist also identified low self-esteem, situational stressors, and poor lifestyle habits as additional factors contributing to her obesity and assumed a collaborative and motivational therapeutic approach initially prioritizing rapport building. Validating Ms. L's desire to achieve healthy weight loss and empathizing with the challenges of being a single, low-income, monolingual Latina mother with scarce social supports residing in a rural, predominantly Caucasian environment facilitated establishment of her trust in the psychologist as a credible health care provider. Once trust was established, Ms. L was receptive to education about health, behavioral, and psychological factors that were contributing to her obesity, and behavioral interventions were then implemented to address these. The psychologist shared impressions with the bariatric surgery team and made culturally sensitive recommendations that included provision of interpreter services at each medical appointment and strategies to assess Ms. L's understanding of her diagnosis and treatment recommendations. The patient soon began to demonstrate openness

(*continued*)

> **Ms. L (*continued*)**
>
> to feedback from her health care providers, efforts to adequately understand and manage her diabetes and make healthy lifestyle changes, and confidence in her ability to successfully manage her weight and model a healthy lifestyle to her children.

Although Ms. L's case did not take place in an inpatient neurorehabilitation setting, it clearly illustrates some of the ways psychologists can integrate cultural brokerage into their role as health care providers. We can also see the multispheric influence of the psychologist's role benefiting the patient by fostering trust toward health care providers, understanding of health issues, and engagement in treatment. The psychologist was able to translate understanding of Ms. L's worldview to other health care providers, who were then able to view her initial noncompliance as a cultural issue rather than refusal to outwardly follow treatment recommendations. This case also exemplifies some of the challenges confronted when language barriers are not properly addressed with the use of qualified medical interpreters.

THE TRANSCULTURAL TRANSDISCIPLINARY REHABILITATION TEAM

Models of rehabilitation service delivery have gradually shifted from single discipline care to what has more recently become recognized as the transdisciplinary rehabilitation team (Karol, 2014). Compared to interdisciplinary and multidisciplinary teams, transdisciplinary teams not only recognize that there is overlap among professional roles, but they assume shared responsibility. This means that, for instance, if one of the treatment goals is to help a traumatic brain injury patient improve attention, then each discipline will address this goal through its interventions. Thus, the speech–language pathologist provides cognitive strategies, and the physical therapist later implements those strategies to help the patient become more spatially aware. Transdisciplinary teams do not draw lines in the sand to define professional territory but rather glide within the sphere of patient care, while respecting their professional limitations.

Following a transdisciplinary framework, we advocate for a shift from multiculturalism to transculturalism because the latter provides more space for a broad conceptualization of cultural issues on a spectrum that minimizes placing our patients into particular categories. We might think of transculturalism as a color wheel, where when one color gradually blends into another color, we can see different shades of each. Similarly, cultural factors may be viewed on a spectrum with overlap into each other. For instance, it would be very difficult to consider race and ethnicity distinct from language, religion, or SES. Therefore, we must first acknowledge that cultural issues affect the rehabilitation experience in one way or another. Second, transcultural transdisciplinary teams recognize that knowledge about the optimal ways to address these issues may lie beyond their professional competence and consult. As such, these teams expand the concept of rehabilitation team to include professionals who can educate them about how to address identified or presumed cultural issues. Because psychologists, social workers, and case managers most commonly

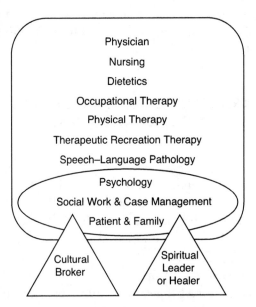

Figure 4.1 *The transcultural rehabilitation team. At their core, rehabilitation teams typically include the patient, the family, and all the disciplines involved in providing direct care. The psychologist, social worker, or case manager provides a connection to external sources for cultural consultation.*

address biopsychosocial issues, it would be most reasonable for these team members to assume the role of obtaining cultural consultation and translating that information to the whole team. Figure 4.1 illustrates how such a team might be structured.

Ms. M

Ms. M, a 54-year-old, Spanish-speaking Mexican woman, was referred after a left hip hemiarthoplasty for psychological evaluation after the inpatient rehabilitation team found that "depression" was becoming an impediment to her participation in therapy. She had a complex medical history significant for osteoporosis, anemia, recurrent urinary tract infections, multiple ankle fractures with surgical intervention, and poorly managed diabetes mellitus, with several secondary complications including nephropathy, neurogenic bladder, gastrointestinal prophylaxis, and orthostatic hypotension (likely due to autonomic neuropathy). Ms. M was native to a province of central Mexico, where she completed 6 years of education. She had relocated to the United States with her husband approximately 30 years ago and now resided with her husband and four adult children. She was a homemaker and described her religious beliefs as those similar to Evangelical Catholics. Ms. M's performance on a cognitive screener was normal, although the psychologist noted that she was a poor historian and could not elaborate much on her medical status. She endorsed sadness about being in the hospital and suggested that she had possibly experienced depression sometime in the past.

With the patient's permission, the Spanish-speaking and bicultural psychologist then attempted to obtain collateral information from her husband, who had arrived during the evaluation. The husband was vague in answering the psychologist's questions, but when the evaluation was interrupted by a nurse for medication administration, he discreetly called the psychologist to step outside the room. He quickly started talking about his wife's health problems, but then stopped abruptly and asked, "You're Catholic, right?" Realizing that

---

(continued)

Ms. M (*continued*)

religion was likely an important aspect in rapport building in this case, the psychologist smiled and stated that she was Christian so as to provide genuine reassurance without entering into a full disclosure. The man hesitantly went on to explain that his wife's real problem was "spiritual possession." He explained, "She throws her hands up shaking and falls on the floor. I just read the Word to her. I don't want her to know." He explained that her "depression" was related to "that disk in the brain that when it runs out of space, this is what happens. You know, like Alzheimer's." He verified that she had been admitted on more than one occasion for suicide attempts but was vague with respect to when these incidents took place and whether she had taken psychotropic medications. He believed that the pharmaceuticals currently provided were in fact making her worse and turned nurses away when they attempted to administer insulin injections. Her husband continued to explain how the family felt and believed that it was more important for his wife to consume a nutritional shake marketed by an herbal supplement company popular among many Hispanics/Latinos.

The psychologist, resisting impulses to correct or educate Ms. M's husband, spent extra time listening attentively to his concerns and beliefs. This interaction facilitated rapport building, which then allowed the psychologist to engage both Ms. M and her husband in several follow-up conversations to provide concrete information about the relationship of health, mood, and cognition. The psychologist was able to inform the rehabilitation team about altered mental status in the context of her medical conditions, made recommendations to rule out possible additional etiologies (e.g., seizures) for altered mental status, provided suggestions for sensitivity to beliefs about the causes of the patient's health problems and most adequate treatment, and facilitated dialogue among the patient, family, and rehabilitation team.

This account barely scratches the surface of the true complexity and length of Ms. M's case; however, the information provided allows us to review several key issues that we have discussed so far in this chapter.

Let us first consider language and communication. Although a bilingual Hispanic/Latina psychologist familiar with traditional Mexican culture and religion conducted this evaluation in the patient's native language, the patient and her husband only spoke Spanish and tended to channel communication with providers through their son. So not only were there literal language barriers that limited direct communication between the patient and the treatment team, but messages were filtered through the son (who had his own ideas about what was best for his mother) that reflected his different levels of acculturation, education, and religiosity.

Interpreter services were widely available at this hospital but were not consistently utilized with this family, a situation easily remedied by a simple recommendation from the psychologist. Second were issues of acculturation. Although Ms. M and her family had resided in the United States for three decades, their limited English proficiency suggested limited exposure or relationships with mainstream culture and may have reflected a distinct subgroup. In this case, the psychologist was not only imperative in explaining the patient's behavior, but she also translated cultural beliefs to the treatment team (e.g., possible seizures versus spiritual possession) and suggested culturally sensitive approaches to addressing family concerns.

CONCLUSIONS

Working in a neurorehabilitation setting allows each of us the privilege of providing psychological services to individuals during what could be the most challenging times of their lives. This chapter gives some examples of patients' experiences with the world of neurorehabilitation and how we can make them positive events rather than challenges. We have seen how some clinicians have integrated the transcultural transdisciplinary neurorehabilitation team model into their daily clinical work.

This chapter also highlights the cultural factors that can affect patient recovery and care, including ethnicity and race, spirituality, generational status, linguistic variables, culture of origin, and experience with medical systems. It presents issues that are likely to be encountered with transcultural and international neurorehabilitation patients with a variety of brain injuries and medical problems that can affect cognition and coping. As providers, we must be aware that it is not necessarily the patients' job to understand us but rather it is up to us to understand our patients so we can help them and ease their transition into this new chapter in their lives.

To be useful, we must increase our awareness of our own limitations, whether these are a lack of knowledge about the ethnicity or cultural background of our patients or our limited experience in using interpreters. It may entail recognizing our clinical limitations and knowing when to consult with both colleagues and individuals outside of our field who may be more familiar with the diversity issue we are facing. We must be willing to go outside our comfort zone and provide treatments in less conventional ways if that makes our patients more comfortable. We have to be able to put ourselves in the patient's position and advocate for the patient when necessary.

As neurorehabilitation psychologists, we are in a unique multispheric position that allows us to have credibility with the neurorehabilitation team as well as with our patients. This allows us to both increase cultural awareness of our teams and help our patients appreciate the novel world and culture of neurorehabiliation and how they can best navigate in it. By using interpreters, arranging consultations, and truly understanding how our patients' educational experiences and diverse backgrounds, spirituality, acculturation, and lifestyles can affect their responses to injuries, acute and chronic disabilities, and the neurorehabilitation experience, we can adjust treatment to the patients' needs.

As a final note, many of the issues we addressed speak to the clinician and frontline provider, but the issues and resources necessary to provide optimal services to our diverse patient population must be supported at all levels in a proactive manner. It requires not only awareness of our own cultural limitations but advocating for our patients' rights and increasing awareness at the institutional level about the need for qualified interpreters and cultural sensitivity trainings when the institutional culture lacks this emphasis. Having a department or resource center whose primary purpose is to provide translation services, cultural services (e.g., culture-related publications, information regarding community organizations), diversity training, and training for interpreter competency can significantly increase our ability to provide linguistically and culturally sensitive neurorehabilitation services and maximize positive patient outcomes. Proactive changes to meet the growing needs of our changing patient populations can help transform our health care system and improve our patients' lives faster.

REFERENCES

American Medical Association. (2013). *Office guide to communicating with limited English proficient patients* (2nd ed.). Retrieved from http://www.multicultural mentalhealth.ca/wp-content/uploads/2013/10/lep_booklet.pdf

American Psychological Association. (2002). *Guidelines on multicultural education, training, research, practice, and organizational change for psychologists.* Washington, DC: American Psychological Association.

Arango-Lasparilla, J. C., & Niemeier, J. (2007). Cultural issues in the rehabilitation of TBI survivors: Recent research and new frontiers. *Journal of Head Trauma Rehabilitation, 222*(2), 73–74.

Baker, D. W., Hayes, R., & Puebla-Fortier, J. (1998). Interpreter use and satisfaction with interpersonal aspects of care for Spanish-speaking patients. *Medical Care, 36*, 1461–1470.

Betancourt, H., & Lopez, S. R. (1993, June). The study of culture, ethnicity, and race in American psychology. *American Psychologist, 48*(6), 629–637.

Boulware, L. E., Cooper, L. A., Ratner, L. F., LaVeist, T. A., & Powe, N. R. (2003). Race and trust in the health care system. *Public Health Reports, 118*, 358–365.

Castillo, L. G., & Caver, K. A. (2009). Expanding the concept of acculturation in Mexican American rehabilitation psychology research and practice. *Rehabilitation Psychology, 54*(4), 351–362.

Chukwuneke, F. N., Ezeonu, C. T., Onyire, B. N., & Ezeonu, P. O. (2012). Culture and biomedical care in Africa: The influence of culture on biomedical care in a traditional African society, Nigeria, West Africa. *Nigerian Journal of Medicine, 21*(3), 331–333.

Cianelli, R., Ferrer, L., & McElmurry, B. (2008). HIV prevention and low-income Chilean women: Machismo, marianismo and HIV misconceptions. *Culture, Health & Sexuality, 10*(3), 297–306.

Coffey, L., Gallagher, P., & Desmond, D. (2014). Goal pursuit and goal adjustment as predictors of disability and quality of life among individuals with a lower limb amputation: A prospective study. *Archives of Physical Medicine and Rehabilitation, 95*, 244–252.

Comstock, D. L., Hammer, T. R., Strentzsch, J., Cannon, K., Parsons, J., & Salazar, II, G. (2008). Relational-cultural theory: A framework for bridging relational, multicultural, and social justice competencies. *Journal of Counseling and Development, 86*, 279–287.

Dezutter, J., Casalin, S., Wachholtz, A., Luyckx, K., Hekking, J., & Vandewiele, W. (2013). Meaning in life: An important factor for the psychological well-being of chronically ill patients? *Rehabilitation Psychology, 58*(4), 334–341.

Eamranond, P. P., Wee, C. C., Legedza, A. T. R., Marcantonio, E. R., & Leveille, S. G. (2009). Acculturation and cardiovascular risk factor control among Hispanic adults in the United States. *Public Health Reports, 124*, 818–824.

Flores, G. (2006). Language barriers to health care in the United States. *New England Journal of Medicine, 355*(3), 229–231.

Glover, N. M., & Blankenship, J. C. (2007). Mexican and Mexican American beliefs about God in relation to disability. *Journal of Rehabilitation, 73*(4), 41–50.

Gottlieb, M. C. (1994a). Ethical challenges when working with Hispanic/Latino families: Familismo. *The Family Psychologist,* 19–20.

Gottlieb, M. C. (1994b). Ethical challenges when working with Hispanic/Latino families: Personalismo. *The Family Psychologist,* 32–34.

Hanson, S. L., & Kerkhoff, T. R. (2007). Ethical decision making in rehabilitation: Consideration of Latino cultural factors. *Rehabilitation Psychology, 52*(4), 409–420.

Hays, P. A. (2008). *Addressing cultural complexities in practice* (2nd ed.). Washington, DC: American Psychological Association.

Helsel, D. G., & Mochel, M. (2002). Afterbirths in the afterlife: Cultural meaning of placental disposal in a Hmong American community. *Journal of Transcultural Nursing, 13*(4), 282–286.

Hunt, D. B. (2007). Language assistance for limited English proficient patients: Legal issues. In P. Walker & E. Barnett (Eds.), *Immigrant Medicine* (pp. 37–56). Philadelphia, PA: Elsevier.

Jacobs, E. A., Lauderdale, D. S., Meitzer, D., Shorey, J. M., Levinso, W., & Thisted, R. A. (2001). Impact of interpreter services on delivery of health care to limited-English-proficient patients. *Journal of General Internal Medicine, 16,* 468–474.

Johnson, S. K. (2002). Hmong health beliefs and experiences in the Western health care system. *Journal of Transcultural Nursing, 13*(2), 126–132.

Karol, R. (2014). Team models in neurorehabilitation: Structure, function and culture change. *Neurorehabilitation, 34,* 655–669.

Lutsey, P. L., Diez-Roux, A. V., Jacobs, D. R., Burke, G. L., Harman, J., Shea, S., & Folsom, A. (2008). Associations of acculturation and socioeconomic status with subclinical cardiovascular disease in the multi-ethnic study of atherosclerosis. *American Journal of Public Health, 98*(11), 1963–1970.

Mainous, A. G., Díaz, V. A., & Geesey, M. E. (2008). Acculturation and health lifestyles among Latinos with diabetes. *Annals of Family Medicine, 6*(2), 131–137.

Mainous, A. G., Majeed, A., Koopman, R. J., Baker, R., Everett, C. J., Tilley, B. C., & Díaz, V. A. (2006). Acculturation and diabetes among Hispanics: Evidence from the 1999–2002 national health and nutrition examination survey. *Public Health Reports, 121,* 60–66.

Masel, M. C., Rudkin, L. L., & Peek, K. M. (2006). Examining the role of acculturation in health behaviors of older Mexican Americans. *American Journal of Health Behavior, 30*(6), 684–699.

National Center for Cultural Competence. (2004). Bridging the cultural divide in health care settings: The essential role of cultural broker programs. Retrieved from http://nccc.georgetown.edu/documents/Cultural_Broker_Guide_English.pdf

Oaksford, K., Frude, N., & Cuddihy, R. (2005). Positive coping and stress-related psychological growth following lower limb amputation. *Rehabilitation Psychology, 50*(3), 266–277.

Pattison, S. (2013). Religion, spirituality and health care: Confusions, tensions, opportunities. *Health Care Analysis, 21*, 193–207.

Pontón, M. O., & Ardila, A. (1999). The future of neuropsychology with Hispanic populations in the United States. *Archives of Clinical Neuropsychology, 14*(7), 565–580.

Rohner, R. P. (1984). Toward a conception of culture for cross-cultural psychology. *Journal of Cross-Cultural Psychology, 15*, 111–138.

Ross, E. D. (2000). Affective prosody and the aprosodias. In M. Mesulam (Ed.), *Principles of behavioral and cognitive neurology* (2nd ed.) (pp. 316–331). New York, NY: Oxford University Press.

Scheermesser, M., Bachmann, S., Schäman, A., Oesch, P., & Kool, J. (2012). A qualitative study on the role of cultural background in patients' perspectives on rehabilitation. *BMC Musculoskeletal Disorders, 13*(5), 1–13.

Sirven, J. I., Lopez, R. A., Vazquez, B., & Haverbeke, P. A. (2005). Qué es la epilepsia? Attitudes and knowledge of epilepsy by Spanish-speaking adults in the United States. *Epilepsy & Behavior, 7*, 259–265.

Sue, D. W., & Sue, D. (2008). *Counseling the culturally diverse—Theory and practice* (5th ed.). Hoboken, NJ: John Wiley & Sons.

Suinn, R. M. (2010). Reviewing acculturation and Asian Americans: How acculturation affects health, adjustment, school achievement, and counseling. *Asian American Journal of Psychology, 1*(1), 5–17.

U.S. Census Bureau. (2010). *Language use in the United States: 2007*. Retrieved from http://www.census.gov/hhes/socdemo/language/data/acs/ACS-12.pdf

U.S. Department of Justice. Retrieved from http://www.justice.gov/crt/about/cor/coord/titlevi.php; http://www.justice.gov/crt/about/cor/13166.php

Zhao, M., Esposito, N., & Wang, K. (2010). Cultural beliefs and attitudes toward health and health care among Asian-born women in the United States. *Journal of Obstetric, Gynecological, & Neonatal Nursing, 39*(4), 370–385.

CHAPTER FIVE

LAYERS OF CULTURE: ITS INFLUENCE IN A MILIEU-ORIENTED HOLISTIC NEUROREHABILITATION SETTING

Kavitha R. Perumparaichallai and Pamela S. Klonoff

I don't much like him. I think I need to get to know him better.
—Abraham Lincoln

Conflict arises not from culture difference itself, but from the ignorance of the difference.
—Yoshitaka Miike

Cultural beliefs have a tremendous influence on a person's perception of disability (Uomoto & Wong, 2000). Individuals from majority cultures in the United States value equality and individualized ability as sources of social identity, which shape their concept of disability. According to the Center for International Rehabilitation Research Information and Exchange's monograph on cultural competency, the rehabilitation system in the United States has been established to enable individuals with disabilities to become self-sufficient through employment. Rehabilitation methodologies are based on the individualistic approach, which encourages the rehabilitation programs to focus on improving self-determination, increasing productivity, and enhancing one's individualism and independence. Self-sufficiency is considered an ideal outcome of these rehabilitation programs (Jezewski & Sotnik, 2001). Conversely, people from minority cultures who mostly follow the collectivistic approach have an entirely different view about rehabilitation (Ingstad & Whyte, 1995). They mostly focus on functioning synchronously within a group (e.g., family) rather than developing individualistic tendencies (Jezewski & Sotnik, 2001). The increased flow of immigrants into the United States and the upsurge in the incidence of brain injuries in minority populations have amplified the demand for culturally competent neurorehabilitation programs.

According to Nora Groce (1999), a medical anthropologist, "Unless programs for individuals with disabilities are designed in a culturally appropriate way, the opportunity to make real and effective change is often lost" (p. 38). Providing culturally competent health services has the potential to improve health outcomes, increase the efficiency of clinical and support staff, and result in greater clinical satisfaction with services (Beach et al., 2005; Brach & Fraser, 2000). Furthermore, the need for culturally competent rehabilitation programs has been well established to improve the brain injury outcomes of individuals from minority cultures (Arango-Lasprilla & Kreutzer, 2010). Viewing culture as a discrete system that encompasses interconnected components should enhance the cultural competence in rehabilitation centers. Some of the important elements of culture that are relevant in rehabilitation planning include food and religious practices; child-rearing practices; verbal and nonverbal aspects of language; problem-solving strategies and coping styles; and family and social relationships (Jezewski & Sotnik, 2001).

The overlap of different layers of culture in a milieu-oriented holistic neurorehabilitation program, including the culture of origin (e.g., the

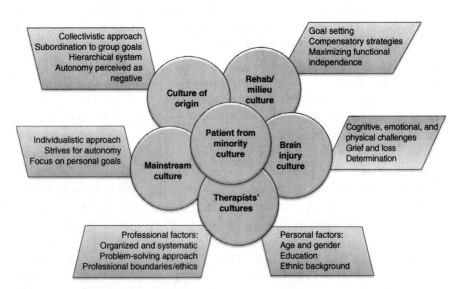

Figure 5.1 *The overlap of different layers of culture in a milieu-oriented holistic neurorehabilitation program.*

Hispanic culture), neurorehabilitation/milieu culture, brain injury culture, therapists' cultures, and mainstream culture (i.e., majority culture) are depicted in Figure 5.1.

CULTURE OF HEALTH CARE PROVIDERS AND REHABILITATION THERAPISTS

With the increased emphasis on cultural sensitivity, health care training programs have been focusing on enhancing the cultural sensitivity and competency of health care providers (Beach et al., 2005). In reality, there is a vast cultural gap between patients and general health care providers regarding understanding health and illness behaviors, styles of functioning, their individual approaches to problem solving, and expectations about the recovery process (Hendson, Reis, & Nicholas, 2015).

In addition to their majority culture, health care providers are molded by the culture of their profession (e.g., beliefs, practices/habits, norms, rituals; Klonoff, 2013). Consequently, therapists personify unique styles of communication, which are often characterized by using medical terminologies or jargons, charting practices (e.g., taking notes in sessions), and applying professional behaviors such as being prompt and organized, setting boundaries, and practicing or advising preventive measures. They also follow various systematic problem-solving methodologies in a given situation (Chang, 2007). These health care provider aspects also very much apply to the therapists in neurorehabilitation settings.

HOW DOES MILIEU-ORIENTED HOLISTIC NEUROREHABILITATION CREATE A LAYER OF CULTURE?

The milieu-oriented neurorehabilitation program creates a unique culture that is different from other cultural influences encountered by an individual. As Nora Groce (2005) perceptively noted, "The rehabilitation system is not 'culture-free.' It is vitally important to keep in mind that when dealing with the interface between immigrant populations and the rehabilitation system, we are dealing with not one but two culturally defined and culturally bounded systems" (p. 3). This very aptly fits the description of milieu-oriented holistic neurorehabilitation offered at the Center for Transitional NeuroRehabilitation (CTN). The therapeutic environment of the program creates an opportunity for people from different socio-cultural backgrounds to form relationships based on empathy, mutual respect, and genuine concern (Klonoff, 2010; Klonoff, Lamb, Henderson, Reichert, & Tully, 2000). The flavor of the milieu setting is drawn from the patients' cultural diversity; the therapists' cultural, educational, and training experiences; and the CTN program principles and philosophy.

The CTN Program Philosophy and Goals

The CTN program is built on the conceptual framework derived from the work of Luria's theory of restoration of higher cognitive functions (Luria, 1963, 1974) and Ben-Yishay's holistic approach to neurorehabil-itation (Ben-Yishay & Diller, 1993). It is beyond the scope of this chapter to review these (for reviews, see Ben-Yishay & Diller, 1993; Ben-Yishay & Prigatano, 1990). The following information is abstracted from a variety of publications relevant to the cultural components of holistic milieu-oriented therapy at the CTN (Klonoff, 2010, 2014; Klonoff, Koberstein, Talley, & Dawson, 2008; Klonoff et al., 2000). First and foremost, the program emphasizes developing a positive working alliance with patients and families (Prigatano et al., 1986) and helping patients improve their levels of awareness, acceptance, and realism about the effects of their brain injuries (Klonoff, 1997, 2010). Other embedded culture-specific CTN goals are to assist patients in improving their emotional reactions to their brain injuries, coping with their losses, and supporting them in their community reintegration. All individual and group therapies focus on skill building through the use of compensatory strategies, cognitive retraining, and other discipline-specific interventions to remediate deficit areas.

The philosophy of the CTN program expects patients to strive toward enhancing their roles and responsibilities in the clinic, as well as in the community (home, school, and/or work). Three programs that help them achieve these goals are home independence, work reentry, and school reentry (Klonoff, 2010). All of these facets are under the umbrella of the cultural diversity and sensitivity of the patients, families, therapists, and the milieu entity itself.

The "Milieu" Environment

The cultural basis of the CTN emanates from the French term *milieu*, which means "community." Interestingly, diversity is in preponderance, yet the holistic culture operates in synchrony. For example, the CTN milieu consists of patients with different types of brain injuries (e.g., traumatic brain injury, cerebrovascular accidents, tumor, anoxia, and neuro-infectious disorders), caregivers, therapists, administrative staff, and others (e.g., taxi drivers, employers). The interdisciplinary team is composed of neuropsychologists, occupational therapists, physical therapists, speech–language pathologists, and recreational therapists, as well as a neurorehabilitation technician, dietician, rehabilitation physician, and psychiatrist. The therapists vary in terms of age, work experience, culture, and ethnic backgrounds. Nonetheless, the team strongly emphasizes cohesiveness, collaboration, and continuity of care.

Vital cultural aspects of the CTN milieu environment are nurturance and empathy, but incorporating structure, accountability, and hope (Klonoff, 2010). Patients have multiple opportunities to relate to and support one another (e.g., group therapies, between-session and lunch breaks, and regular milieu sessions). Circumstances that foster empathy are inherent in a variety of activities in the milieu setting (Klonoff, 2010). Milieu sessions set the tone of community feeling (e.g., concern and commitment). They are usually 15 minutes in length and occur four times a week. All patients, therapists, and family members, if possible, attend these milieu sessions. Patients are given the rotating opportunity to lead the milieu sessions, and they are responsible for calling on those individuals who wish to contribute. The purpose of the meeting is to discuss the business, progress, and the concerns of milieu members in a community fashion. Furthermore, the milieu sessions are used to monitor the patients' progress—for example, the use of compensatory strategies (including completing weekly checklists and datebook use) and updates about work or school (Klonoff, 2010).

Milieu meetings also have certain traditions, including the "circle of positives"; expressing acknowledgments for fellow milieu members; the "song of the week"; and "cake days." To inculcate an optimistic attitude, patients participate in a weekly "circle of positives," in which they proudly share accomplishments related to their therapies and/or recovery process. Milieu members (patients, caregivers, and therapists) take turns sharing an inspiring song that symbolizes their neurorehabilitation journey. It is noteworthy to mention that patients/caregivers and therapists from minority cultural backgrounds are encouraged to present culturally diverse music and songs, which facilitates the milieu members' sensitivity and acceptance of cultural differences. Other aspects that nurture the relationship among the milieu members include celebrating birthdays and graduations in the milieu sessions. Mutual care and consideration are exemplified by patients receiving get well cards from the entire milieu when they are ill. "Cake day" is a ceremony that represents the graduation of a patient from his or her neurorehabilitation program. As a token of recognition, patients are presented with a cake, fruit, vegetables, or a book, according to their personal interests and appeal, in addition to verbal accolades from therapists and other patients (Klonoff, 2010).

The Working Alliance

Another cultural emphasis of the CTN milieu is the saliency of developing a positive working alliance with patients and families. Patients and therapists agree to work together in an integrated and cohesive manner to maximize patients' community independence and productivity. The working relationship is built upon mutual respect, collaboration, and trust (Bordin, 1979; Klonoff, 2010). The working alliance for patients consists of "the bonds," or the relationship between the patient and therapist founded on rapport, trust, and respect; the "tasks," which are the substance of the counseling process, including specific therapeutic activities (e.g., home independence checklist [HIC], datebook training); and the "goals," which are the outcomes and targets of the therapy (e.g., achieving independence in the home, returning to work or school). The patients and families are assisted in understanding this working model to maximize outcome (Bordin, 1979; Klonoff, 2010). However, to achieve this, therapists require cultural competency to work with patients from different backgrounds (Liu & Pope-Davis, 2005).

The nature of the working relationship in the CTN milieu is a "two-way" street, which empowers the patients to play an active role in building the relationship with their therapists. The quality of the working alliance among the therapists, patients, and families is reviewed on a monthly basis as part of program documentation. Therapists rate their perceptions of the working alliance with patients and families independently, and patients and families independently rate their impressions of their relationships with the therapists. It is noteworthy to mention that outcome research in the milieu-oriented holistic neurorehabilitation center strongly supports the influence of a positive working alliance between patients (and families) and therapists on better neurorehabilitation outcomes. Higher working alliance ratings of the therapists, patients, and their families were associated with better school and work status (Klonoff, Lamb, & Henderson, 2001; Klonoff, Lamb, Henderson, & Shepherd, 1998; Klonoff et al., 2007). Given the important role of the working alliance, one of the objectives of psychotherapy is to develop and maintain the best working alliance possible among patients, families, and therapists. This requires knowledge and sensitivity about the patients' families/cultural backgrounds and belief systems. By extension, apart from educating the team regarding the neurological and psychological aspects of brain injury, neuropsychologists also help the team to understand the cultural aspects of the patients/family systems and modify treatment approaches accordingly.

In the milieu environment, the therapists' enhanced knowledge about the neurological recovery process, compensatory strategies, and expectations are mostly different from that of the patients and their families, in part due to cultural disparities (Klonoff, 2013). Extensive hours of treatment are focused on bridging this gap through exploration of cultural components relevant to psychoeducation for patients and families; the choice of culturally sensitive compensatory strategies for patients and family members, also through relevant group therapies (e.g., cognitive group, community outings, relatives' group); and family meetings to discuss treatment recommendations as well as goals (for more information on group therapy techniques, see Klonoff, 2010, 2014).

The cultural dialogue and competency within the CTN milieu program allows interactions among therapists from different disciplines through conjoint therapy sessions, staff meetings, and retreats. Therapists (e.g., occupational therapists, physical therapists, speech–language pathologists, and recreational therapists) in the CTN milieu are aware of relevant discipline-specific cultural influences. For example, speech–language pathologists are knowledgeable about the impact of bilingualism on aphasia, which guides them to modify their evaluations and therapy tasks. Occupational therapists visit patients' homes to help design patients' home independence programs so as to increase their functional independence. Through home visits, the occupational and physical therapists' sensitivity and awareness about patients' cultural needs enables them to interactively devise home exercise programs that are applicable to patients from minority cultures, including their unique family structure and routines.

Role of the Neuropsychologist

Neuropsychologists in the CTN milieu program play an important role in fostering a culturally sensitive and competent interdisciplinary team and in translating cultural considerations into concrete treatment approaches and goals. Neuropsychologists work closely with patients and their support network to grasp the impact of the brain injury on patients and their families, their coping styles, and their family values. This working knowledge allows the neuropsychologist to adopt the role of a "cultural broker" to educate therapists from other disciplines about cultural variations and their impact on the working alliance, follow-through, and community outcomes. According to Jezewski (1990), culture-brokering is "the act of bridging, linking, or mediating between groups or persons of differing cultural backgrounds for the purpose of reducing conflict or producing change" (p. 497). Cultural broker is a relatively new concept for neurorehabilitation therapists and is borrowed from anthropology (http://culturalbroker.info/2_role/index.html). Cultural brokers' responsibilities and abilities include, but are not limited to, assessing and understanding their own cultural identities and value systems (self-awareness); recognizing the values that guide and mold patients'/families' attitudes and behaviors; understanding a community's traditional health beliefs, values, and practices, as well as changes that occur through the patients'/families' acculturation; understanding and practicing the tenets of effective cross-cultural communication, incorporating the cultural nuances of both verbal and nonverbal communication; and advocating for the patient to ensure the delivery of effective health services (http://culturalbroker.info/2_role/index.html).

In addition to the traditional role of a cultural broker, neuropsychologists also help the team recognize the influences of cultural beliefs on an individual's coping following a brain injury (e.g., family role changes associated with a brain injury). Changes in family roles secondary to the aftermath of a brain injury are a commonly reported phenomenon.

Consequently, patients lose their major roles in their families (e.g., breadwinner) and gain minor roles such as home maintainer and religious participant (Hallett, Zasler, Maurer, & Cash, 1994). Based on the brain injury alone, patients struggle to embrace these changes. Cultural beliefs often complicate this process for patients from a minority culture operating in the majority culture. When designing neurorehabilitation programs targeting skills related to home independence, awareness about the cultural issues and changes in family roles is critical for creating culturally sensitive interventions. A list of the principles that can enhance the cultural competency of the neurorehabilitation programs is provided in Exhibit 5.1.

Exhibit 5.1 *Principles That Enhance Cultural Competency*

At the administration level, programs should
- Employ qualified mental health workers from different ethnic backgrounds
- Survey clients and workers to elicit their comprehension of cultural competence and culturally competent practice
- Understand the cultural biases of staff and provide training to address educational needs
- Recognize cultural biases in program designs
- Evaluate procedures and programs for cultural sensitivity and effectiveness
- Identify resources within the community, which will help individuals from minority cultures
- Obtain feedback from patients and families about the cultural sensitivity of the program

Therapists should
- Examine their own attitudes and belief systems because these may affect their decisions and practices
- Be aware of their own culture and personal biases before attempting to understand cross-cultural issues
- Learn to view unfamiliar situations without assumptions, judgments, or expectations
- Modify intake and assessment documentation, as well as policies and procedures, to be more inclusive of the needs of individuals from minority cultures
- Design and implement culturally sensitive treatment plans

http://culturalbroker.info/2_role/2_role.html; http://www.dhs.state.or.us/caf/safety _model/procedure_manual/ch01/chapter1-section5.pdf

COLLECTIVISM AND THE HISPANIC CULTURE

The construct of collectivism facilitates the understanding of cultural variations in behavior, values, attitudes, cognitions, and family structures, and organizes them into general cultural themes. Core characteristics of the collectivistic approach include, but are not limited to, people are loyal to the groups they belong to; "we" consciousness, in which individuals endeavor to maintain the harmony of the units they belong to (e.g., family); transgression from group norms leads to shameful feelings; education focuses on learning how to do activities (e.g., hands-on training); and conflicts are usually solved within the minority group (e.g., family or extended families; Hofstede, 2012).

Rehabilitation therapists strive to be aware of all the facets of these different cultural subgroups. In addition to the variability related to their geographical location, patients' cultural values are influenced by the degree of acculturation, age, gender, socioeconomic status, and education (Klonoff, 2014). Patients from both majority and minority cultures attend the CTN milieu program, which adds another stratum to the already existing diverse layers of cultures in the program. Among them, patients of Hispanic background are the most commonly represented minority group. The Hispanic culture encompasses people from different racial backgrounds (including Black and White) from regions spanning thousands of miles. The Centers for Disease Control and Prevention (CDC) define Hispanic in the United States as "any person of Cuban, Mexican, Puerto Rican, South or Central American, or other Spanish culture of origin, regardless of race" (www.cdc.gov/nccdphp/dch/programs/healthycom munitiesprogram/tools/pdf/hispanic_latinos_insight.pdf).

The Hispanic culture, like most other minority cultural groups, incorporates the attributes of collectivism. Other characteristics more specific to the Hispanic culture are that responsibilities are shared among the members of a family. Accountability is collective, and group-oriented activities dominate the society (Gudykunst, 1998). Consequently, harmony and cooperation among the group tend to be emphasized more than individual functions and responsibilities (Gudykunst, 1998).

With regard to the Hispanic family structure, the patriarchal system grants the father or oldest male relative the greatest power, whereas women are expected to show submission (Kemp & Rasbridge, 2004). Men are assumed to adopt the traditional gender role of *machismo*, denoting that the male is the breadwinner of the family and has more power and control over family affairs (Galanti, 2003). Diminished independence at home and in the community secondary to a brain injury often exacerbates the narcissistic insult to a Hispanic male's pride, shattering his sense of self. Nonetheless, family bonds are very durable. A family member who has a disability is seen as someone who needs to be "taken care of," so the family can become overprotective. They may begin to make decisions on behalf of the disabled individual. Independence is considered unrealistic to the family and also to the patient (U.S. Department of Health and Human Services, 2001).

The Hispanic collectivistic culture also has an entirely different view about rehabilitation. The focus is on functioning synchronously within a group (e.g., family) rather than developing individualistic tendencies. Furthermore, Hispanic individuals are less likely to use professional psychiatric or psychological services to treat mental health conditions, such as depression. They mostly rely on natural healers (e.g., curanderos/curanderas) and family support systems, which reduces the reliance on formal health and mental health care providers (Vega, Kolody, Aguilar-Gaxiola, & Catalano, 1999).

Case Study

This case study demonstrates the common challenges and possible solutions when treating an individual from a minority culture (i.e., Hispanic) in a holistic milieu program. It answers two questions: First, what are the common obstacles to successful follow-through, and how can therapists use this knowledge to more effectively support individuals with brain injuries and their families? Second, what cultural and other strengths might individuals with brain injuries and their families have that enhance community reintegration?

Background Information

CR was a 38-year-old Hispanic male who sustained a severe traumatic brain injury (TBI) secondary to a motor vehicle accident. At the time of his accident, CR was working as a supervisor for a landscape company. He started his job as a landscape gardener and was soon promoted to a supervisor position because of his hard work. Social history indicated that after completing high school, he emigrated from Mexico to the United

States, where he learned to speak fluent English. He had been married for 8 years and had two young children. His wife was employed as a sales associate in a retail store. It is noteworthy that his wife was also of the Hispanic cultural background, but she was born and raised in the United States. Her cultural values were somewhat different from her husband's beliefs, secondary to differences in their acculturation stages.

Following his acute inpatient neurorehabilitation, CR started the CTN work reentry program. CR obtained financial support from the Vocational Rehabilitation (VR) services, which was sponsored by the Department of Economic Security of Arizona, to participate in the CTN milieu program. CR's TBI impacted his cognitive functioning in the domains of language (expressive and receptive), attention, speed of information processing, visuospatial skills, learning and memory, and aspects of executive functioning. Mood assessment revealed a moderate level of depression. Subsequent to his TBI, he was not able to drive or work. His wife became the primary breadwinner for their family. The primary goal of his rehabilitation was to develop the necessary skills to return to competitive employment.

The principles and philosophy of the CTN milieu program complemented the values of VR services, and particular care was taken to address CR's unique cultural factors. For example, when planning CR's neurorehabilitation program, the therapy activities were modified to fit his values and beliefs. His family's assistance was obtained when planning his therapy sessions, home visits, situational assessments, and work site visits. Some sessions exclusively focused on educating him and his family about the importance of improving their awareness about CR's strengths and challenges related to his TBI and its impact on his functioning. Culturally relevant educational material was meticulously prepared so CR and his family could relate his therapy activities to his return-to-work goals. This included Spanish material, which then enabled the non-English-speaking extended family to participate in the psychoeducation process. The team decided to enlist male therapists (some of whom were bilingual) to treat CR, because this increased his comfort level, especially at work. In addition, the team helped CR and his family relate to the differences between Mexico and their current living situation in the United States. This required discussion about acculturation factors in the majority culture pertinent to community reintegration (e.g., driving and work).

What are the common obstacles to successful follow-through? How did therapists use this knowledge to more effectively support CR and his family?

Some of the challenges observed during CR's program participation included organic unawareness and limited acceptance about the difficulties posed by his injury; expecting the men and women in his life to have traditional roles in the neurorehabilitation setting; difficulties with speaking two languages and the terminology related to TBI; reduced comfort with English-speaking therapists; a tendency to be dependent on his support network; disparities in the acculturation status between him and his wife; challenges in accepting role changes in his family; and difficulty relating therapy tasks to "real-life" activities.

CR had limited awareness regarding the impact of his injury on his ability to function well at home. He was also miffed about his nondriving status and having to depend on his wife or other family members for his transportation needs. Initially, he also had difficulty grasping the relevance of his neurorehabilitation within the context of his return to work goals. Being dependent on his wife was not consistent with his *machismo* values, which caused annoyance as well as friction between CR and his wife. A neuropsychologist worked with CR and his wife in psychotherapy to reduce the conflict in their relationship. Due to his wife's familiarity with the dominant cultural values of individualism and independence, she encouraged CR to follow the CTN therapists' recommendations. The neuropsychologist emphasized the importance of CR and his wife working in harmony not only to achieve his neurorehabilitation goals but also to fulfill their culturally relevant family needs. The neuropsychologist reminded CR to prioritize his family's needs, honor his role as a father and husband, and regain his status as a breadwinner. This helped CR to see how his wife's support was important in the process of returning to his prior roles. Given his memory challenges, CR took notes in his psychotherapy sessions and reviewed them whenever he had difficulty coping with the changes in his family status.

Another challenge that impacted CR's participation in his program was his language difficulties, which were related to the location of his brain injury as well as his bilingual status. To accommodate his bilingual status, his speech and language evaluation was conducted in both English and Spanish. His language abilities related to Spanish recovered faster than English. Consequently, he preferred to converse in Spanish rather than

English. This was taken into account when developing his compensatory strategies. When feasible, he was encouraged to take notes in Spanish, and then his bilingual therapists would check the accuracy of his notes. As his note-taking skills developed, his functional independence and confidence improved. Consequently, he was willing to use his compensatory strategies, including a datebook and note taking, at his situational assessment.

In the milieu environment, CR initially appeared shy, and his interactions with other milieu members were very limited. Typically, experienced patients in the milieu monitor other patients' comfort levels and help new patients and others who have social skill challenges ease into the milieu. In addition, involvement in daily milieu meetings, lunch breaks, and group therapy sessions help patients appreciate one another's life experiences. As CR became more involved in the milieu and group sessions, he slowly came out of his shell. At first, he gravitated toward other Hispanic patients and therapists. However, gradually, CR forged new bonds with other patients of different ages, education levels, and sociocultural backgrounds. He was able to relate to other patients' experiences after their brain injuries. He stated in his individual psychotherapy session that he could empathize with other patients based on the commonalities (e.g., losses and challenges) associated with their brain injuries. As his emotional well-being improved, he volunteered to lead the milieu meetings more often, which helped him practice his expressive language skills. He also shared the "song of the week" in one of the Thursday milieu meetings. He chose a Spanish song, and everyone in the milieu relished the selection. It became evident that the culture developed by patients with brain injuries had penetrated the layers of his personal sociocultural background.

CR had difficulty with abstract thinking, secondary to his brain injury, as well as his preinjury learning style, which was mostly hands-on learning. This impacted his ability to translate the traditional speech and occupational therapies that utilized paper-and-pencil tasks. His therapists modified his clinic-based therapies to mimic his work tasks. For example, in occupational therapy, to work on his attention and working memory, exercises involving landscaping/gardening tasks were generated. To improve his upper extremity strength, tasks that imitated landscaping skills (e.g., filling and carrying hod boxes; shoveling gravel) were utilized. These practical activities made it easier for CR and his family to understand the purpose of his therapies, particularly within the context of his return-to-work goals. As CR's therapy tasks were modified, his acceptance of the therapies clearly increased.

CR's challenge with following through with treatment recommendation stemmed from his cultural beliefs regarding treatment for depression. Initially, as part of the *machismo* image, he denied experiencing depression and was not able to link his frustrations, irritability, and other mood-related symptoms to depression. He was also reticent to meet with the program psychiatrist. Based on the fortified working alliance with his male neuropsychologist, and at his wife's urging, he agreed to meet with the CTN program psychiatrist in the presence of his neuropsychologist and wife. Several follow-up psychotherapy sessions and subsequent meetings with the psychiatrist were dedicated to helping CR and his wife learn about the symptoms of depression, the strong prevalence of depression in patients with TBIs, and the role of medications in treating mood problems. His brother also attended some of these educational sessions. In addition to these sessions, CR also learned about emotional challenges following brain injury from his peer patients in the group psychotherapy sessions.

It is noteworthy that during this process, CR's wife was more open to psychoeducation, most likely related to her advanced stage of acculturation. His wife and other family members had the opportunity to gather similar information in the relatives' group meetings, which is a support group for caregivers. All of this psychoeducation helped to normalize CR's emotions and reduce his shameful feelings. As CR and his family obtained concordant messages from different sources in the milieu, they became more willing to try medications and other behavioral strategies to manage CR's depression. Overall, his wife was a "bridge" between multiple layers of culture both inside and outside his neurorehabilitation.

What cultural and other strengths might an individual with an acquired brain injury and his family have that can enhance community reintegration?
After his injury, CR's status in his family changed, secondary to his cognitive challenges related to the injury. He was no longer "the head of the family." He required his wife's assistance with making higher level decisions (e.g., managing finances), which impacted his self-esteem and self-confidence. In addition, he also expressed his guilt related to not being

able to provide financial support for his family. More important, during his program participation, CR displayed admirable qualities emanating from his cultural beliefs. He became more cooperative and respectful toward his therapists; he did not display argumentative behavior; he exhibited a very strong work ethic; and he had excellent family support and participation in his neurorehabilitation process, including extended family involvement. His observed strengths were incorporated in his therapeutic interventions to enhance the program's cultural competency, which intensified CR's "buy-in" to treatment and community transitions.

As a case in point, usually the HIC consists of traditionally female household chores (e.g., loading and emptying the dishwasher, cooking twice a week, cleaning the bathroom, doing laundry for the entire family; for more details, see Klonoff, 2010, 2014). In this situation, including standard household activities on CR's HIC would cause more damage to his self-esteem and further erode his sense of self. His therapists encouraged him to generate a list of HIC activities that he was interested in. It was evident that CR was motivated to do activities that mimicked his traditional husband/father role and his work tasks (e.g., taking care of the family's garden, landscaping their front yard). To ensure the tasks he chose were feasible to do at home, his occupational therapist collaborated with CR and his wife to generate a modified HIC. The interdisciplinary therapists built his compensatory strategies around these activities (e.g., developing checklists and using his datebook to plan and organize his tasks). CR gradually developed his ability to use his checklists and datebook to accomplish his modified HIC tasks (e.g., shopping for materials, estimating the cost, dividing his work tasks, and scheduling them in his datebook). Other meaningful stepping-stones included participating in bill paying and playing soccer with his son. All of this information was used when planning the next stages of his therapy.

Another strength that was incorporated in CR's treatment planning was his family support to help him follow through with his treatment recommendations. Given CR's severe injury, he experienced challenges in higher level balance and endurance. His physical therapist recommended that CR attend workouts at a nearby gym. To reduce his embarrassment related to his nondriving status, CR's brother agreed to accompany him to the gym on a regular basis. Going to the gym with his brother felt more normal to him because he often did that before his injury. His occupational therapist prioritized his return to driving as a treatment goal by focusing on driving simulator exercises, as well as assisting him in securing an adaptive driving assessment, and meeting state requirements to resume driving.

CR's brother's help was also utilized in the return to work. He offered CR a volunteer position at his family business (i.e., maintaining gardens for large commercial businesses). This was considered a "situational assessment" (i.e., an unpaid position as a stepping-stone to competitive employment) to evaluate his work skills in the "real world." This position provided CR with the opportunity to practice his gardening and landscaping skills. Although CR had retained his basic job skills, his memory challenges impacted his ability to perform optimally at his situational assessment. He failed to take detailed notes, which negatively impacted his ability to complete his job duties. CR relied on his coworkers for the information he needed to complete his job tasks, such as his customers' addresses and specific jobs to be done for each of the garden projects. His coworkers, mostly from the same cultural background, helped him complete his job duties. They also helped him increase his awareness about his challenges with using his compensations (e.g., shared their note-taking approaches, which encouraged CR to take his own notes). Gradually, CR realized the power of using his compensations, which increased his functional independence as well as his confidence.

As CR showed progress in his ability to complete his job duties, his therapy sessions turned to helping him acquire a paid position. Given CR's exemplary work ethic and solid past work history, he was able to obtain a paid position as a landscaper with assistance from his occupational therapist. His male physical and occupational therapists attended his work site to help him develop written strategies in the form of Spanish notations to increase his competency and efficiency. The physical therapist assisted CR in regaining the necessary balance skills to be on a short stepladder, which then normalized CR's job functions. His brother remained a strong ally, and he continued to be involved in encouraging CR to use his compensations at work. As CR started earning money and regaining his productive status, his depression waned and his follow-through with the treatment recommendations blossomed. The therapists followed his progress for 3 months. At that time, he was discharged from the CTN milieu program, and VR considered his case as a successful closure. On his cake day, in the milieu meeting, a cake was presented to CR to honor his accomplishments. CR and his family proudly participated in the celebration, and they expressed their deep gratitude by sharing burritos and conchas with the milieu members.

CONCLUSIONS

Multiple layers of culture influence the experience, adjustment, and outcomes of individuals from minority cultures seeking neurorehabilitation. The manifold layers of culture include the: culture of origin, mainstream culture, brain injury culture, therapists' culture, and the culture of the neurorehabilitation program. It is important to enhance the awareness of neurorehabilitation professionals regarding the interaction and impact of these multiple layers when treating individuals from minority cultures. Developing culturally competent treatment programs for individuals from minority cultures is vital for successful outcomes. Neuropsychologists and psychologists, in general, play a role as a cultural broker in bridging the gap between the different layers of culture and promoting culturally sensitive intervention programs.

REFERENCES

Arango-Lasprilla, J. C., & Kreutzer, J. S. (2010). Racial and ethnic disparities in functional, psychosocial, and neurobehavioral outcomes after brain injury. *Journal of Head Trauma Rehabilitation, 25*(2), 128–136.

Beach, M. C., Price, E. G., Gary, T. L., Robinson, K. A., Gozu, A., Palacio, A., . . . Cooper, L. A. (2005). Cultural competency: A systematic review of health care provider educational interventions. *Medical Care, 43*(4), 356–373.

Ben-Yishay, Y., & Diller, L. (1993). Cognitive remediation in traumatic brain injury: Update and issues. *Archives of Physical Medicine and Rehabilitation, 74*(2), 204–213.

Ben-Yishay, Y., & Prigatano, G. P. (1990). Cognitive remediation. In M. Rosenthal, E. R. Griffith, J. S. Kreutzer, & B. Pentland (Eds.), *Rehabilitation of the adult and child with traumatic brain injury* (pp. 393–409). Philadelphia, PA: F. A. Davis.

Bordin, E. S. (1979). The generalizability of the psychoanalytic concept of the working alliance. *Psychotherapy: Theory, Research & Practice, 16*(3), 252–260.

Brach, C., & Fraser, I. (2000). Can cultural competency reduce racial and ethnic disparities? A review and conceptual model. *Medical Care Research and Review, 57*(Suppl. 1), 181–217.

Chang, M. (2007). Patient education: Addressing cultural diversity and health literacy issues. *Urologic Nursing, 27*(5), 411–417.

Galanti, G. A. (2003). The Hispanic family and male–female relationships: An overview. *Journal of Transcultural Nursing, 14*(3), 180–185.

Groce, N. (1999). Health beliefs and behavior towards individuals with disability cross-culturally. In R. Leavitt (Ed.), *Cross-cultural rehabilitation: An international perspective* (pp. 37–47). Philadelphia, PA: W. B. Saunders.

Groce, N. (2005). Immigrants, disability and rehabilitation. In J. H. Stone (Ed.), *Culture and disability: Providing culturally competent services* (pp. 1–14). Thousand Oaks, CA: Sage.

Gudykunst, W. B. (1998). *Bridging differences: Effective intergroup communication.* Newbury Park, CA: Sage.

Hallett, J. D., Zasler, N. D., Maurer, P., & Cash, S. (1994). Role change after traumatic brain injury in adults. *American Journal of Occupational Therapy, 48*(1), 241–246.

Hendson, L., Reis, M. D., & Nicholas, D. B. (2015). Health care providers' perspectives of providing culturally competent care in the NICU. *Journal of Obstetric, Gynecologic, & Neonatal Nursing, 44,* 17–27.

Hofstede, G. (2012). Dimensionalizing cultures: The Hofstede Model in context. In L. A. Samovar, R. E. Porter, & E. R. McDaniel (Eds.), *Intercultural communication: A reader* (13th ed.) (pp. 19–33). Boston, MA: Wadsworth Cengage Learning.

Ingstad, B., & Whyte, S. R. (1995). Disability and culture: An overview. In B. Ingstad & S. Whyte (Eds.), *Disability and culture* (pp. 3–32). Berkeley, CA: University of California Press.

Jezewski, M. A. (1990). Culture brokering in migrant farmworker health care. *Western Journal of Nursing Research. 12*(4), 497–513.

Jezewski, M. A., & Sotnik, P. (2001). *Culture brokering: Providing culturally competent rehabilitation services to foreign-born persons.* Retrieved from http://cirrie.buffalo.edu/culture/monographs/cb

Kemp, C., & Rasbridge, L. A. (2004). Mexico. *In refugee and immigrant health: A handbook for health professionals* (pp. 260–270). Cambridge, MA: Cambridge University Press.

Klonoff, P. S. (1997). Individual and group psychotherapy in milieu-oriented neurorehabilitation. *Applied Neuropsychology, 4*(2), 107–118.

Klonoff, P. S. (2010). *Psychotherapy after brain injury: Principles and techniques.* New York, NY: Guilford Press.

Klonoff, P. S. (2013). Practitioner traits in neurorehabilitation. In C. A. Noggle & R. S. Dean (Eds.), *Neuropsychological rehabilitation* (pp. 275–290). New York, NY: Springer Publishing Company.

Klonoff, P. S. (2014). *Psychotherapy for families after brain injury.* New York, NY: Springer Science & Business Media.

Klonoff, P. S., Koberstein, E. J., Talley, M. C., & Dawson, L. K. (2008). A family experiential model of recovery after brain injury. *Bulletin of the Menninger Clinic, 72*(2), 109–129.

Klonoff, P. S., Lamb, D. G., & Henderson, S. W. (2001). Outcomes from milieu-based neurorehabilitation at up to 11 years post-discharge. *Brain Injury, 15*(5), 413–428.

Klonoff, P. S., Lamb, D. G., Henderson, S. W., Reichert, M. V., & Tully, S. L. (2000). Milieu-based neurorehabilitation at the Adult Day Hospital for Neurological Rehabilitation. In A.-L. Christensen & B. P. Uzzell (Eds.), *International handbook of neuropsychological rehabilitation* (pp. 195–213). New York, NY: Kluwer Academic/Plenum Publishers.

Klonoff, P. S., Lamb, D. G., Henderson, S. W., & Shepherd, J. (1998). Outcome assessment after milieu-oriented rehabilitation: New considerations. *Archives of Physical Medicine and Rehabilitation, 79,* 684–690.

Klonoff, P. S., Talley, M. C., Dawson, L. K., Myles, S. M., Watt, L. M., Gehrels, J., & Henderson, S. W. (2007). The relationship of cognitive retraining to neurological patients' work and school status. *Brain Injury, 21*(11), 1097–1107.

Liu, W. M., & Pope-Davis, D. B. (2005). The working alliance, therapy ruptures and impasses, and counseling competence: Implications for counselor training and education. In R. T. Carter (Ed.), *Handbook of racial-cultural psychology and counseling, training and practice* (pp. 148–166). Hoboken, NJ: John Wiley & Sons.

Luria, A. R. (1963). *Restoration of function after brain injury.* New York, NY: Macmillan.

Luria, A. R. (1974). *The working brain.* London, UK: Penguin.

Prigatano, G. P., Fordyce, D. J., Zeiner, H. K., Roueche, J. R., Pepping, M., & Wood, B. C. (1986). *Neuropsychological rehabilitation after brain injury.* Baltimore, MD: The Johns Hopkins University Press.

Uomoto, J. M., & Wong, T. M. (2000). Multicultural perspectives on the neuropsychology of brain injury assessment and rehabilitation. In E. Fletcher-Janzen, T. L. Strickland, & C. R. Reynolds (Eds.), *Handbook of cross-cultural neuropsychology* (pp. 169–184). New York, NY: Kluwer Academic/Plenum Publishers.

U.S. Department of Health and Human Services. (2001). *Mental health: Culture, race, and ethnicity—A supplement to mental health. A report of the Surgeon General.* Rockville, MD: U.S. Department of Health and Human Services, Substance Abuse and Mental Health Services Administration, Center for Mental Health Services.

Vega, W. A., Kolody, B., Aguilar-Gaxiola, S., & Catalano, R. (1999). Gaps in service utilization by Mexican Americans with mental health problems. *American Journal of Psychiatry, 156*(1) 928–934.

CHAPTER SIX

THE EFFECTS OF ACCULTURATION ON NEUROPSYCHOLOGICAL REHABILITATION OF ETHNICALLY DIVERSE PERSONS

Janet P. Niemeier, Joseph Keawe'aimoku Kaholokula, Juan Carlos Arango-Lasprilla, and Shawn O. Utsey

The acculturation process experienced by many racial and ethnic populations in the United States has the potential to complicate adjustment to daily incidental or chronic stressors, and is further complicated by disability related to neuropsychological illness and injury. Researchers tell us that the range of values, beliefs, customs, and views of disability among acculturating patients (i.e., native people, immigrants, and refugees) is reflected in significant differences in mental health symptom expression, attitudes toward treatment, adherence to treatment recommendations, coping, and outcomes (Myers & Rodriguez, 2002). Rehabilitation psychologists and counselors working with neuropsychological disorders, such as cognitive difficulties due to stroke and traumatic brain injury, can enhance the potential benefit, relevance, and effectiveness of their services for people of ethnically and culturally diverse backgrounds by understanding the process of acculturation and how it impacts their assessment and treatment.

The acculturation process can differ remarkably across cultural groups, a phenomenon embedded in the theory of segmented assimilation (Rogers-Sirin, 2013). In this chapter, we explore the impact of acculturation on three diverse U.S. populations: Hispanics, represented by a specific focus on Mexican immigrants; African Americans; and Native Hawaiians. We review relevant acculturation theories developed to explain cultural and psychological changes occurring in racial and ethnic populations in the United States as a result of interactions with the majority racial/ethnic population. We present Berry's (2001, 2003) model of acculturation in particular, as a helpful theoretical model for clinicians working in neuropsychological rehabilitation to use for understanding psychological issues related to acculturation pressures. We also highlight the unique historical context of acculturation for each ethnic group and its effect on their acculturation experience as well as mental and physical health outcomes. Finally, we provide rehabilitation psychologists and counselors with culturally relevant assessment and intervention recommendations for working with ethnically diverse clients.

ACCULTURATION THEORIES: FROM UNIDIMENSIONAL TO MULTIDIMENSIONAL

Theorists have advanced models of acculturation far beyond the writings of early social anthropologists. Acculturation was once simply described as a gradual process of coercing or effecting changes in customs and beliefs, through direct contact between a dominant society and another society, resulting in the two becoming similar to each other over time (Kroeber, 1948). This early position promoted two basic, unidirectional, assumptions. First, acculturating individuals were viewed as "assimilating" toward the mainstream or host culture. Second, this assimilation was seen as occurring simultaneously with a lessening of affiliations and identification with their traditional cultural groups (Zane & Mak, 2003). Models of acculturation later began adopting more psychologically and behaviorally complex explanations. For example, Landrine and Klonoff (1996, 2004) provided a behavioral model to explain acculturation processes and changes. Their earlier dynamic process theory (Landrine & Klonoff, 1996) evolved toward a model using operant conditioning terminology, such as differential reinforcement and extinction. They explained adherence to or distance from customs and behaviors of country or culture of origin, in terms of what was experienced most frequently in daily life or seen as most rewarding. A test of this model (Corral & Landrine, 2008) revealed that health-enhancing behaviors characteristic of the indigenous, Hispanic culture (exercise, no smoking, eating five or more servings of fruit and vegetables daily) were extinguished through acculturation. In their place, health-damaging behaviors characteristic of the dominant-host culture (smoking, diets high in meat and cholesterol, sedentary lifestyles) were acquired or learned in the assimilated groups.

Newer theories of acculturation challenge the older, unidirectional assumptions and conceptualize the process on a more individual and psychological level. For these reasons, these newer models of acculturation are most helpful for rehabilitation psychologists and counselors in enhancing their understanding of the social and psychological situations of their clients. In particular, Berry (2003) presents a multidimensional approach to understanding how acculturating individuals experience and adapt to the mainstream or host cultural group. In Berry's view, acculturating individuals can identify and affiliate with both their traditional cultural group and the new host culture, independent of each other and to varying degrees. His view allows for the possibility of some flexible and alternating movement between traditional and dominant cultural group influences. Berry describes four adaptation strategies of acculturation—integration, separation, assimilation, and marginalization—that acculturating individuals could eventually adopt in response to the acculturation process. Berry characterizes a person with a preference for maintaining his or her ethnic cultural group identity, while also having a preference toward identifying with the mainstream cultural group, as having an integration strategy of acculturation. A person is said to have a separation strategy of acculturation when he or she has a preference to maintain his or her ethnic cultural group identity with little to no preference to identify with the mainstream cultural group; the inverse would be an example of a person with an assimilation strategy. Finally, a person with little to no preference in maintaining his or her cultural group identity and no reference toward adopting the mainstream cultural group identity is said to have a marginalized acculturation strategy.

Berry also describes four strategies the larger mainstream cultural group might take in its promotion of policies and attitudes that impact acculturating peoples. A multiculturalism strategy can be taken in which acculturating peoples are encouraged to maintain their ethnic cultural identities, while also embracing the larger mainstream cultural identity. A segregation strategy can be taken in which acculturating peoples prefer to maintain their ethnic cultural heritage and identity because the larger society encourages the segregation of different social groups. A melting pot strategy can be taken in which acculturating peoples are encouraged to give up their ethnic cultural identities for adoption of the mainstream cultural group identity. Finally, an exclusion strategy can be taken in which there is neither a support for acculturating groups to maintain their ethnic cultural heritage or identity nor a support for relationships to be developed across groups.

Stress, crisis, and conflict can occur prior to these acculturation stages or choices (Berry & Kim, 1988) because of communication, educational, and economic barriers, and the experience of ethnic discrimination. Berry hypothesized that physical and mental health status can thus differ across the acculturation strategies. Berry identified several other mediating and moderating factors, including type of acculturating group (voluntary vs. involuntary group), reason for entering into an acculturation situation (e.g., conquered vs. immigrant), and the dominant group's attitude toward the acculturating group (Berry & Kim, 1988, 2003; Landrine & Klonoff, 1996, 2004). All of these factors and pressures for change can result in depression, abuse of substances, and other health compromising behaviors that place individuals at risk for psychological and medical disability (Kaholokula, 2007; Myers & Rodriguez, 2002). Psychologists and counselors can become more culturally competent providers through increased understanding of the role and impact of acculturation in the lives of ethnically and culturally diverse clients. For example, the stresses and implications of acculturation are additional pressures for clients because they are already coping with mental health symptoms that are disrupting their daily lives.

MEASURES OF ACCULTURATION

Measures of acculturation are an additional resource for improving cultural appropriateness of rehabilitation psychology and counseling services when working with persons of diverse cultural backgrounds. These validated measures and culturally informed interviewing techniques evolved from the multicultural and health disparities research. When chosen for relevance to a particular ethnic group, the measures can help clinicians identify the kinds of acculturative experiences, stressors, and other related factors that may be affecting their clients. Acculturation measures can also help to identify culturally based strengths that will enhance progress in therapy. The scientific literature tells us that acculturation indices are strongly linked to performance on neuropsychological testing (Boone, Victor, Wen, Razani, & Ponton, 2007), access to health care (Oliveira et al.,

2006; Steffen, Smith, Larson, & Butler, 2006), chronic disease prevalence (Kaholokula, Nacapoy, Grandinetti, & Chang, 2008), depression (Leung, LaChapelle, Scinta, & Olvera, 2014), risk factors for a variety of health problems (Conway, Swendsen, Dierker, Canino, & Merikangas, 2007; Eamranond, Marcantonio, Patel, Legedza, & Leveille, 2006), recovery rate, adherence to medical advice, health habits, and addictions (Conway et al., 2007; Niemeier, Burnett, & Whitaker, 2003). However, providers should acknowledge the capacity of their clients to demonstrate the multidimensional ability to move flexibly from one cultural influence to another, as theorized by Berry.

Professional boards that license and certify mental health providers are increasingly recommending the use of acculturation measures as one way of demonstrating ethical, culturally competent, and effective medical and mental health practice (American Psychological Association, 2002; American Psychological Association, Council of Representatives, 2002; U.S. Department of Health and Human Services, 2001). As Zane and Mak (2003) discussed, each of the multiple acculturation measures that are available reflects the foci and assumptions of its developers related to the acculturation process. The individual items of existing acculturation measures also often reflect the psychosocial characteristics of the population for which they were developed. Content domains within acculturation measures include language; affiliation preference; cultural identification; cultural traditions; communication style; perceived discrimination; generational status; family socialization; and cultural knowledge, beliefs, or values (Zane & Mak, 2003). The discussions about each cultural group in this chapter include information about the most relevant and psychometrically sound acculturation measures for use with that group.

Multicultural scholars have a variety of approaches to studying and describing acculturation. However, mental health clinicians in many settings should heed their overarching recommendations. Experts in multicultural studies who have focused on disparities in medical outcomes in the United States are united in urging clinicians to consider the impact of culture during testing, interpretation of scores, selection of diagnoses, making treatment recommendations, and providing interventions for their clients from diverse ethnic and cultural backgrounds (Alegria et al., 2004; Chené et al., 2005; Dana, 1993, 2000; Hansen & Kerkhoff, 2007; Niemeier et al., 2003; Ponton & León-Carrión, 2001; Reynolds, 2000; Sandoval, 1998).

ACCULTURATION AND MEXICAN IMMIGRANTS, AFRICAN AMERICANS, AND NATIVE HAWAIIANS

We now examine acculturation from the lens of persons within three ethnic groups residing in the United States: Mexican immigrants, African Americans, and Native Hawaiians. It is important to consider the cultural histories, values, beliefs, and experiences of each of these U.S.-dwelling populations prior to discussing potential similarities and differences in their acculturation reactions and choices. Table 6.1 contains primary historical occurrences leading to acculturation, as well as core values for each of our populations of focus.

Mexican Immigrants and Acculturation

Mexicans were the first group of people referred to as Hispanics to become part of the U.S. culture. When compared to immigrants from such South American countries as Colombia and Venezuela, Mexicans' early history in the United States, as shown in Table 6.1, is unique in terms of linkage to wars, U.S. land acquisition, and economic and labor issues. They also have a strong history of political activism rooted in their more recent reactions to U.S. governmental labor policies and practices (Castillo & Cano, 2008). Mexican immigrants tended to be less well educated and poorer than Colombian immigrants, but both have struggled against negative views by the dominant culture in the United States (Delgado-Romero, Rojas-Vilches, & Shelton, 2008). Table 6.1 also contains several values and beliefs, some of which are shared with other Hispanic cultures that affect the acculturation reactions of Mexican immigrants and influence their psychological responses to illness or injury-related disabilities. Among the most prominent are specific cultural values that strongly influence the daily social and psychological lives of Mexican immigrants. The first of these, familismo, is a strong identification with and attachment to one's nuclear and extended family (Castillo & Cano, 2008). Components of familismo include reliance on relatives, belief in obligation to provide support, and the perception that relatives are important anchors for behavior and attitudes. Machismo and mariaismo capture the prescribed and preferred gender roles involving differential, traditional and conservative responsibilities for men and women. Finally, Mexican immigrants value personalismo, or a behavioral preference for giving relationships

Table 6.1 *Cultural History and Core Values: U.S.-Dwelling Mexican Immigrants, African Americans, and Native Hawaiians*

	Population		
	Mexican Immigrants	**African Americans**	**Native Hawaiians**
History and Social Experiences	Arrived 17th century, seeking economic opportunity War, land acquisition Labor, economic issues Exploitation for labor Exclusion Discrimination 15.8% of U.S. population	Arrived 17th century, through chattel slavery; businessmen Deracination Exploitation for labor Forced to adopt new religion and language Lost basic social structures Emancipation Exclusion, discrimination 12.9% of U.S. population	18th century U.S. occupation, businesspeople, missionaries Sovereign ruler overthrown Decimation by diseases Forced to adopt new religion and language Exploitation for tourism Multiple immigrants Now in minority Exclusion, discrimination 0.2% of U.S. population
Core Values and Customs	Church, religious faith Family *Familismo* *Machismo* *Marianismo* *Personalismo* Close communities Beliefs in folk illnesses, folk healing practices	Church, religious faith Family, parents and extended Close communities Self-expression Determination Strong reliance on prayer for healing	Family Balance between human needs and preserving nature Strong identification with Native Hawaiian heritage Preservation of cultural customs and values Health = Balance and harmony among spirituality, physical well-being, and relational well-being

Source: Castillo & Cano, 2008; Coffman, 2009; Degruy-Leary, 2005; Eyerman, 2002; Hardy, 2007; Herskovits, 1958; Kuykendall, 1965; Pinkney, 1993; Stannard, 1989; State of Hawaii Data Book, 2005; U.S. Census Bureau, 2001; U.S. Department of Health and Human Services, 2001.

145

and relating more importance than individual or institutional needs. An additional cluster of influential beliefs is associated with health and curative factors. Mexicans have a strong belief in the existence of folk illnesses and often rely on healers, spirituality, or remedios caseros (home remedies; Arbona & Virella, 2008; Castillo & Cano, 2008) for recovery. Finally, Mexicans often favor living within circumscribed neighborhoods populated exclusively by Spanish-speaking Mexicans. Using Berry's (2003) model, the amount of acculturative pressure to change felt by Mexican immigrants depends on where they live and the amount and frequency of interaction they have with the dominant culture. Mexican immigrants who live in Spanish-speaking neighborhoods will potentially have less acculturative stress because most people there will speak Spanish and engage in traditional behaviors and customs. Furthermore, Mexican immigrants living in Mexican neighborhoods will be less likely to notice or be affected by any dominant culture negative views or behaviors toward them. However, obtaining a college degree or employment that requires travel or residence outside a traditional Mexican neighborhood could increase their acculturative stress. They may then have conflict between identification with cultural customs and values and the values of the wider dominant culture. Selecting from Berry's (2003) eight possible kinds of acculturation outcomes or modes, Mexican immigrants who leave traditional neighborhoods may opt for loss of heritage culture but need and want to build relationships with other groups. Their cultural group would thus see them as assimilating, and society as a whole would view them as having joined the U.S. "melting pot." If they opt to separate and stay in their exclusively Mexican, Spanish-speaking neighborhood, as well as remain immersed in their culture and customs, and do not take work outside, the larger society would see them as segregated. If the choice is to maintain Mexican heritage and identity but reside and work outside the traditional neighborhoods, the minority group would view them as integrated, and the larger society would view them as multicultural. A choice to lose cultural heritage but minimally seek relationships with other groups is considered marginalization by the minority group and exclusion by the larger society. Crisis and conflict at each choice point create stress and can lead to changes in physical and mental health status. In terms of Berry's (2003) identified mediating and moderating factors, Mexican immigrants might be seen as less at risk for acculturative stress than African Americans or Native Hawaiians because their history includes voluntary immigration versus conquest or occupation by outsiders. However, Mexican immigrants who are attracted to the promise of a better life in America often experience trauma and betrayal after arriving (Nava, 1983). Those who separate or segregate and remain in poorer, more insulated neighborhoods are less likely than Whites to have health care coverage, a regular health care provider, a regular clinic to visit for medical care (Chowdhury, Balluz, Okoro, & Strine 2006), and access to preventive medical care such as cancer screenings and vaccinations. In addition, Mexican immigrants who choose to separate or segregate are more likely to live in poverty, have limited education, and have higher rates of illness and injuries than Whites. Compared to Whites, Mexicans who isolate in this manner are at greater risk for heart disease, cancer, stroke, diabetes, traumatic brain injuries, depressive symptoms, and general psychological stress (McGruder, Malarcher, Antoine, Greenlund, & Croft, 2004; O'Brien et al., 2003). However, despite the apparent disadvantages of not assimilating or integrating, research is showing that assimilation can be a double-edged sword for Mexican immigrants. For example, when more traditional Mexican immigrants transition toward the values and behaviors of the dominant population in their adopted country, they also move to a more sedentary lifestyle, a reduction in healthy traditional dietary patterns, and ultimately toward greater risk for certain illnesses. Assimilating Mexican immigrants are also more at risk for obesity (Gordon-Larsen, Harris, Ward, & Popkin, 2003; Himmelgreen et al., 2004; Kaplan, Huguet, Newsom, & McFarland, 2004), hypertension, smoking, and increased alcohol intake (Abraido-Lanza, Chao, & Florez, 2005). Gender differences have been found in these changes, with more highly assimilated Mexican immigrant women more apt to smoke or drink than men of their ethnic group (Corral & Landrine, 2008). In terms of predictors for psychological problems such as depression, a recent survey (Leung et al., 2014) revealed increased self-report of depression symptoms in Mexican Americans who were concerned about discrimination, had a loss of income, or were worried about access to medical care. The Leung et al. study also confirmed that Latinos prefer to seek help with mental health issues from a medical doctor or indigenous community resources. These findings were not related to acculturation. Gonzalez, Haan, and Hinton (2001) found that older Mexican Americans with the least acculturation were more likely to be depressed. The authors speculated that cultural barriers encountered by immigrants and less acculturated older Mexicans may lead to poorer health status and depression.

Acculturation Scales for Use With Mexican Immigrant Clients

Acculturation measures that have been validated for use with Mexicans in particular include the Acculturation Rating Scale for Mexican Americans–Revised (ARSMA-II; Cuellar, Arnold, & Maldonado, 1995) and the Children's Acculturation Scale (CAS; Franco, 1983). The ARSMA-II measures the respondent's extent of involvement in Mexican culture and Anglo culture by rating how frequently he or she engages in certain behaviors. Internal consistency of the subscales ranges from 0.68 to 0.91. Test–retest reliability ranges from 0.72 to 0.96. Concurrent validity was evident in the positive relationship of the ARSMA to the Behavioral Acculturation Scale ($r = 0.76$, $p < 0.001$) (BAS; Szapocznik, Scopetta, Kurtines, & de los Angeles Aranalde, 1978). The BAS measures the degree to which a respondent has adopted American cultural practices relative to those of Spanish or Cuban culture. The CAS (Franco, 1983) consists of 10 items measuring aspects of language usage, cultural identification, and social affiliation, and has a test–retest reliability of 0.97 as well as a 0.76, significant ($p < 0.01$) correlation with the ARSMA. The CAS scores increase with education and age and successfully differentiate Mexican American from Anglo students.

African Americans and Acculturation

Got one mind for White folks to see, 'Nother for what I know is me.
(Author unknown)

The African American acculturation experience contrasts with that of Hispanics and most other racial and ethnic groups living in the United States. The social and historical analysis for African Americans in Table 6.1 includes the forced removal of African Americans from their land of origin, imposed deracination and acculturation, and continued exclusion and discrimination in the United States. Rehabilitation psychologists and counselors should be aware of the mental health issues related to these several separate, but similarly influential, phenomena of acculturation among African Americans. First, the acculturative experience of African Americans is inextricably linked to the institution of chattel slavery (DeGruy-Leary, 2005; Eyerman, 2002; Hardy, 2007; Pinkney, 1993; Utsey, Bolden, & Brown, 2000). Both the culture and the cultural identity of the enslaved Africans were forcibly erased. Expression and outward manifestations of such keystones as native language, social structure, and customs, religion, and worldview (Frazier, 1964; Herskovits, 1958; Pinkney, 1993; Stampp, 1956) were forbidden, and they were made to incorporate their oppressors' culture. A breaking in or "seasoning period" was used to facilitate the process (Frazier, 1964; Pinkney, 1993). The slaves were taught enough rudiments of the English language to enable them to understand the commands of the master and overseer (Frazier, 1964). Rudiments of this language can be observed in present-day "Black English," "Ebonics," or African American vernacular (Herskovits, 1958; Holloway, 1990). Survival required enslaved Africans to develop competencies in both the culture of the White slave master and a creolized African culture created by the amalgamation of the various West and Central African subgroups living together on the plantations (Lovejoy, 1997). Although the creolized culture gave the enslaved Africans a sense of connectedness (Holloway, 1990; Lovejoy, 1997), a fusing of cultural patterns created out of the enslaved Africans' necessity to survive under the brutal system of U.S. slavery (Lovejoy, 1997; Pinkney, 1993) set the course for an African American bicultural identity development. The implications of this identity for health behaviors and outcomes for African Americans are unclear because of limited research. Second, the amount of contact between slave and master affected the African Americans acculturation process. Enslaved Africans who had more intimate contact with Whites experienced the most direct route for adopting European cultural values and behavior. The amount of contact with the slave master was determined by the size of the plantation, the ratio of enslaved Africans to Whites, and, most important, whether the individual(s) was a house servant or field hand (Herskovits, 1958). Third, rather than acceptance of servitude as an inescapable fate because of their debased condition, Lovejoy (1997) points out that the cultural pliability of the enslaved Africans allowed them to reinterpret their cultural and religious practices in the context of their oppression. On this subject, Blassingame (1979) stated, "In the process of acculturation, the slaves made European forms serve African functions" (pp. 20–21). For example, African religious beliefs and practices were often disguised and/or merged with Christian rites of worship to conceal them from the White slave master (Herskovits, 1958). Fourth, postemancipation forms of racism, oppression, and exclusion persist and are factors in the acculturation of modern-day African Americans.

Berry's (2003) model of acculturation is, in some respects, complementary to the concept that African Americans developed a bicultural identity as a result of the potent aspects of their history and social experience in this country. Berry sees acculturating individuals as able to identify and affiliate with both their traditional cultural group and with the new host culture, independent of each other and to varying degrees. However, the access to indigenous cultural customs and beliefs is often not possible for African Americans who have lived in the United States for many generations, in comparison with persons who have recently immigrated from Africa or other countries. The loss of records and resulting lack of knowledge about original family and national ties, customs, language, and social connections at the time of slavery hinder African Americans' acculturation choice of strong identification and affiliation with their traditional cultural group (Hardy & Laszloffy, 1995). Furthermore, stress, crisis, and conflict are likely to occur not only because of acculturation choice dilemmas (Berry and Kim, 1988) for African Americans but because of their continued experience of social and economic barriers and ethnic discrimination (Carter, 1995). Berry's (2003) model (Berry & Kim, 1988) describes the additional unique acculturation stressors for African Americans, including the involuntary and forced aspects of their acculturation process, as well as the dominant culture's continued oppressive attitudes and behaviors toward them. Additional acculturation theorists have attempted to adequately describe the African American acculturation experience. For example, Landrine and Klonoff (1996, 2004) provided two models of African American acculturation. Their early theory (1996) includes four descriptive principles. First, the principle of return refers to a dynamic process that can take several forms. Individuals may seek cultural roots as they grow older due to feelings of nostalgia, a longing for communal ties, and pending mortality. African American parents may be more likely to expose their children to customs and views of their ethnic group to strengthen their child's sense of self. Discrimination and racism may lead to a return to the culture of origin after a rejection of the dominant culture. The second and third principles, fractionization and allopatricity, emphasize the individual's possible "split" from the culture of origin. African Americans who are split off and less involved with their ethnic group may experience fewer challenges while acculturating. Allopatricity refers to the impact of the nature and length of contact with the dominant culture on the acculturation process. African Americans who have positive and prolonged contact may experience rapid acculturation, whereas individuals who experience negative prolonged contact may experience failed acculturation. These terms equate with Berry's (2003) descriptors—assimilation and marginalization. Landrine and Klonoff's (1996) Principle of Ethnic Socialization refers to the role of the acculturating individual's perception of the dominant group in choice of acculturation strategy. If the perception of the dominant group is "all bad," individuals are unlikely to assimilate to the dominant group. In a later theory, Landrine and Klonoff (2004) used operant conditioning terminology, such as differential reinforcement and extinction, to explain this gradual change in adherence to Afrocentric customs and behaviors. The authors proposed that compared to African Americans living in mixed or predominantly White areas, individuals living in African American enclaves will be reinforced for continuing to exhibit the behaviors and linguistic habits of that community. Psychologists and counselors should note that all acculturation theorists attempting to describe the African American acculturation experience share a belief that African Americans may have "acculturative stress." According to Anderson (1991), threats to racial identity, cultural values, and patterns of living are particular stressors for African Americans that contribute to vulnerability for distress and compromised health. African American acculturative stress, as well as that of Latinos and other culturally diverse populations, has also been found to be associated with depression and suicidal ideation (Walker, Wingate, Obasi, & Joiner, 2008). However, a recent study examined the relationship between acculturative stress, mental health, and attitudes toward psychotherapy and found that a negative view of psychotherapy was mediated by mental health symptoms for immigrants of color but not White immigrants from European countries (Rogers-Sirin, 2013). Attitudes toward psychotherapy became increasingly negative as mental health symptoms increased for immigrants of color only. Although the participants in the study were immigrants rather than persons of color born and living in the United States, the Rogers-Sirin study finding is concerning because it suggests that culturally and racially diverse persons may avoid the very support they need when they are depressed. This study also underscores an additional theory of acculturation—"segmented assimilation"—which holds that there are important differences in the ways racial groups experience the immigration process. Anderson (1991) asserts that an understanding of core Afrocentric values can help social and medical scientists and theorists more comprehensively examine acculturative (Eurocentric) influences that negatively impact African American people.

In summary, we contend that current models of acculturation may be inadequate to describe the process of second culture acquisition for

African Americans. Not only is there a dearth of both theoretical and empirical literature on the topic, but what is available fails to take into account African Americans' experience during slavery, Jim Crow segregation, and current forms of societal racism and oppression. It is our position that a new model delineating the psychology of the African American bicultural experience needs to be developed. This model must take into account the social and historical experiences of African Americans, including but not limited to the African genesis of African American culture, slavery, Jim Crow segregation, and modern forms of racism and oppression.

Acculturation Scales for Use With African American Clients

Among the reliable and valid acculturation scales used with African Americans are the African American Acculturation Scale (AAAS; Landrine & Klonoff, 1994) and the African American Acculturation Scale (AfAAS; Snowden & Hines, 1999). The 74-item AAAS measures engagement in African American behaviors and knowledge about African American culture. The AAAS has a split-half reliability of 0.93. The AfAAS has ten items and measures behaviors and attitudes of respondents related to media preferences, social interactions, and race relations. Internal consistency of the AfAAS is 0.75, and it has a unidimensional factor structure as well as an observed, significant gender and acculturation level interaction.

Native Hawaiians and Acculturation

Native Hawaiians (Kānaka ʻŌiwi) are the indigenous people of Hawaii whose ancestors were the first Polynesians to settle in the Hawaiian archipelago some 2,000 years ago (Bushnell, 1993). Although ancient Hawaiians made frequent open ocean voyages to other Polynesian islands, they lived in relative isolation for a period of time until 1778, when European explorers first arrived in the Hawaiian Islands. Native Hawaiians have since experienced drastic sociopolitical and sociocultural changes, which have resulted in acculturation experiences that contrast significantly with those of African Americans and Mexican immigrants. These pivotal historical and traumatic sociocultural experiences are listed in Table 6.1 and include decimation from diseases introduced by foreigners, forced changes in their spiritual practices from Calvinist missionary activity in the 1800s, and U.S.-supported illegal overthrow of their sovereign ruler and nation, with U.S. occupation, in the late 1800s. Militarization of the islands and cultural exploitation through the tourism industry followed in the 1900s. Finally, the United States declared statehood for Hawaii in 1959 (Coffman, 2009; Dougherty, 1992; Osorio, 2002). As a result of all these traumatic events, the Kānaka 'Ōiwi population declined, and they became a minority in their own homeland (Stannard, 1989).

Many scholars believe that the U.S. occupation of Hawaii and the acculturation process experienced by Native Hawaiians, which diminished their social standing and devalued their cultural beliefs and practices, are responsible for their negative social and health statistics. This phenomenon is often referred to as historical or cultural trauma (Brave Heart, Chase, Elkins, & Altschul, 2011). For example, Hawaiians experience high rates of death and disability due to chronic illnesses, such as obesity, diabetes, heart disease, and certain types of cancers (Braun, Fong, Gotay, Pagano, & Chong, 2005; Johnson, Oyama, LeMarchand, & Wilkens, 2004), and higher rates of depression compared to the other major ethnic groups of Hawaii (Cho et al., 2006; Kaholokula, 2007; Rezentes, 1996). Despite the many losses experienced by Native Hawaiians from U.S. occupation of their islands, many still hold strong to their fundamental cultural values and practices that can serve as supports for the duration of their therapy sessions. Among these values and practices are 'ohana (the importance of the family and kin group), mālama 'āina (the ancestral connection to their islands), pono (sense of justice and fairness), and lōkahi (maintaining harmony among the self, humankind, and their ancestral connections). Rezentes (1996) and Pukui, Haertig, and Lee (1972) provide a detailed explanation of these values and their relevance to psychological services with Native Hawaiians.

Using the four acculturation strategies theorized by Berry (2003), it is estimated that 77% of Native Hawaiians can be categorized as integrated (bicultural), 17% as separated, 2% as assimilated, and 4% as marginalized (Kaholokula et al., 2008). Studies have linked these four acculturation strategies to the prevalence of depressive symptoms and type 2 diabetes in Native Hawaiians (Kaholokula, 2007). Findings in Native Hawaiian youth also suggest that those with a stronger Hawaiian identity are most at risk for attempted suicide compared to youth of other ethnic groups (Yuen, Nahulu, Hishinuma, & Miyamoto, 2000). In contrast, Native Hawaiians with a stronger American identity may feel alienated from the Hawaiian community but also have difficulty "fitting into" the American mainstream. Subsequent studies have identified acculturation strategies as a possible marker of discrimination in Native Hawaiians. Studies also have found a positive correlation between a stronger Hawaiian ethnic identity and perceived ethnic discrimination and that discrimination is associated with higher risk for hypertension (Kaholokula, Iwane, & Nacapoy, 2010) and cortisol dysregulation (Kaholokula et al., 2012) in Native Hawaiian adults.

What is clear from empirical studies of Native Hawaiians is that acculturation modes and ethnic discrimination are associated with their psychological and physical health and well-being. Psychologists and counselors providing services to Native Hawaiians or other indigenous U.S. populations (i.e., Alaska Natives and American Indians) or other Pacific Islanders (e.g., Samoans and Tongans) would be wise to explore how acculturative stressors may be impacting a person's disability burdens and their recovery from disability. Psychologists and counselors who know how to facilitate putting cultural strengths and supports in place to assist in recovery will be perceived as providing the most culturally relevant services.

Acculturation Scales for Use With Native Hawaiian Clients

Several valid and appropriate acculturation measures are available for use with the Native Hawaiian client. For adolescents, the Hawaiian Culture Scale–Adolescent Version (HCS) is a 50-item inventory with seven subscales that assess traditional lifestyle (eight items), customs (11 items), activities (10 items), folklore (five items), sociopolitical causes (five items), and language proficiency (two items), using a 5-point rating scale (1 = not at all to 5 = very much). Hishinuma et al. (2000) published a study of the HCS's psychometric properties. The Nā Mea Hawai'i Scale, or "Hawaiian Ways" scale, is a 21-item questionnaire that assesses knowledge of Hawaiian vocabulary, customs, history, and participation in cultural activities. Using two response styles, respondents either answer yes, no, or don't know to closed-ended questions or provide definitions of Hawaiian phrases or cultural terms to open-ended questions. Rezentes (1993) published a study of its psychometric evaluation. The Kohala Health Research Project's Cultural Affiliation Questionnaire is an eight-item acculturation scale with two subscales. Four items assess ethnic cultural identity and four items assess Western cultural identity. Based on the assumption that acculturation and retention of a person's ethnic identity are independent of each other, the four items in each subscale are nearly identical (with only the reference cultural group changing) to assess degree of identity/affiliation with, feelings toward, and knowledge about each cultural group and the impact each group has on lifestyle on a 5-point rating scale (e.g., 1 = very knowledgeable to 5 = not knowledgeable at all). No formal psychometric evaluation has been published on this questionnaire, but it has been found to predict health outcomes in adult Native Hawaiians (Kaholokula et al., 2008).

CONCLUSIONS

This chapter explores three unique perspectives on the impact of acculturation and the variety of experiences of this process to enrich the understanding of psychologists and counselors who provide care to people of diverse ethnic and cultural backgrounds in the United States. In applying the understanding to practice, two factors emerge as key to improving cultural effectiveness of psychological and counseling services. We must practice with the knowledge that the history, customs, beliefs, worldviews, and acculturation choices of our clients will influence what kinds of help they want from us and whether they will view our services as relevant and helpful. Some of our ethnically and culturally diverse clients have daily experiences of discrimination and live in poverty, are at risk for injury, and have substandard or no health care. Prior experiences with medical health care providers in the United States may have been negative, and clients may seek treatment with mistrust of the system and its representatives on board. Providers will need to gather history from clients and available family so both acculturation choice and stressors can be more clearly understood. In particular, psychologists should consider possible conflicts related to acculturation strategy choice that are underlying and complicating the presenting problems. For example, a Mexican client with a separatist strategy may prefer a doctor–patient relationship that is more traditional and expect that the doctor will provide specific advice rather than conduct open-ended, uncovering methods of psychotherapy. A more acculturated or assimilated individual may prefer exploring his or her own feelings and preferences but still have some discomfort about foregoing family responsibilities to realize individual goals. Sensitivity to these issues will help avoid outcomes or treatment goals that could place the client in an untenable or potentially unhelpful position. With regard to treatment and follow-up recommendations, psychologists and counselors should consider relevance, appropriateness, and feasibility for their Mexican clients. In addition, psychologists and counselors should be aware that their ethnically diverse clients have acculturation experiences based not only on their history in the United States but on their contemporary experiences as well. Many African Americans and Native Hawaiians still feel the impacts of slavery and dispossession, respectively, and the associated attempts to erase their culture and cultural identity today. In addition, although these terrible early conditions and treatment are now part of history, modern-day racism continues to place these and other U.S.-dwelling ethnic groups at risk for poverty, injury, illness, unemployment, substandard health care, and social alienation. Our review of the multicultural and acculturation literature tells us that, although each group has a unique experience and stressors, the consequences to physical and mental health are similar and often transgenerational.

A Blended and Tailored Therapeutic Approach

The study of acculturation and consideration of its impact on the health status of a people is important for psychologists, counselors, and other mental health and medical professionals for the reasons reviewed here. However, we encourage researchers and providers to go further and develop solutions that reflect awareness of differences between ethnically and culturally diverse patient groups, taking into account their history, experience, views, and current situations. Development of culturally sensitive psychotherapeutic interventions will depend on providers' understanding of sources of acculturative stress, awareness of adaptive coping strategies each population has already devised, and knowledge of mechanisms of relief. This foundation of knowledge should be coupled with goals to provide health education, preventive mental and physical health care services, and increased access to culturally relevant, quality psychological services for ethnically and culturally diverse persons in the United States.

Although many forms of psychotherapy were developed and tested within White European populations, there are promising new evidence-based interventions that may, with culturally sensitive tailoring, be helpful and considered meaningful by clients of diverse cultural backgrounds.

For example, motivational interviewing (MI) techniques (Arkowitz, Westra, Miller, & Rollnick, 2007), which can assist the client in directing his or her own changes toward improved health, have inherent components and foundational concepts that are potentially more sensitive to cultural differences and preferences than traditional psychotherapy approaches. The MI approach trains psychotherapists to employ several key principles in helping clients to identify changes they wish or need to make and then support their individual journeys toward achieving them. In MI, the clients, not the therapist, are considered experts on themselves. Therapists' MI work is guided by four principles: expressing empathy, developing discrepancy so clients can see how their situations do not necessarily fit their values or beliefs, rolling with resistance, and supporting self-efficacy. When the therapy dyad includes persons from two different racial or ethnic groups, MI may be more helpful for therapists who wish to grow in their cultural understanding and sensitivity. The potential for enhancement of cultural effectiveness of MI therapists working with culturally diverse clients has not been studied. Adherents of MI (Miller & Rollnick, 2012) have researched general effectiveness and have found evidence to support MI with addictions, intimate partner violence, depression, medication adherence, and those adjustment and stressful life problems that involve some possibly uncomfortable changes. Evidence has shown that culturally modified MI can be effective with African American and Hispanic groups who are depressed or struggling with chronic health problems (Breland-Noble, 2012; Hu, Juarez, Yeboah, & Castillo, 2014; Lewis-Fernandez & Aggarwal, 2013; Venner, Feldstein, & Tafoya, 2008). Hu et al. (2014) found that interventions lasting longer than 6 months that involved human contact rather than online or telephone methods and provided tangible incentives and skill building for self-management were most likely to produce positive change for diverse clients. However, in their review of the literature related to interventions to increase medication adherence in culturally diverse groups, Hu et al. found no evidence for effectiveness of MI with Native Hawaiians or Pacific Islanders. Clearly, more research needs to be done to determine which of the more nontraditional and change-focused therapies are most effective for which groups and whether acculturation moderates effectiveness. Table 6.2 contains some general suggestions for providing culturally sensitive and tailored psychological and counseling services for ethnically diverse clients.

Table 6.2 Providing Rehabilitation Psychology and Counseling Services to Ethnically Diverse Clients

Clinical Guidelines	Assessment/Treatment Strategies
Assess cultural identity and acculturation level	• Use validated self-report measures of acculturation and ethnic/racial identity. • When validated measures are not feasible, inquire about client's degree of identification with his or her ethnic/racial group and the mainstream culture; language preference, fluency, and proficiency. • Conceptualize acculturation and ethnic identity using a multidimensional framework such as Berry's model (i.e., client can strongly identify with his or her ethnic group as well as the mainstream cultural group). • Therapist determines whether he or she is competent to continue working with the client, whether a referral is necessary, or whether consultation is needed.
Assess cultural identity and acculturation level of client's family and/or primary support group	• Same strategies as preceding. • Inquire about the family and community systems, such as family relationships and differences in acculturation levels and cultural and social expectations.
Clinician should be familiar and competent	• Overall, the clinician needs to have a working knowledge about the ethnic/racial background of the client. This should include knowing the client's historical background in the United States (i.e., how the client and his or her ancestors came to the United States), the cultural and social challenges often faced by the ethnic/racial group, the scientific literature relevant to both the client's ethnic/racial group and the specific mental health symptoms he or she is reporting.
Assess causal/ explanatory model and preferred treatment strategies/ modalities	• The client's perspective of the causal mechanisms involved in his or her mental health problems, such as stressors due to perceived discrimination, family discord, financial worries, discriminatory work policies, and/or lack of culturally relevant treatment options. • Greater emphasis should be placed on the client's explanatory model. • Ask the client how his or her symptoms would be addressed within his or her own cultural/ community context. Who are the recognized healers, and what are the appropriate treatment approaches supported by the client's culture/community?

Assess the role of ethnocultural and acculturation-related factors on the client's disability and rehabilitation process	• Specify how cultural factors might either serve as barriers or facilitators to rehabilitation. Some facilitators to recovery might include a strong and supportive family environment, existing traditional health beliefs and attitudes, and the availability of traditional healers. Barriers might include lack of cultural supports and unsafe work and living conditions. • Conducting a functional analysis to identify and specify the causal mechanism can be very helpful, culturally appropriate, and focus on assets rather than deficits.
Negotiate treatment goals	• After initial assessment and identification of factors related to the client's psychological and psychosocial challenges, negotiate treatment goals with the client and his or her family (if desired by client). • Pay careful attention to how the acquisition of new skills or attitudes might be viewed by or operate within the client's cultural context. For example, a Western notion of assertiveness (e.g., making direct eye contact, questioning the intention of others) might not be acceptable in another cultural context. • Consider a more transtheoretical therapeutic approach, such as embodied in motivational interviewing.
Collaborate on treatment variables	• Ensure that treatment goals, target behaviors, agents of change, and methods of treatment are culturally appropriate and acceptable to the client and his or her family. • Ongoing assessment of the treatment process and identified goals (i.e., outcomes) should be conducted to inform the modification of failing treatments and/or iatrogenic effects. • Ensure that the data collection procedures and measures are culturally relevant and valid.
Collaborate on assessment of and conclusions about treatment outcomes	• Ensure that client perceptions and goals have as large a role in evaluating treatment outcomes as analysis and findings of data collected before, during, and after treatment. • Ensure that proper sampling techniques have preceded data collection prior to making conclusions related to use of a particular treatment method with the client's entire ethnic group. • Ensure that recommendations for follow-up or treatment goal or intervention changes are culturally relevant and meaningful.

The authors hope that these recommendations will assist psychologists, counselors, and cross-field neurorehabilitation providers to select and deliver services that will be viewed as relevant and valuable by their ethnically and culturally diverse patients and clients. If this goal is achieved, culturally diverse clients and their family members will be less likely to drop out of their behavioral health, targeted therapeutic, and neurorehabilitation treatment prematurely. Clients who perceive their therapy providers to be respectful, sensitive, and caring are more likely to trust their clinicians and health systems. As a result, these clients may stay the course of their treatments and potentially achieve improved adjustment and functional status. The results will help reduce neurorehabilitation and mental health treatment outcome disparities.

AUTHORS' NOTE

The authors would like to thank Aukahi Austin, PhD, from the I Ola Lāhui: Rural Behavioral Health Program for her valuable comments on Native Hawaiians.

REFERENCES

Abraido-Lanza, A. F., Chao, M. T., & Florez, K. R. (2005). Do healthy behaviors decline with greater acculturation? Implication for the Latino mortality paradox. *Social Science and Medicine, 61,* 1243–1255.

Alegria, M., Takeuchi, D., Canino, G., Duan, N., Shrout, P., Meng, X. L., . . . Gong, F. (2004). Considering context, place and culture: The National Latino and Asian American Study. *International Journal of Methods of Psychiatric Research, 13,* 208–220.

American Psychological Association. (2002). *Ethical principles of psychologists and code of conduct.* Washington, DC: American Psychological Association.

American Psychological Association, Council of Representatives. (2002). *Guidelines on multicultural education, training, research, practice, and organizational change for psychologists.* Washington, DC: American Psychological Association.

Anderson, L. P. (1991). Acculturative stress: A theory of relevance to black Americans. *Clinical Psychology Review, 11,* 685–702.

Arbona, C., & Virella, B. (2008). Psychological issues with Puerto Ricans: A review of research findings. In C. Negy (Ed.), *Cross-cultural psychotherapy: Toward a critical understanding of diverse clients* (2nd ed.) (pp. 103–132). Reno, NV: Bent Tree Press.

Arkowitz, H., Westra, H. A., Miller, W. R., & Rollnick, S. (2008). *Motivational interviewing in the treatment of psychological problems.* New York, NY: Guilford Press.

Berry, J. W. (2001). A psychology of immigration. *Journal of Social Issues, 57,* 615–631.

Berry, J. W. (2003). Conceptual approaches to acculturation. In K. M. Chun, P. B. Organista, & G. M. Marín (Eds.), *Acculturation: Advances in theory, measurement, and applied research* (pp. 17–37). Washington, DC: American Psychological Association.

Berry, J. W., & Kim, U. (1988). Acculturation and mental health. In P. Dasen, J. W. Berry, & N. Sartorius (Eds.), *Health and cross-cultural psychology: Towards application.* Newbury Park, CA: Sage.

Blassingame, J. (1979). *The slave community.* New York, NY: Oxford University Press.

Boone, K. L., Victor, T. L., Wen, J., Razani, J., & Ponton, M. (2007). The association between neuropsychological scores and ethnicity, language, and acculturation variables in a large patient population. *Archives of Clinical Neuropsychology, 22,* 355–365.

Braun, K. L., Fong, M., Gotay, C., Pagano, I. S., & Chong, C. (2005). Ethnicity and breast cancer in Hawaii: Increased survival but continued disparity. *Ethnicity and Disease, 15,* 453–460.

Brave Heart, M. Y. H., Chase, J., Elkins, J., & Altschul, D. B. (2011). Historical trauma among indigenous peoples of the Americas: Concepts, research, and clinical considerations. *Journal of Psychoactive Drugs, 43,* 282–290.

Breland-Noble, A. M., Bell, C. C., & Burriss, A. (2012). The significance of strategic community engagement in recruiting African America youth & families for clinical research. *Journal of Child and Family Studies, 21,* 273–280.

Bushnell, O. A. (1993). *Germs and genocide in Hawai'i.* Honolulu, HI: University of Hawai'i Press.

Carter, R. T. (1995). *The influence of race and racial identity in psychotherapy.* New York, NY: John Wiley & Sons, Inc.

Castillo, L. G., & Cano, M. A. (2008). Mexican American psychology: Theory and clinical application. In C. Negy (Ed.), *Cross-cultural psychotherapy: Toward a critical understanding of diverse clients* (2nd ed.) (pp. 8–102). Reno, NV: Bent Tree Press.

Chené, R., Garcia, L., Goldstrom, M., Pino, M., Roach, D. P., Thunderchief, W., & Waitzkin, H. (2005). Mental health research in primary care: Mandates from a community advisory board. *Annals of Family Medicine, 3,* 70–72.

Cho, S., Salvail, F., Gross, P., Crisanti, A., Gundaya, D., & Smith, J. (2006). Depression and anxiety among adults in Hawai'i: A focus on gender and ethnicity. Retrieved from Hawaii.gov/health/statistics/brfss/reports/nri_samhsa_poster_hi.pdf

Chowdhury, P. P., Balluz, L., Okoro, C., & Strine, T. (2006). Leading health indicators: A comparison of Hispanics with non-Hispanic Whites and non-Hispanic Blacks, U.S. 2003. *Ethnicity and Disease, 16*, 534–541.

Coffman, T. (2009). *Nation within: The history of the American occupation of Hawaii.* Kihei, HI: Koa Books.

Conway, K. P., Swendsen, J. D., Dierker, L., Canino, G., & Merikangas, K. R. (2007). Psychiatric comorbidity and acculturation stress among Puerto Rican substance abusers. *American Journal of Preventive Medicine, 32*(Suppl. 1), S219–S225.

Corral, I., & Landrine, H. (2008). Acculturation and ethnic-minority health behavior: A test of the operant model. *Health Psychology, 27*, 737–745.

Cuellar, I., Arnold, B., & Maldonado, R. (1995). Acculturation rating scale for Mexican Americans—II: A revision of the original ARSMA Scale. *Hispanic Journal of Behavioral Sciences, 17*, 275–304.

Dana, R. H. (1993). *Multicultural assessment perspectives for professional psychology.* Boston, MA: Allyn & Bacon.

Dana, R. H. (2000). *Handbook of cross-cultural and multicultural personality assessment.* Mahwah, NJ: Erlbaum.

Degruy-Leary, J. (2005). *Post traumatic slave syndrome: America's legacy of enduring injury and healing.* Milwaukie, OR: Uptone Press.

Delgado-Romero, E. A., Rojas-Vilches, A., & Shelton, K. L. (2008). Immigration history and therapy considerations with Hispanics from Cuba, Central and South America. In C. Negy (Ed.), *Cross-cultural psychotherapy: Toward a critical understanding of diverse clients* (2nd ed.) (pp. 133–160). Reno, NV: Bent Tree Press.

Dougherty, M. (1992). *To steal a kingdom: Probing Hawaiian history.* Waimanalo, HI: Island Style Press.

Eamranond, P. P., Marcantonio, E., Patel, K., Legedza, A., & Leveille, S. G. (2006). The association of acculturation with prevalence of undiagnosed hypertension among older Hispanic adults. *Journal of General Internal Medicine, 21*, 136–137.

Eyerman, R. (2002). *Cultural trauma: Slavery and the formation of African American identity.* Cambridge, UK: Cambridge University Press.

Franco, J. N. (1983). An acculturation scale for Mexican-American children. *Journal of General Psychology. 108*, 175–181.

Frazier, E. F. (1964). *The Negro church in America.* New York, NY: Schocken Books, Inc.

Gonzalez, H. M., Haan, M. N., & Hinton, L. (2001). Acculturation and the prevalence of depression in older Mexican American: Baseline results of the Sacramento Area Latino Study on Aging. *Journal of the American Geriatric Society, 49*, 948–953.

Gordon-Larsen, P., Harris, K. M., Ward, D. S., & Popkin, D. M. (2003). Acculturation and overweight related behaviors among Hispanic immigrants to the

U.S.: The national longitudinal study of adolescent health. *Social Science and Medicine, 57,* 2023–2034.

Hanson, S. L., & Kerkhoff, T. R. (2007). Ethical decision making in rehabilitation: Consideration of Latino cultural factors. *Rehabilitation Psychology, 52,* 409–420.

Hardy, K. V. (2007). *Psychological residuals of slavery.* San Francisco, CA: Psychotherapy.net.

Hardy, K. V., & Laszloffy, T. A. (1995). Therapy with African Americans and the phenomenon of rage. *In Session-Psychotherapy in Practice, 1*(4), 57–70.

Herskovits, M. J. (1958). *Myth of the Negro past.* Boston, MA: Beacon Press.

Himmelgreen, D. A., Perez-Escamilla, R., Martinez, D., Bretnall, A., Eeels, B., Peng, Y., & Bermudez, A. (2004). The longer you stay, the bigger you get: Length of time and language use in the U.S. are associated with obesity in Puerto Rican women. *American Journal of Physical Anthropology, 125,* 90–96.

Hishinuma, E. S., Andrade, N., Johnson, R. C., McArdle, J. J., Miyamoto, R. H., Nahulu, L. B., & Yates, A. (2000) Psychometric properties of the Hawaiian Culture Scale—Adolescent Version. *Psychological Assessment, 12,* 140–157.

Holloway, J. E. (1990). The origins of African-American culture. In J. E. Holloway (Ed.), *Africanisms in American culture* (pp. 1–18). Bloomington, IN: Indiana University Press.

Hu, D., Juarez, D. T., Yeboah, M., & Castillo, T. P. (2014). Interventions to increase medication adherence in African-American and Latino populations: A literature review. *Journal of Medicine and Public Health, 73,* 11–18.

Johnson, D. B., Oyama, N., LeMarchand, L., & Wilkens, L. (2004). Native Hawaiian mortality, morbidity, and lifestyle: Comparing data from 1982, 1990, and 2000. *Pacific Health Dialog, 11,* 120–130.

Kaholokula, J. K. (2007). Colonialism, acculturation and depression among Kānaka Maoli of Hawaii. In P. Culbertson, M. N. Agee, & C. Makasiale (Eds.), *Penina Uliuli: Confronting challenges in mental health for Pacific peoples.* Honolulu, HI: University of Hawai'i Press.

Kaholokula, J. K., Iwane, M. K., & Nacapoy, A. H. (2010). Effects of perceived racism and acculturation on hypertension in Native Hawaiians. *Hawaii Medical Journal, 69*(Suppl. 2), 11–15.

Kaholokula, J. K., Nacapoy, A. H., Grandinetti, A., & Chang, H. K. (2008). Association between acculturation modes and type 2 diabetes among Native Hawaiians. *Diabetes Care, 31,* 698–700.

Kaholokula, J. K., Stefan, K., Mau, M. K., Nacapoy, A. H., Kingi, T. K., & Grandinetti, A. (2012). Association between perceived racism and physiological stress indices in Native Hawaiians. *Journal of Behavioral Medicine, 35,* 27–37.

Kaplan, M. S., Huguet, N., Newson, J. T., & McFarland, B. H. (2004). African American acculturation and neuropsychological test performance following traumatic brain injury. *Journal of the International Neuropsychological Society, 10,* 566–577.

Kroeber, A. L. (1948). *Anthropology: Race, language, culture, psychology, prehistory.* New York and Burlingame: Harcourt, Brace & World.

Kuykendall, S. R. (1965). *The Hawaiian Kingdom: 1778–1854.* Honolulu, HI: University of Hawai'i Press.

Landrine, H., & Klonoff, E. A. (1994). The African American Acculturation Scale: Development, reliability, and validity. *Journal of Black Psychology, 20,* 104–127.

Landrine, H., & Klonoff, E. A. (1996). *African American acculturation: Deconstructing race and reviving culture.* Thousand Oaks, CA: Sage.

Landrine, H., & Klonoff, E. A. (2004). Culture change and ethnic-minority health behavior: An operant theory of acculturation. *Journal of Behavioral Medicine, 27,* 527–552.

Leung, P., LaChapelle, A. R., Scinta, A., & Olvera, N. (2014). Factors contributing to depressive symptoms among Mexican Americans and Latinos. *Social Work, 59,* 42–51.

Lewis-Fernández, R., & Aggarwal, N. K. (2013). Culture and psychiatric diagnosis. *Advances in Psychosomatic Medicine, 33,* 15–30.

Lovejoy, P. E. (1997). The African diaspora: Revisionist interpretations of ethnicity, culture, and religion under slavery. *Studies in the world history of slavery, abolition, and emancipation, II.* Toronto, ONT: York University.

McGruder, H. F., Malarcher, A. M., Antonie, T. L., Greenlund, K. J., & Croft, J. B. (2004). Racial and ethnic disparities in cardiovascular risk factors among stroke survivors: United States 1999 to 2001. *Stroke, 35,* 1557–1561.

Miller, W. R., & Rollnick, S. (2012). *Motivational Interviewing: Helping people change* (3rd ed.). New York, NY: Guilford Press.

Myers, H. F., & Rodriguez, N. (2002). Acculturation and physical health in racial and ethnic minorities. In K. M. Chun, P. B. Organista, and G. Marin (Eds.), *Acculturation: Advances in theory, measurement, and applied research* (pp. 165–163). Washington, DC: American Psychological Association.

Nava, G. (1983). *El norte* [Motion picture]. New York, NY: Cinecom.

Niemeier, J. P., Burnett, D. M., & Whitaker, D. A. (2003). Cultural competence in the multidisciplinary rehabilitation setting: Are we falling short of meeting needs? *Archives of Physical Medicine and Rehabilitation, 84,* 1240–1245.

O'Brien, K., Cokkinides, V., Jemal, A., Cardinez, C. J., Murray, T., Samuels, A., . . . Thun, M. J. (2003). Cancer statistics for Hispanics. *California Cancer Journal Clinic, 53,* 208–226.

Oliveira, J. M., Austin, A. A., Miyamoto, R. E., Kaholokula, J. K., Yano, K. B., & Lunasco, T. (2006). The Rural Hawai'i Behavioral Health Program: Increasing access to primary care behavioral health for Native Hawaiians in rural settings. *Professional Psychology: Research & Practice, 37,* 174–182.

Osorio, J. K. (2002). *Dismembering Lahui: A history of the Hawaiian nation to 1887.* Honolulu, HI: University of Hawai'i Press.

Pinkney, A. (1993). *Black Americans* (4th ed.). Englewood Cliffs, NJ: Simon & Schuster.

Ponton, M. O., & Leon-Carrion, J. (2001). *Neuropsychology and the Hispanic patient: A clinical handbook.* Mahwah, NJ: Erlbaum.

Pukui, M. K., Haertig, E. W., & Lee, C. A. (1972). *Nānā I Ke Kumu: Look to the source, vols. I & II.* Honolulu, HI: Queen Lili'uokalani Children's Center.

Reynolds, C. R. (2000). Methods for detecting and evaluating cultural bias in neuropsychological tests. In E. Fletcher-Janzen, T. L. Strickland, & C. R. Reynolds (Eds.), *Handbook of cross-cultural neuropsychology* (pp. 249–285). New York, NY: Kluwer Academic.

Rezentes, W. C. (1996). *Ka Lama Kukui: Hawaiian psychology: An introduction.* Honolulu, HI: 'A'ali'i Books.

Rogers-Sirin, L. (2013). Segmented assimilation and attitudes toward psychotherapy: A moderated mediation analysis. *Journal of Counseling Psychology, 60,* 329–339.

Sandoval, J. (1998). Critical thinking in test interpretation. In J. Sandoval, C. L., Frisby, K. F., Geisinger, J. D., Scheuneman, & J. R. Grenier (Eds.), *Test interpretation and diversity: Achieving equity in assessment* (pp. 31–49). Washington, DC: American Psychological Association.

Snowden, L. R., & Hines, A. M. (1999). A scale to assess African American acculturation. *Journal of Black Psychology, 25,* 36–47.

Stampp, K. M. (1956). *The peculiar institution: Slavery in the ante-bellum South.* New York, NY: Random House.

Stannard, D. (1989). *Before the horror: The population of Hawai'i at the eve of Western contact.* Honolulu, HI: Social Science Research Institute, University of Hawai'i.

State of Hawaii Data Book. (2005). *State of Hawai'i data book: A statistical abstract.* Honolulu, HI: Hawai'i State Department of Health.

Steffen, P. R., Smith, T. B., Larson, M., & Butler, L. (2006). Acculturation to Western society as a risk factor for high blood pressure: A meta-analytic review. *Psychosomatic Medicine, 68,* 386–397.

Szapocznik, J., Scopetta, M. A., Kurtines, W., & de los Angeles Aranalde, M. (1978). Theory and measurement of acculturation. *Inter-American Journal of Psychology, 12,* 113–130.

U.S. Census Bureau. (2001). *The Native Hawaiian and other Pacific Islander population: 2000.* Washington DC: U.S. Department of Commerce, Economics and Statistics Administration.

U.S. Department of Health and Human Services. (2001). *National standards for culturally and linguistically appropriate services in health care. Final report.* Retrieved from http://minorityhealth.hhs.gov/assets/pdf/checked/final report.pdf

Utsey, S. O., Bolden, M. A., & Brown, A. (2000). Vision of revolution from the spirit of Frantz Fanon: A psychology of liberation for counseling African Americans confronting societal racism and oppression. In J. Ponterotto, J.

Casas, L. Suzuki, & C. Alexander (Eds.), *Multicultural counseling handbook* (2nd ed.). Thousand Oaks, CA: Sage.

Valdez, J. S. (2000). Psychotherapy with bicultural Hispanic clients. *Psychotherapy, 37,* 240–246.

Venner, K. L., Feldstein, S. W., & Tafoya, N. (2008). Helping clients feel welcome: Principles of adapting treatment cross-culturally. *Alcohol Treatment Quarterly, 25,* 11–30.

Walker, R. L., Wingate, L. R., Obasi, E. M., & Joiner, T. E. (2008). An empirical investigation of acculturative stress and ethnic identity as moderators for depression and suicidal ideation in college students. *Cultural Diversity and Ethnic Minority Psychology, 14,* 75–82.

Yuen, N. Y. C., Nahulu, L. B., Hishinuma, E. S., & Miyamoto, R. H. (2000). Cultural identification and attempted suicide in Native Hawaiian adolescents. *Journal of the American Academy of Child and Adolescent Psychiatry, 39,* 360–367.

Zane, N., & Mak, W. (2003). Major approaches to the measurement of acculturation among ethnic minority populations: A content analysis and an alternative empirical strategy. In K. M. Chun, P. B. Organista, and G. Marin (Eds.), *Acculturation: Advances in theory, measurement, and applied research* (pp. 30–60). Washington, DC: American Psychological Association.

PART THREE

SPECIAL TOPICS IN MULTICULTURAL NEUROREHABILITATION

CHAPTER SEVEN

DISABILITY CULTURE:
AN ETHICS PERSPECTIVE

Thomas R. Kerkhoff and Stephanie L. Hanson

*I*n the 2002 revision of the American Psychological Association's (APA) *Ethical Principles of Psychologists and Code of Conduct*, "culture" was added to Ethical Standard 2.01: Boundaries of Competence (APA, 2002). Although it was always aspirational, the revision made cultural competence an enforceable practice standard; therefore, understanding the significance of cultural differences became mandatory for competent, ethical medical practice. In that same year, the APA (2002) released *Guidelines on Multicultural Education, Training, Research, Practice, and Organizational Change for Psychologists* and, in 2013, *Guidelines for Psychological Practice in Health Care Delivery Systems.* All of these publications reflected the broader sociopolitical climate, changing demographics, and need for psychology to pay more attention to cultural issues and the meaning of cultural competence. Cultural competence is a complex construct that has traditionally focused on ethnicity, race, and social and economic disadvantage. With changes in federal policy supporting the rights of individuals with disabilities and the growth of the disability rights movement, disability has been increasingly recognized as a distinct cultural concept (Brown, 2002; Lotan & Ells, 2010). Brain injuries can result in significant impairments and make it necessary for both patients and their families to redefine their identities internally and in relation to one another. In this chapter, we examine disability identity as a unique area in which the clinician working with individuals with brain injuries must become culturally competent. We begin with an overview of the disability rights movement and its influence on disability identity as a construct. We then discuss critical issues in cultural competence and how these intersect with ethical practice in working with individuals and families with neurorehabilitation needs. We conclude with suggestions regarding cultural competence that transcend individual diagnoses, although we clearly recognize that disability is not a uniform construct and that cultural differences can create unique challenges in acquiring a skill set consistent with competent ethical practice.

THE DISABILITY RIGHTS MOVEMENT

The civil rights of individuals with disabilities have been influenced by a broad range of legislative, regulatory, and social efforts throughout U.S. history, from the founding of the School for the Deaf in 1817, to the creation of Social Security Disability Insurance in 1956, to the passing of the Americans with Disabilities Act (ADA) in 1990. Although advocacy efforts can be dated back to at least the early 19th century, people with disabilities generally have been marginalized by society as a whole for much of U.S. and world history. People with certain disabilities did not have access to buildings, mainstream schools, varied social strata, competitive employment, or appropriate health care. Eugenics, or forced sterilization of individuals with disabilities, was ruled constitutional in 1927, and 30 states subsequently implemented eugenics-related laws (Disability Justice, 2015). Individuals with disabilities were often treated as noncitizens and locked away in institutions (Anti-Defamation League, 2005). As Longmore (1985) stated, "Stigma is the assumption that stigmatized persons are less human than the rest of us" (p. 421). As recently as 50 years ago, there were no handicapped parking spaces, no power doors or ramps to make it easier for individuals in wheelchairs to enter buildings, no bus lifts for wheelchairs, and no auditory floor markers or Braille labels in elevators. It was not until the mid-20th century that the disability rights movement gained significant sociopolitical momentum. This intersected with advances in technology that improved the survival rates for individuals who sustained catastrophic injuries, especially after World Wars I and II, and who demanded better care and access to public places.

Shapiro (2012) credits the birth of the modern disability rights movement to Edward Roberts, who was left quadriplegic after having polio. In 1962, Edwards had to go to court to win the right to attend the University of California, Berkeley, and his efforts led to the breakdown of the structural and attitudinal barriers that many individuals with disabilities had to face at that time. (Ten years later, Roberts founded the Center for Independent Living.) When President Lyndon Johnson signed the Civil Rights Act into law in 1964, grass-roots organizational efforts by and for people with disabilities really caught fire. Although the Act did not include disability as a basis for protection from discrimination, the legislation served as a catalyst for people with disabilities to expect and demand equal rights, shifting the disability model from medical to social. (See Olkin, 2002, for a comparison of disability models.) These efforts broadened the sociocultural landscape from perceiving people with disabilities based primarily on medical diagnoses and physical limitations to being a minority group oppressed by external circumstances and societal barriers that could be fundamentally changed (Lee & Ramsey, 2006; Welch & Palames, 1995; Tables 7.1 and 7.2; for examples of expanded time lines of events, see San Francisco State University, 2015; Federal Transit Administration, 2015.)

Two pieces of landmark legislation, the Rehabilitation Act of 1973 and the ADA of 1990, are considered victories for the disability rights movement and reflect the change in focus from medical limitations to limitations imposed by societal barriers. Section 504 of the Rehabilitation Act, which was modeled after the Civil Rights Act, defined disability as a

Table 7.1 *Historical Legislative Actions*

Year	Action	Result
1920	The Smith–Fess Act (Civilian Rehabilitation Act)—amended multiple times since to broaden services, such as the 1943 Barden–LaFollette Act and the 1954 VR amendments	The role of the Federal Board of Vocational Rehabilitation (VR) expands the Soldiers Rehabilitation Act to include all individuals with disabilities; therefore, federal dollars for vocational training for people with disabilities was guaranteed for the first time. 1943 Amendment: Physical rehabilitation added to federally funded VR programs and made states accountable for VR plans. 1954 Amendment: Funding authorized for university-based rehabilitation programs; increased funding for training rehabilitation professionals and research and demonstration grants

(continued)

Table 7.1 *Historical Legislative Actions (continued)*

Year	Action	Result
1935	Social Security Act passed (amended multiple times since 1935 to clarify disability benefits; most notably 1956, when Social Security Disability Insurance was implemented, 1958 when dependent benefits were added, and 1965 when Medicaid and Medicare were established)	Initially provided funds to states for vocational rehabilitation for individuals with physical disabilities, aid to needy individuals who were blind, and "crippled" children to access reasonable medical services. Amendments established disability benefits and Medicaid and Medicare established to provide federally subsidized health care coverage to people with disabilities.
1943	Barden–LaFollette Act (amended from the Smith–Fess Act)	Physical rehabilitation added to federally funded vocational rehabilitation programs.
1946	Hill–Burton Act	Funding established to build rehabilitation hospitals.
1964	Civil Rights Act	Major discrimination protection based on race, gender, national origin, and religion; disability not included but laid groundwork for Rehabilitation Act.
1968	Architectural Barriers Act	Previous acts to facilitate employment had not addressed structural barriers; this act requires all federal buildings to be accessible.
1973	Rehabilitation Act, including Section 504, was passed and subsequently amended multiple times to expand and clarify who qualifies (definition of disability) and the types of services provided	Civil rights of persons with disabilities legally protected in federally funded programs; supported removal of transportation, architectural, and employment barriers.
1975	Education for All Handicapped Act	Children with disabilities given equal access to education; included provision for support services.
	Renamed Individuals with Disabilities Education Act in 1990	Added covered services. Parents have right to be included in educational programming via individualized education plans (IEPs).

(continued)

Table 7.1 *Historical Legislative Actions (continued)*

Year	Action	Result
1990	Americans with Disabilities Act— amended in 2008 (referred to as the ADA Amendments Act [ADAAA] of 2008)	Sweeping antidiscrimination protection for persons with disabilities; equal access to employment and government services, including transportation, public accommodations, telecommunications; reasonable accommodations required; amended to clarify and broaden definition of disability to return to inclusiveness intended in 1990 after restrictive judicial rulings.

Table 7.2 *Grass-Roots Activism and Advocacy Efforts*

Year	Action	Result
1817	Connecticut Asylum for the Education and Instruction of Deaf and Dumb Persons (renamed American School for the Deaf) established by Thomas Gallaudet in response to a need raised by Mason Cogswell, whose daughter became deaf from scarlet fever in 1807	One of first American schools organized to provide education to people with disabilities, with financial support being substantially provided by the state.
1948	National Paraplegia Foundation, established by members of Paralyzed Veterans of America	Serves as strong advocate for disability rights.
1948	Howard Rusk establishes the Institute of Rehabilitation Medicine in New York	Establishes "whole person" treatment model for rehabilitation and uses interdisciplinary approach, establishing foundation for modern rehabilitation practice.
1962	Ed Roberts, who had quadriplegia as a result of polio as a child, admitted to University of California, Berkeley	Exerted pressure on university to become more accessible; credited with beginning the modern disability rights (and independent living) movement in which people with disabilities empower themselves as change agents.

(*continued*)

Table 7.2 *Grass-Roots Activism and Advocacy Efforts (continued)*

Year	Action	Result
1962	President's Committee on Employment of the Physically Handicapped is renamed, removing the word *Physically*	Places more focus on people with cognitive and mental health issues.
1977	Sit-in protests in federal buildings across the country mobilized in response to slow implementation of Section 504 of the Rehabilitation Act	Brought together different disability groups; after 100 protestors staged a sit-in at the U.S. Department of Health, Education, and Welfare (HEW) in San Francisco, the HEW secretary endorsed the regulations 28 days later.
1978	19 protesters block a nonaccessible city bus in Denver	Raised awareness of inaccessible public transportation; credited with starting the American Disabled for Accessible Public Transportation (ADAPT) civil rights movement and influencing passage of the Americans with Disabilities Act (ADA).
1978	National Council on Disability established (became an independent agency in 1984)	Formal recognition within the Department of Education of the importance of advocacy for persons with disabilities; responsibilities include promoting policies and programs supporting equal opportunity; involved in drafting the ADA of 1990 and passage of amendments in 2008; responsible for monitoring the effectiveness of the ADA.
2004	First Disability Pride parade organized	Organized to break down attitudinal barriers; 1,500 to 2,000 people were estimated to have attended when only 500 to 600 were predicted.
2006	West Virginia Youth Disability Caucus champions House Bill 4491 to establish Disability History Week in all West Virginia public schools	Spurs a youth movement in other states to create similar foci on disability history in the public school system.

civil rights issue. In other words, some of the challenges people with disabilities faced in their daily lives were no longer considered characteristics of the disability itself but instead were the result of discriminatory practices resulting in exclusion. That said, equal treatment under the law was not the same as for other minority groups covered under the Civil

Rights Act, because people with disabilities still faced accessibility issues. Section 504 of the Rehabilitation Act required that all federally supported programs must provide reasonable access to individuals with disabilities. It took another 17 years and the successful passage of the ADA to expand that right to persons with disabilities in both the public and private sectors. The ADA states, "The continuing existence of unfair and unnecessary discrimination and prejudice denies people with disabilities the opportunity to compete on an equal basis and to pursue those opportunities for which our free society is justifiably famous." The ADA is considered the most powerful civil rights legislation affecting disabilities because it established the constitutional right of equal protection. It has also had an impact on disability rights laws around the globe. Mayerson (2007) described its basic principles as "the rejection of paternalism, the right to self-determination, and the dignity of making choices about risks" (p. 267). These grass-roots and legislative efforts focused attention squarely on the need for societal transformation, even as discrimination continued and funding for services was limited.

Today, although significant progress has been made, the summit of the mountain has not yet been reached. Civil rights protections have been eroded to a certain extent, and entrenched cultures have been slow to change. Mpofu, Chronister, Johnson, and Denham (2012) stated, "Sociocultural understanding influences how those with disabilities are categorized and the nature of services they are provided" (p. 543). Surprisingly, it has been the U.S. Supreme Court that has negatively impacted some of the progress of the disability rights movement. Under the ADA, the definition of "disability" encompasses three parts: the person must have a physical or mental impairment that limits one or more major activities of daily living, and the person must either have a record of impairment or must be regarded as having such impairment (ADA, Article I). Being "regarded as having such impairment" is when an individual is fired just because the employer sees the individual as disabled, even though he or she is capable of doing the job. This three-part definition has proven critical in discrimination cases brought by individuals with disabilities, several of which are highlighted in Mayerson (2007), Mayerson and Mayer (2000), and the National Council on Disability (see, for example, Frieden, 2005). In essence, the Court began considering whether one meets the definition of disability when compensatory strategies or assistive devices ameliorate its physical effects and what the demands of the disability have to be. In *Sutton v. United Airlines, Inc.,* for example, the airline refused to hire two individuals who did not meet the company's vision requirements without eyeglasses, although glasses improved their vision sufficiently to meet the requirements. The court dismissed the case, stating that the plaintiffs did not meet the second part of the definition in which a major life activity was impaired. So, in essence, the company used disability as an excuse not to hire the plaintiffs, but, according to the court, the plaintiffs were not disabled enough to win their case. Mpofu et al. (2012) explained that disability is often defined partly by the individual's functional limitations compared to those without disabilities in a similar environment, which may offer one conceptual basis for evaluating this type of decision. The ADA was amended in 2008 to correct the effects of the Supreme Court rulings, including eliminating consideration of items such as medications and assistive devices in determining whether impairment is truly disabling. The successful passage of the amendments required activism and advocacy by a number of citizen, governmental, and legislative groups, proving that the public was ahead of the courts in accepting disability as a civil rights issue across a broad range of individuals and circumstances. That said, full implementation of the ADA has been challenging, limited by both lack of knowledge and continuing attitudinal barriers. In its 2007 report entitled *The Impact of the Americans with Disabilities Act: Assessing the Progress Toward Achieving the Goals of the Americans with Disabilities Act*, the National Council on Disability (2007) said the following:

> Many people with disabilities credit the ADA with improving their lives. As consumers, Americans with disabilities have greater access to goods and services from businesses, state and local governments, and their local communities. . . . As workers, people with disabilities are more likely to receive accommodations and less likely to be terminated due to their disabilities. Many people with disabilities, employers, and businesses, however, still do not understand major provisions of the ADA, particularly the employment provisions. (p. 9)

> Many Americans with disabilities remain frustrated that disability discrimination has not been eliminated, despite ADA implementation. People with disabilities report that the ADA has not been fully enforced and that the barriers they face remain primarily attitudinal. Additionally, the backlash against disability rights and the ADA has been growing. The lack of national consistency of access makes it difficult for people with disabilities to carry out daily activities. (p. 10)

Significant disparities [also] exist in access to health insurance and health care for people with disabilities, . . . and economic self-sufficiency remains elusive for too many people with disabilities. (pp. 105–106)

These findings are echoed worldwide. See the 2011 World Health Organization's (WHO) *World Report on Disability*.

In addition, although access to education is improving, graduation rates and subsequent employment for persons with disabilities are lower than for their peers. Davis (2011) reported that colleges have not effectively integrated disability as a construct in diversity discussions. He explains, "If diversity rejects the idea of a normal ethnicity, it has no problem with the notion of the normal in a medical sense, which means, of course, it has no problem with branding some bodies and minds normal and some abnormal. As long as disability is seen in this medical sense, it will therefore be considered abnormal and outside the healthy, energetic bodies routinely depicted in celebrations of diversity" (p. 3). Davis questions whether disability can ever be recognized as a valid human identity, given the way our society looks at diversity. This, of course, assumes that our values and definitions of diversity are nonmalleable, which is not the case. Concepts formed by theoretical constructs can clearly be challenged by practical experience, wherein negative perceptions of persons with disabilities are shown to be decreasing (WHO, 2011). Wright (1983) explained that "the positive context of a person constrained the negative spread" (p. 56), meaning someone's personal biases against people with disabilities based on individual characteristics can be eliminated by personal contact with such people. Also, as practical experience gains social footing, the concept of what diversity represents can shift, which has been the case over time in our social characterization of disability. For example, people who are unable to find employment are no longer considered "the problem," and the impact of this shift in public policy has been fairly broad. The disability rights movement has had a significant impact on the protections against discrimination that now exist, which have largely followed traditional patterns of other minority groups toward inclusion.

Although we still have a long way to go, other movements have had an impact. For example, Page, Castillo-Page, Poll-Hunter, Garrison, and Wright (2013) found that approximately 30% of academic health centers now include persons with disabilities among their targeted groups for diversity programs. This percentage is not what it should be, but it was presented no differently than the inclusion of any other group. The focus of this survey was not on medical diagnosis but on service to an under-served population. From this perspective, the focus is on the benefits we gain from cultural diversity, not on medical diagnoses that create physical or cognitive limitations. This is progress. The disability rights movement also has undergone a fairly recent paradigm shift, focused not just on an absence of discrimination but on the advantages of having a disability and how it can actually enrich one's life. Embracing disability is also reflected in the change from person-first language to the use of the term Disabled Person. In other words, instead of defining someone as "disabled," "person with a disability" demonstrates that the disability does not define the person but reflects a social construct (Olkin, 2002). From a human rights perspective, this position is consistent with actions of social justice supporting diversity, thereby reducing stigma and marginalization based on disability. Brown (2002) pointed out that difference is to be celebrated, but to do so, we must move beyond the social construct of oppression toward a viewpoint in which living with disability is valuable in and of itself.

The sociocultural shift has also directly impacted the role of health care providers and counselors. Gill, Kewman, and Brannon (2003) pre-sented an excellent discussion on the impact of sociopolitical change on psychology policy, advocacy, and practice. Psychologists working in neurorehabilitation increasingly serve as patient advocates and change agents who help individuals with disabilities remove social and organi-zational barriers as part of maximizing independence. Therefore, the psy-chologist is balancing the intrapersonal identity of the individual and the broader cultural identity within the social context. In essence, professional practice has been significantly influenced by social justice—for example, the psychologist must supply information to the client about access to work, school, and further health care after discharge. However, how an individual defines herself and her disability affects her receptivity to such advocacy. In the case of stroke or traumatic brain injury, this can be further complicated by the occurrence of denial as a coping mechanism in post-injury adaptation. Therefore, to facilitate maximum independence, we must understand how the individuals we serve shape their own disability identity in the health care system, in both their preexisting and emerging cultural experiences, and in a shifting social landscape and inconsistent judicial system. We consider the health care system's influence as a cultural factor in the next section.

Disability Culture

Fyffe and Lequerica (2013) define "culture" as shared beliefs and practices within shared attributes. Mpofu et al. (2012) present a similar definition and describe "culture" as a "major prism through which social perceptions are formed and applied unto others, which in turn, categorizes persons on a single or few qualities" (p. 544). Therefore, at any given time, an individual is viewed and acquires self-efficacy via intersecting cultures (e.g., race, gender, geography); in neurorehabilitation, a primary one is disability culture. Disability culture is especially relevant to exercising professional responsibility in the context of the neurorehabilitation environment, which is tasked with justifying its social worth to health care policy makers with measures of success in posttreatment community (cultural) reintegration. (See Ashing-Giwa, 2005, for a contextual model of health-related quality-of-life, in which culture, demographics, social-ecological, and health care contexts are shown to be interrelated.)

To clarify the concept of disability culture, let us first consider familiar "niche cultures" that are contextually defined and often layered over ethnic/racial cultural foundations. Some examples of niche cultures are individuals with developmental and acquired disabilities, individuals in active military service or who qualify for veterans benefits, individuals who are incarcerated, survivors of geographically localized natural disasters, individuals who play collegiate or professional sports, and even the employees of corporations that emphasize the development of culture kinship among their staff. (See Tilley, Fredricks, and Hornett, 2012, regarding corporate kinship; see Galer, 2012, and Budd, 2011, regarding the role of employment in the formation of disability identity.) The members of these niche cultures share common social and personal experiences (narratives) by virtue of what they have in common and the group they belong to. These experiences in turn guide the acquisition of adaptive behaviors, including (a) the start of cultural immersion (injury/illness onset, induction into military service or the VA health care system, recruitment into a sports program); (b) learning to navigate the social nuances of these varied niche cultures to improve the chances of successful membership, advancement, and sometimes survival; and (c) reconciling preexisting social beliefs/values and behavioral patterns related to identifying with new niche cultural expectations that can affect inclusion. Culturally competent health care professionals who work in such niche populations must become thoroughly familiar with the social characteristics of daily living within those cultural contexts. For example, the psychologists who worked with military personnel who sustained catastrophic injuries in Iraq and Afghanistan had to become familiar with war-related terminology (e.g., Operation Iraqi Freedom, Operation Enduring Freedom) to be credible to their clients. Acquisition of cultural knowledge, experience, and evaluative/intervention competencies pertinent to these niche cultures during training are fundamental to culturally relevant practice. (See Mpofu et al., 2012, for descriptions of various cultural conceptualizations of disability and rehabilitation.)

In the case of the acquired disability culture, immersion of the individual is often abrupt and can be both physically and emotionally traumatic. Preimmersion preparation is rare, because inclusion in the acquired disability culture is usually unexpected. Thus, the introduction to disability cultural immersion occurs in various segments of the health care system continuum, each of which represents its own subculture, from emergency or trauma services/intensive care units, to inpatient acute or subacute rehabilitation programs, to home health services, to outpatient treatment, until the initial rehabilitative treatment course is completed. In the case of cognitive impairment, the individual's ability to understand all these changes may be difficult or take longer than usual. Thus, the introduction to disability culture is often inextricably intertwined with the health care system, often in the context of an initially dependent relationship. In addition, long-term intermittent contact with the health care system is often required to maintain health. Contact with health maintenance resources can serve as a reminder of the differences the individual has experienced in functional ability as a result of the disability-producing event. Whether this ongoing contact takes on negative or positive emotional valence depends on the degree to which the individual secures a stable postinjury or postillness disability identity and an adaptive relationship with key health care professionals, which actively fosters the process of identity formation and maintenance.

Most important, according to Mpofu, et al. (2012), there are "cultural ways of defining functioning, disability, and health and culturally driven approaches to addressing the health and rehabilitation needs of persons with disabilities" (p. 545). While the disability rights movement detailed earlier in this chapter emphasizes the social construct of disability, the foundations of rehabilitation psychology embrace an interaction model in which the medical and social models converge and on which the WHO's definition of "disability" is based. Psychologists in rehabilitation settings operate from the fundamental premise that disability is shaped by a combination of the effects of one's state of health, diagnosis, and functional abilities (physical, cognitive, etc.); coping skills; caregiver and broader social support; and environment, which is broadly defined as the structures within which one lives (e.g., community, recreation, work). In addition, as Mpofu et al. (2012) pointed out, having an impairment is only one of the several factors that impact social reengagement after injury. In this conceptual orientation, disability identity involves an integration of multiple components and an evaluative process of finding meaning in inconsistencies in social messages, comparisons with familial and personal perceptions of one's self both before and after the injury, and identification as a member of a specific minority group with social constructions of what disability and humanness attached to it represent. This perspective necessitates the recognition that both the patient and his or her family have grown up with specific beliefs and stereotypes about disability shaped by social mores within their support systems and communities, personal experience, and knowledge of disability issues. The changes in functional ability—probably including the ability to reason— that the individual with stroke or traumatic brain injury experiences during the long rehabilitation process can complicate matters further. Considering that one of our rehabilitation goals is to facilitate patient autonomy, as psychologists we need to understand the redevelopment of the patient's self as an individual with a disability nested in the broader societal context.

Acceptance of the reality of physical and cognitive functional changes in persons served by health care professionals is virtually universal in the social context of the health care system. Indeed, such change is the focus of evaluation, intervention, and care. However, upon return to the community, transitional identity conflict related to "cultural fit" can occur. For example, what is the practical applicability of a new set of functional and social skills that are adaptive in the context of the neurorehabilitation environment to home and community environments? It is important to remember that recovery is often tacitly defined by both patients and family members as the degree of return to preinjury or preillness functional, cognitive, and social capacities. Acculturation (seeking readmission to the dominant culture) is considered a social requirement by some, but others consider it as potentially forfeiting disability identity and disability culture affiliation. The process of discovering a position of social equilibrium within transition to the community after rehabilitation remains a key focus of intervention regarding emotional adjustment to disability and associated identity intertwined with this adjustment.

Sue and Sue (2008) presented a comprehensive model for counseling the culturally diverse that includes consideration of persons with disabilities in a cultural context. Gill (1997), on the other hand, presented a more topically focused and compelling model that consisted of four types of integration. In his model, integration represents the discovery of who one is and where one belongs—forming both individual and group identities that involve "at least temporary relinquishment of self, and reconfiguration of relationships to others and society" (p. 42). The four types of integration include the following:

- Coming to feel we belong (integrating into society). This represents the patient's right to be considered an equal in society. Rehabilitation psychologists and neuropsychologists contribute to this process by conducting school or work reentry assessments and cognitive evaluations in the context of activities of daily living and by offering accessibility recommendations.
- Coming home (integrating with the disability community). This represents the patient's discovery of commonality and the benefits of being with others who have disabilities. It also involves letting go of negative stereotypes regarding people with disabilities as a group and/or inferiority by association. Rehabilitation psychologists, in particular, contribute to this by facilitating contacts with peers to assist with coping and discharge referrals to community support groups and resources. This represents a proactive effort in small communities where individuals with disabilities and disability support resources may exist but without an established integration network.
- Coming together (internally integrating our similarities and differences). This represents the discovery of self-identity as a whole, not just the part that is not disabled (e.g., physical strength when one has a brain injury). This requires rejecting the devaluation of oneself based on negative social messages and embracing both the similarities and differences within oneself, with one's own previous

self, and with others. Psychologists contribute to this through interventions aimed at normalizing grief for losses of previous self, rebuilding self-esteem, facilitating self-discovery and autonomous decision making, and addressing the person's changed roles within the family.

- Coming out (integrating how we feel about presenting ourselves). This represents the blending of the ideal and the real selves, with internal conflict and social discomfort about one's identity removed. The psychologist facilitates this discovery by helping determine reasonable expectations for performance based on cognitive recovery, encouraging exploration of social roles individually and with the family, encouraging return to daily routines (work, school, etc.) with or without any needed compensatory strategies, and reaching out to others. This complex socialization process is often facilitated in postacute rehabilitation programs.

Individuals with neurorehabilitation needs may look the same as before the injury but think and act very differently. Learning to become an autonomous person usually occurs only after everyone's world is turned upside down, from having to relearn common tasks to interacting with one another and redefining familial roles. While the acute care environment reveals the changes that have occurred, the rehabilitation environment becomes the first step in the integration process. It is critical to note that we are not conceptualizing integration as an adaptation to the majority culture but rather as a process of centering one's life in a way that has personal meaning and value, resulting in benefit to both the individual and society.

Cultural Competence

This brings us back to the concept of cultural competence—impacting the psychologist's skills in supporting disability identity development and cultural integration in new ways for those we serve. The 2013 American Psychological Association *Guidelines for Psychological Practice in Health Care Delivery Systems* addressed cultural competence in Guideline 9:

It is important that they [psychologists in health care practice] maintain cultural competence for health care delivery to diverse patient groups, including specific competence for working with patients of varying gender, race and ethnicity, language, culture, socioeconomic status, sexual orientation, religious orientation and disabilities. (p. 5)

Additionally, in the APA's multicultural care clinician's guide, Comas-Diaz (2012) emphasized that the most important factor motivating well-trained psychologists to engage with multicultural individuals is the desire to do so. Fortunately, in the field of neurorehabilitation, the members of the treatment team are singularly dedicated to providing high-quality evaluation, intervention, and care to individuals with neurological disabilities, affecting not only recovery of central nervous system function but ultimately influencing adaptive lifestyle and social role viability.

The importance of cultural competence cannot be overstated. Cultural competence is not simply a critical part of the training process for psychologists because of the changing U.S. demographics and the prevalence of disability (e.g., one in four Americans, 1.7 million traumatic brain injuries and 795,000 strokes each year; Centers for Disease Control and Prevention [CDC], 2013). It may, however, be a key factor in being able to successfully close the health disparities gap. Despite significant efforts to address health disparities in our country (and throughout the world), they still exist in large numbers among minority populations. Our failure to systematically educate psychologists and other health care providers to incorporate culture as a core tenet of service delivery may be a crucial piece of this puzzle. If a psychologist is not able to provide culturally appropriate evaluations and treatment to clients with disabilities, it may lead to cultural insensitivity (e.g., to others' beliefs, practices, and worldviews), ineffectiveness (e.g., inappropriate language, poorly adapted tools), or, worst of all, unethical practices that may actually cause harm (e.g., missed diagnoses, mismatched treatment recommendations). The end result is that consumers do not access new and/or continuing psychological services that are needed, particularly if the provider is seen as lacking cultural credibility. Instead, as Salter and Salter (2012) stated, "Psychologists are charged to push the boundaries of their comfort zones and act as true agents of change in promoting fairness, justice, and access to exemplary professional services" (p. 235).

Cultural Competence Defined

Now that we know cultural competence is integral to contemporary psychological practice, we still need to understand exactly what cultural competence is. Many definitions of cultural or multicultural competence have been promulgated in the literature. (See, for example, the classic work by Sue, Arrendondo, and McDavis, 1992, on competence with ethnic minorities, and the summative work by Mollen, Ridley, and Hill, 2003.) As an example of critical components of cultural competence in the counseling field, Lee and Ramsey (2006) suggest that providers (a) consider each person as a unique individual; (b) simultaneously consider shared experience as a human being; (c) take into account the cultural backgrounds of the individual; and (d) pay attention to one's own cultural experiences. They caution not to use "the one-size-fits-all" approach, which can lead to unintended stereotyping, and to be aware of cultural dynamics to prevent ethical pitfalls in providing treatment. In the case of acquired disability, reconciling the individual's cultural background with new niche culture expectations represents an important factor to guide the health care professional in treatment plan development.

A somewhat different, yet common, conceptualization of cultural competence is aligned with psychology's broader competency movement. That is, psychologists must have the knowledge, skills, and awareness of cultural similarities and differences to practice competently. Balcazar, Suarez-Balcazar, and Taylor-Ritzler (2009) offered evidence that supported these three components in one of the few empirically validated models of competence. They analyzed the literature to identify common components among cultural competence models that were based on some type of conceptual framework. These overlapping components served as the basis for the creation of their own synthesized model that consisted of three components: critical awareness and knowledge, skills development, and a new factor called organizational support. It was hypothesized that organizational support emerged because psychologists' skills, knowledge, and actions are influenced by organizational policies and procedures in the context of the practice environment. In other words, it is easier to undergo the journey of becoming culturally competent if the organization has a supportive environment in which to do so. Psychologists' intentions and actions are indeed influenced by organizational structures and processes that can be either facilitative or hindering. However, even within restrictive organizations, psychologists can potentially practice in a culturally competent, ethical manner at the individual practice level. This would not be the case, however, if the psychologist lacked self-awareness regarding biases, beliefs, and attitudes; knew little about the client; and did not have the skills to effectively implement her services in a culturally sensitive manner.

Others have argued that sensitivity, knowledge, and skills are not enough to acquire intercultural competence. For example, Bennett (Hammer, Bennett, & Wiseman, 2003) developed the Developmental Model of Intercultural Sensitivity (DMIS), in which an individual's behavior and attitudes reflected his worldview. He proposed a worldview orientation ranging from three ethnocentric (e.g., defining one's worldview/value by one's own culture only) to three ethnorelative (e.g., evaluating and integrating information at multiple levels) stages, based on how a person evaluates and incorporates other cultures into his own identity. The underlying principle is that as "one's experience of cultural differences becomes more complex and sophisticated, one's potential competence in intercultural relations increases" (p. 423).

Bourjolly et al. (2005) and Pernell-Arnold, Linley, Sands, Bourjolly, and Stanhope (2013) applied Bennett's worldview model to demonstrate that intercultural sensitivity training can facilitate movement from ethnocentricity (avoiding cultural differences; entrenched in one's own worldview) to ethnorelativity (appreciating cultural differences; embracing differences in one's own identity). These two studies employed the PRIME training model in which participants described their cultural experiences in between training sessions. The stages reflected in these logs were then rated using Bennett's cultural worldview stages. The majority of participants, who were all mental health providers, showed positive change but in a nonlinear manner, suggesting that experiential integration is an important component for true transformation to occur. Pernell-Arnold et al. concluded that training models that target only first-order change (i.e., increasing sensitivity and knowledge) are insufficient for providers to transform their worldview to ultimately reduce health disparities. Training has to address second-order change (transforming the structure of one's worldview).

To further complicate this already complex process of attaining performance-validated cultural competency, two studies speak to the potentially different perceptions of the clinician and the client as necessary metrics of therapist cultural competence. Fuertes et al. (2006) discovered that therapist self-perceived multicultural competency was correlated with education and training. Clients, on the other hand, rated the therapists' professionalism, attractiveness, and trustworthiness as separate from perceived multicultural competence. Thus, in this study, a conceptual disconnect existed between the therapist's self-appraisal and the client's other-perception regarding multicultural competence. A study by Tummala-Narra, Singer, Li, Esposito, and Ash (2012) found that the UDO (universal-diverse orientation) of clinicians was related to access to and experience with training and resources (consultation with peers, open exploration of cultural values and beliefs)—a clinician-centered appraisal. This seems consistent with Pernell-Arnold et al.'s (2012) work given that the logs offered the opportunity for open exploration, and interpersonal group processes were believed critical to worldview change. However, in neither work was competency validated with persons served, although Pernell-Arnold et al.'s training included activities with social networks. Perhaps one can think about awareness and attitudes, knowledge, skills, and ultimately one's worldview as primary factors (part of competence) and organizational systems, inclusive of components such as peer review and open dialogue, as secondary factors (in support of developing competence) in shaping the psychologist's development as a culturally competent professional. However, the validation of the clinician's self-perceived cultural competence, even in an organizational environment that promotes, evaluates, and approves such preparation, must ultimately include the perceptions of persons served in the context of the treatment milieu.

So how does the psychologist fulfill his or her ethical obligations to provide culturally competent care, thereby facilitating a constructive therapeutic relationship and development of a culturally relevant integrated identity in individuals with cognitive deficits and neurorehabilitation needs? This requires behavior consistent with the principles and standards of the American Psychological Association's *Ethical Principles of Psychologists and Code of Conduct* (also called the Ethics Code; 2002).

The APA Ethics Code and Disability Culture

The APA Ethics Code addresses disability and cultural issues in both principles and standards. The Ethics Code provides the practitioner with field-tested guidelines for ethical professional conduct. As can be seen in the following breakdown of the Code as it relates to culture and disability, the guidelines are, for the most part, straightforward and relevant to daily practice.

Principle E: Respect for People's Rights and Dignity. This cites the importance of psychologists' awareness of and need for respecting cultural, individual, and role differences, including disability, among a variety of differentiating factors. The principle further acknowledges individual practitioner biases related to prejudices that should be eliminated from affecting professional activities.

Standard 2.01(b): Related to Boundaries of Competence. This requires that psychologists obtain the training, experience, consultation, or supervision necessary to ensure competence in delivering services to those individuals with disabilities (among other cultural factors).

Standard 3.01: Unfair Discrimination. This enjoins psychologists not to engage in unfair discrimination on the basis of disability (among other cultural factors) or any other basis proscribed by law.

Standard 3.03: Other Harassment. This prohibits psychologists from knowingly engaging in behavior that is harassing or demeaning to persons with whom they interact in their work based on cultural factors, including disability.

In more global terms, other standards within the Ethics Code require psychologists to accommodate the needs of the individuals they serve, including seeking the help of other professionals, and provide effective and appropriate service (Standard 3.09). Regarding informed consent for individuals with decisional capacity, the information provided must use language that the individual can understand (3.10[a]). In the case of individuals who are unable to make decisions, the psychologist must provide an appropriate explanation, seek the individual's assent, consider personal preferences (substituted judgment) and best interests, and obtain permission from a legally authorized person (if such permission is permitted or required by law) (3.10[b]).

In the case of assessment of individuals with disabilities, psychologists must document the efforts they made when instruments were subject to procedural modifications to accommodate the person served, clarifying the probable impact of those accommodations on reliability and validity, conclusions, and recommendations (9.01[b]). When assessment instruments do not have published reliability and validity data regarding use with individuals with disabilities, psychologists must describe the strengths and limitations of test results and limitations (9.02[b]). Regarding broader issues of language preference, psychologists must keep in mind alternative language relevance to the assessment (9.02[c]). In Standard 9.03(b)—a standard of special relevance to intellectual disabilities—psychologists must inform persons with questionable capacity to consent or for whom testing is mandated by law or governmental regulation about the nature of the proposed assessment, using language that is reasonably understandable by the person. In test construction, developers must use techniques that are appropriately validated on target populations (accounting for cultural factors) and reduce or eliminate bias (9.05). When interpreting assessment results, culture is acknowledged as a characteristic of the person served that must be formally addressed regarding interpretive judgments and interpretation accuracy.

Standards in the Ethics Code related to therapy are less directly prescriptive regarding cultural issues, including disability. Salter and Salter (2012) stated, "Psychologists are encouraged to ask themselves what personal and professional qualities and abilities are necessary for a positive interaction to occur" (p. 235). Indeed, the question of applicability of various psychotherapeutic techniques to individuals with disabilities has not yet been adequately addressed in the literature (see Woidneck, Pratt, Gundy, Nelson, and Twohig, 2012, for a discussion of acceptance and commitment therapy outcomes and cultural competence). Cartwright and Fleming (2010) suggested that the competent rehabilitation practitioner must develop services that are congruent with the values and cultural context of individuals with disabilities as interventional approaches evolve.

Using the preceding Ethics Code provisions regarding culturally sensitive practice in the context of neurorehabilitation, we can construct an ethically guided clinical process. The principle related to autonomy provides us with overarching guidance regarding an emphasis on patient-centered care and ensuring that the rights related to self-determination of those persons we serve are center-focused. Ethics standards enjoin us to be aware of the boundaries of our practice competencies, driving us to expand our clinical repertoire as necessary to meet the needs of individuals with disabilities, especially when they involve diagnoses with which we are not familiar. Included in the boundaries issue is the encouragement to seek peer consultation when faced with challenges. It appears on the surface that rehabilitations psychologists and neuropsychologists would have received adequate training to avoid situations involving discrimination or harassment. However, these concepts often consider personal values and biases that are sometimes not readily evident to us until a situation arises where our initial reactions may cause personal dismay, which can certainly occur when working with clients with different cultural values and traditions. When such circumstances occur, opportunities to self-evaluate become paramount. Such eye-opening situations remind us that both personal and professional growth are infinite processes.

Regarding the continuum of decisional capacity, the process of person-centered care demands preservation of adequate self-determination regarding health decisions. Evaluations revealing the extent of decisional capacity lead to clinical decisions that heavily influence rehabilitation team intervention at all levels of care. When capacity is rendered inoperative, ensuring that an adequately informed surrogate is in place is critical to reflecting the preferences and values of the person served.

When evaluating individuals whose cultural heritage and values differ from the normative group upon whom the test was validated, the clinician must carefully consider both language and culturally based factors in instrument selection (including language-validated parallel forms, using translators, etc.). In a special issue of *Neuropsychological Review* devoted to cultural considerations, Manly (2008) stated that "neuropsychological testing among culturally and linguistically diverse people is an area of critical vulnerability in the theoretical and empirical foundation for neuropsychological practice" (p. 179). Ongoing awareness of the development of new instruments that address such issues is paramount. When conducting evaluations with individuals with disabilities, the clinician should utilize the most technically and culturally relevant instruments available. However, many assessment instruments have not been sufficiently validated with the disability population to be directly applicable without functional modification (see Caplan and Shechter, 1995, for an excellent treatment of this topic). Caplan and Shechter state that the extent to which the clinician varies from normative administration and interpretation rubrics will be dictated by the functional needs of the person served. The effect that such accommodations have upon the interpretation of data generated must be guided by the environmental and cultural contexts in which the patient is living. It is incumbent upon the clinician to present justifications of accommodations made during assessment (regarding assessment and interpretation) that turn on the functional needs of the person served and the cultural context in which the test data will potentially have influence.

Finally, in treatment situations, cultural context is a fundamental factor that will influence both the treatment approach utilized and the culture-relevant data comprising treatment outcome evaluation. Culturally sensitive treatment approaches account for language and cultural preferences. This may entail the use of a translator when necessary, matching the complexity of conceptualization requirements to the cognitive skill level of the patient, and evaluating the language facility of the patient vis-à-vis the technical-conceptual demands of the treatment approach used. Additionally, the utility of any treatment approach is measured against the degree to which therapeutic strategies are successfully employed in the patient's everyday living environment and lead to adaptive behavior change, inferring acceptance by and support of the patient's family/social unit.

The authors recommend that the next iteration of the Ethics Code should specifically address the issue of utilizing culturally appropriate and validated therapy techniques targeted at the needs of the individuals and families served, especially those families with individuals who have disabilities. This recommendation is echoed by Gauthier, Pettifor, and Ferrero (2010), who call for a universal declaration of ethics principles and an ethics code that provides principles based on shared human values across cultures. Those authors acknowledge that the current Eastern and Western concepts of individual and family values are nested within different cultural traditions and are in need of reconciliation regarding applied ethics.

Applied Ethics and Culture

The literature on rehabilitation and psychology in general has not been silent on the issue of ethnic/racial and disability cultural relevance and professional activities. However, much more consideration of the former than the latter has been noted in published works. For example, Hanson and Kerkhoff (2007) dealt with ethical issues and the use of medical translators in the context of accurate representation of Latino cultural values during rehabilitation treatment. Gauthier et al. (2010) stated that psychologists are working in a globalizing world, where traditional boundaries (geographic, ethnic/racial, etc.) are losing relevance. In the context of professional training in rehabilitation psychology, a seminal paper by Stiers et al. (2012) details curriculum training guidelines (5.1) stating that "overarching competencies that are important for all psychologists also include . . . issues of cultural and individual diversity" (p. 272). Of critical importance in this discussion, however, are the specific ethical considerations relevant to disability culture.

Perhaps the well-developed literature regarding culture, stigma, and disability identity existing in the area of intellectual and developmental disabilities can help us clarify issues of relevance. While this literature focuses on a population with varied developmental disabilities, the ethical and cultural concepts parallel those affecting individuals with acquired disability. McDonald and Patka (2012) and McDonald and Kidney (2012) frame varied ethical issues related to research models (and, by extension, to clinical treatment models) pertinent to intellectual disability. They cite three principles that inform research: respecting autonomy and protecting those with reduced autonomy, minimizing harm and maximizing benefits, and equally distributing the risks and rewards of participation in research and other interventions. The gist of their arguments centers on the concepts of reducing barriers to active decision-making participation, eliminating marginalization, and reducing barriers that inhibit access to varied opportunities that may potentially advance persons' with disabilities life situations. Finally, they present cogent rationales for participation in research (and clinical) activities as a right, reflecting a strengths-based socioecological model of disability. Inclusion/participation is a matter of justice and respect, whereas exclusion as a protective measure is described as an outmoded social concept. An abrupt transition from a social role built upon autonomy (as we see with acquired disability), to an altered social role based on diminished decision-making capacity via illness or injury, should be addressed by health care providers in a manner that emphasizes preserved strengths and the potential to contribute to the decision-making process within ethical concept assent and substituted judgment. The latter decision-making approach places the responsibility on a surrogate to reflect the incapacitated person's preferences.

Lotan and Ellis (2010) introduced the concepts of person-centered planning, asymmetrical power, outer directedness, and social-relational context. These concepts describe social-relational factors that can either facilitate or inhibit development of personal identity and integration into the disability culture. These concepts provide a frame of reference for psychological assessment and intervention toward the establishment and maintenance of disability identity. Thus, the psychologist's awareness of and incorporation of these concepts into practice can either enhance or deter from ongoing cultural competence and highlight potential areas of needed training. The concepts are as follows:

- Person-centered planning is a process that involves promoting self-determination and understanding/accounting for each person's specific social/cultural context, goals, and aspirations. Emphasis is centered on empowerment, participation in decision making, and respect for persons—the last being the overarching ethical principle that drives serving persons with disabilities.
- Asymmetrical power is often noted in congregate living arrangements (by extension, an inpatient neurorehabilitation unit) where the individual is in a "one-down" relationship with the health care staff. That position is often tacitly accepted as the norm, deferring to the expertise of the health care professional. However, this attitude can cascade into staff-dominated decision making on behalf of the persons served—by analogy, perceived best interests versus substituted judgment. Psychologists must guard against static power differentials as the individual's recovery progresses and she defines and shapes her cultural frames of reference.
- Outer-directedness refers to the tendency across time to develop external cue dependence by virtue of the treatment relationship between patient and health care professional. Initially, cues are proffered to assist the person with cognitive disability in reasoning, decision-making, and problem-solving activities. Once successful outcomes are derived from this cue-based method of dealing with reasoning tasks, the individual can become dependent on others for such cues. Without active cue weaning built into the treatment plan, this dependency can become an unintended by-product of the treatment process. According to Lotan and Ellis (2010), "A good decision-making process does not end with the decision made. Debriefing with the client (patient) is important to assess the client's understanding of the decision, what actions will be taken and the time frame, and the client's experience of the steps that led to the decision" (p. 122). Emphasizing autonomy in cognitive processes, as well as the conduct of activities of daily living, employment, and broader societal

involvement, is a highly desirable focus of the ethical practice of rehabilitation and supports the individual's journey regarding cultural definition and immersion.

CONCLUSIONS

This chapter presents information that is critical to the consideration of disability identity and culture in the context of ethical multicultural practice. Legislative and regulatory scaffolding for societal responsiveness to and acceptance of individuals with disability exists, but it requires further refinement. Social agencies have been created to support the process of adaptation to disability culture and are attempting to foster development of disability identity through networking resources for employment and socialization. Private nonprofit organizations (typically defined by broad diagnostic categories) are in place to support individual and family adaptation to established disability cultures through education and social networking. Social broadcast media have increasingly offered positive characterizations of individuals with disabilities, helping to broaden cultural exposure and, hopefully, acceptance. Ethics codes in varied health care disciplines demand multicultural competence of their membership. However, an attitudinal gulf between the individual with a disability and societal accommodation of functional needs appended to disability continues to exist, to the frustration of those focused on fully engaging in a personally and societally meaningful manner and with hopes of occupying a societally meaningful role.

Achieving an effective mastery of multicultural practice competence is rapidly becoming a foundational skill for all rehabilitation professionals, including psychologists. As an example, "Individual and Cultural Diversity" is included as a foundational competency for specialty board certification in rehabilitation psychology as described by Cox, Cox, and Caplan (2013), and they offer an excellent discussion and referencing regarding disability as a cultural construct. Similarly, the APA has recently published a two-volume series on multicultural psychology (Leong, Comas-Diaz, Nagayama Hall, McLoyd, & Trimble, 2014a, 2014b). Although it is disappointing that disability did not garner its own chapter in the series and Division 22 was not listed as a division concerned with diversity issues in the chapter by David, Okazaki, and Giroux (2014, p. 85), the series is nevertheless a useful resource that highlights important considerations regarding competent practice. We have much to learn from one another both within and across our disciplines, particularly given that evolving demographics point toward worldwide multiculturalism as the societal norm, independent of traditional geographic boundaries. Most important, disability populates all ethnic/racial cultures, creating a common bond among disparate groups based on shared functional characteristics and challenges and the need to find meaningful disability identity and adaptive lifestyles within dominant cultures. To this end, we offer in this chapter some theoretical constructs and intervention strategies for the rehabilitation professional that speak to initiating the development of disability identity and to supporting immersion in disability culture for those individuals and families we serve in neurorehabilitation (Table 7.3).

In essence, we highlight two intersecting paths toward culturally competent practice. First, psychologists undergo a developmental process in which they assess and shift their worldview based on their perceptions of their own culture, other cultures, and an awareness of and a sensitivity to one's values, biases, and behaviors. As part of this process, and to serve our clients in a fully actualized manner, psychologists must be cognizant of their own cultures and worldview shaped by those cultures. Second, psychologists develop culturally relevant practical (technical) skills applicable to the practice setting, such as assessment addressing

Table 7.3 *Intervention Strategies*

Disability Culture Issues	Adaptive Strategies
Altered personal and social roles after injury or illness	Assess effects of preexisting culture on self-efficacy in context of disability postinjury.
	Acknowledge abrupt change in function, with focus on continuity of the person.
	Facilitate emphasis on preserved strengths and adaptation to change.
	Facilitate development and incorporation of "new" personal, social, and cultural roles in the contexts of acute care.
	Consultation and liaison and inpatient neurorehabilitation.
	Extend role adaptation to family and community contexts with initial education and later guided immersion activities.

(continued)

Table 7.3 *Intervention Strategies (continued)*

Disability Culture Issues	Adaptive Strategies
Disability cultural identity	Promote dialogue with patient and family regarding cultural differences that could impact trust.
	Assess rejection/acceptance of disability as a personal construct.
	Pay attention to language used by the individual, family, and self in referring to disability.
	Provide guided peer interactions among neurorehabilitation inpatients, emphasizing meeting challenges to everyday living in new and adaptive ways.
	Utilize formally trained peer mentors to support and help prepare the individual for personal and community transition.
	Arrange for community outings with team members and with family/friends that emphasize the validity and functional applicability of disability identity within the broader social community context:
	a) Ensure linkages with community, state, and national socialization resources to continue the process of disability cultural adaptation post discharge
	b) Invite socialization-support group membership prior to neurorehabilitation discharge and continuing afterward
	c) Support disability rights advocacy activities of rehabilitation team members and persons with disabilities at the local, state, and national levels
Transition from dependence to independence	Ensure dependence-producing treatment approaches are discontinued as early as possible; educate patient and family regarding expectations for the natural healing course and incremental movement toward independence.
	Negotiate acceptable functional outcomes with the individual served.
	Provide self-management tools to replace established dependent behavioral patterns.
	Train to mastery, weaning cues in the process.
	Evaluate outcomes in the contexts of applicability to disability culture and the home/community environments.

(continued)

Table 7.3 *Intervention Strategies (continued)*

Disability Culture Issues	Adaptive Strategies
Decisional participation	Determine extent of decisional capacity. If accommodations can produce adequately informed decisions, promote autonomy. If accommodations can produce limited informed decisions, utilize surrogates and obtain individuals' informed assent. If accommodations cannot produce adequately informed decisions, utilize surrogates with substituted judgment as the decisional rubric; gain understanding of surrogate's values and views of disability to support awareness in decision making.

disability culture based on the client's preinjury and postinjury experiences, intervention addressing disability identity development, and discharge planning recognizing community and family nuances. In the next iteration of the APA Ethics Code, we hope an even more concrete commitment to mastery of multiculturally sensitive practice is evident. The individual rehabilitation practitioner is encouraged to augment the broadly defined concept of multiculturally sensitive practice to prioritize disability identity and culture. To the extent that rehabilitation professionals introduce and foster exploration of disability culture and disability identity in persons and families served, we prepare the individual and family for return to the community. Having mastered the basics regarding acceptance of and identification with the disability population, we proactively provide adaptive behavioral tools for eventually reaching the goal of social equilibrium within different cultures. The emotional and social adjustment process must now adopt the mantle of cultural contextual relevance as a crucial validating factor, with outcomes meeting the credibility threshold via feedback from individuals served and community peers with disabilities. Finally, psychologists remain key advocates for positive change on behalf of persons with disabilities and the broader community, with the ultimate goal being fully integrated, accessible social systems that facilitate participation by all citizens.

REFERENCES

ADA Amendments Act of 2008. Retrieved from http://en.wikipedia.org/wiki/ADA_Amendments_Act_of_2008

American Psychological Association. (2002). Ethical principles of psychologists and code of conduct. *American Psychologist, 57*, 1060–1073. doi:10.1037/0003-066X.57.12.1060

American Psychological Association. (2013). Guidelines for psychological practice in health care delivery systems. *American Psychologist, 68*, 1–6. doi:10.1037/a0029890

Anti-Defamation League. (2005). *A Brief History of the Disability Rights Movement.* Retrieved November 27, 2012, from http://archive.adl.org/education/curriculum_connections/fall_2005/fall_2005_lesson5_history.asp

Ashing-Giwa, K. (2005). Contextual model of health-related quality-of-life: A paradigm for expanding the HRQoL framework. *Quality of Life Research, 14,* 297–307.

Balcazar, F., Suarez-Balcazar, Y., & Taylor-Ritzler, T. (2009). Cultural competence: Development of a conceptual framework. *Disability & Rehabilitation, 31,* 1153–1160. doi:10.1080/09638280902773752

Bourjolly, J., Sands, R., Soloman, P., Stanhope, V., Pernell-Arnold, A., & Finley, L. (2005). The journey toward intercultural sensitivity: A non-linear process. *Journal of Ethnic and Cultural Diversity in Social Work, 14,* 41–62.

Brown, S. (2002). What is disability culture? *Disability Studies Quarterly, 22,* 34–50. Retrieved March 27, 2013, from http://dsq-sds.org/article/view/343/433

Budd, J. (2011). *The thought of work.* Ithaca, NY: ILR Press.

Caplan, B., & Shechter, J. (1995). The role of nonstandard neuropsychological assessment in rehabilitation: History, rationale and examples. In L. Cushman & M. Scherer (Eds.), *Psychological assessment in medical rehabilitation* (pp. 359–391). Washington, DC: American Psychological Association.

Cartwright, B., & Fleming, C. (2010). Multicultural and diversity considerations in the new Code of Professional Ethics for Rehabilitation Counselors. *Journal of Applied Rehabilitation Counseling, 41,* 20–24.

Centers for Disease Control and Prevention. (2013). Get the stats on traumatic brain injury in the United States. Retrieved from www.cdc.gov/traumaticbraininjury/pdf/BlueBook_factsheet-a.pdf

Colorado State University. (2015). *A brief history of legislation.* Retrieved from http://www.rds.colostate.edu/history-of-legislation

Comas-Diaz, L. (2012). *Multicultural care: A clinician's guide to cultural competence.* Washington, DC: American Psychological Association. doi:10.1037/a0029403

Cox, D., Cox, R., & Caplan, B. (2013). *Specialty competencies in rehabilitation psychology.* Specialty Competencies in Professional Psychology. New York, NY: Oxford University Press.

David, E. J. R., Okazaki, S., & Giroux, D. (2014). A set of guiding principles to advance multicultural psychology and its major concepts. In F. T. L. Leong, L. Comas-Diaz, G. C. Nagayama Hall, J. E. Trimble, & V. C. McLoyd (Eds.), *APA handbook of multicultural psychology: Vol. 1. Theory and research* (pp. 85–104). Washington, DC: American Psychological Association. doi:10.1037/14189-005

Davis, L. J. (2011, September 25). Why is disability missing from discourse on diversity? Retrieved from http://chronicle.com/article/why-is-disability-missing-from/129088

Disability Justice. (2015). *The right to self-determination: Freedom from involuntary sterilization.* Retrieved from http://disabilityjustice.org/right-to-self-deter mination-freedom-from-involuntary-sterilization

Frieden, L. (2005, November 8). *Goodman and United States v. Georgia:* The Supreme Court hears another case challenging the constitutionality of Title II of the Americans with Disabilities Act. Retrieved from http://www.ncd.gov/publi cations/2005/11082005

Fuertes, J., Stracuzzi, T., Bennett, J., Scheinholtz, J., Mislowack, A., Hersh, M., & Cheng, D. (2006). Therapist multicultural competency: A study of therapy dyads. *Psychotherapy: Therapy, Research, Practice, 43,* 480–490. doi:10.1037/0033-3204.43.4.480

Fyffe, D., & Lequerica, A. (2013). *Clinical and research perspectives on cultural issues in rehabilitation.* Presentation at APA Division 22 15th Annual Conference, Expanding the Boundaries of Rehabilitation Psychology, February 22, 2013, Jacksonville, Florida.

Galer, D. (2012). Disabled capitalists: Exploring the intersections of disability and identity formation in the world of work. *Disability Studies Quarterly; Society for Disability Studies.* Retrieved March 27, 2013, from http://dsq-sds.org/arti cle/view/3277/3122

Gauthier, J., Pettifor, J., & Ferrero, A. (2010, May). The universal declaration of ethics principles for psychologists: A culture-sensitive model for creating and reviewing a code of ethics. *Ethics and Behavior, 20,* 179–196.

Gill, C. (1997). Four types of integration in disability identity development. *Journal of Vocational Rehabilitation, 9,* 39–46.

Gill, C., Kewman, D., & Brannon, R. (2003, April). Transforming psychological practice and society: Policies that reflect the new paradigm. *American Psychologist, 58,* 305–312. doi:10.1037/0003-066X.58.4.305

Hammer, M., Bennett, M., & Wiseman, R. (2003). Measuring intercultural sensitivity: The intercultural development inventory. *International Journal of Intercultural Relations, 27,* 421–443.

Hanson, S., & Kerkhoff, T. (2007). Ethical decision-making in rehabilitation: Considerations of Latino cultural factors. *Rehabilitation Psychology, 52,* 409–422.

Lee, C., & Ramsey, C. (2006). Multicultural counseling: A new paradigm for a new century. In C. C. Lee (Ed.), *Multicultural issues in counseling: New approaches to diversity* (3rd ed., pp. 3–11). Alexandria, VA: American Counseling Association.

Leong, F. T. L., Comas-Diaz, L., Nagayama Hall, G. C., McLoyd, V. C., & Trimble, J. E. (Eds.). (2014a). *APA handbook of multicultural psychology: Vol. 1. Theory and research.* Washington, DC: American Psychological Association. doi:10.1037/ 14189-000

Leong, F. T. L., Comas-Diaz, L., Nagayama Hall, G. C., McLoyd, V. C., & Trimble, J. E. (Eds.). (2014b). *APA handbook of multicultural psychology: Vol.2. Applications and training.* Washington, DC: American Psychological Association. doi:10 .1037/14187-000

Longmore, P. (1985). A note on language and the social identity of disabled people. *American Behavioral Scientist, 28*, 419–423.

Lotan, G., & Ells, C. (2010). Adults with intellectual and developmental disabilities and participation in decision making: Ethical considerations for professional-client practice. *Intellectual and Developmental Disabilities, 48*, 112–125. doi:10 .1352/1934-9556-48.2.112

Manly, J. (2008). Critical issues in cultural neuropsychology: Profit from diversity. *Neuropsychological Review, 18*, 179–183. doi:10.1007/s11065-9068-8

Mayerson, A. (2007, September–October). Disability rights law: Roots, present challenges, and future collaboration. *Clearinghouse Review: Journal of Poverty Law and Policy, 41*, 265–271.

Mayerson, A. B., & Mayer, K. S. (2000). Defining disability in the aftermath of Sutton: Where do we go from here? *Human Rights, 27*, 13–16. Retrieved from http://www.heinonline.org/HOL/Page?handle=hein.journals/huri27& collection=journals&index=journals/huri&id=15

McDonald, K., & Kidney, C. (2012, September). What's right? Ethics in intellectual disabilities research. *Journal of Policy and Practice in Intellectual Disabilities, 9*, 27–39.

McDonald, K., & Patka, M. (2012, September). There is no black or white: Scientific community views on ethics in intellectual and developmental disability research. *Journal of Policy and Practice in Intellectual Disabilities, 9*, 206–214.

Mollen, D., Ridley, C. R., & Hill, C. L. (2003). Models of multicultural counseling competence: A critical evaluation. In D. B. Pope-Davis, H. L. K. Coleman, W. Ming Lu, & R. L. Toporak (Eds.), *Handbook of multicultural competencies in counseling and psychology* (pp. 21–38). Thousand Oaks, CA: Sage Publications.

Mpofu, E., Chronister, J., Johnson, E., & Denham, G. (2012). Aspects of culture influencing rehabilitation and persons with disabilities. In P. Kennedy (Ed.), *The Oxford handbook of rehabilitation psychology* (pp. 543–553). New York, NY: Oxford.

National Consortium on Leadership and Disability for Youth. (2007). Disability history timeline: Resource and discussion guide. Retrieved from http:// www.ncld-youth.info/Downloads/disability_history_timeline.pdf

National Council on Disability. (2007, July 26). The impact of the Americans with Disabilities Act: Assessing the progress toward achieving the goals of the ADA. Retrieved from http://www.ncd.gov/publications/2007/0726 2007

Olkin, R. (2002). Could you hold the door for me? Including disability in diversity. *Cultural Diversity and Ethnic Minority Psychology, 8*, 130–137. Special Section: Reports on the National Multicultural Conference and Summit II.

Page, K., Castillo-Page, L., Poll-Hunter, N., Garrison, G., & Wright, S. (2013). Assessing the evolving definition of underrepresented minority and its application in academic medicine. *Academic Medicine, 88*, 67–72.

Pernell-Arnold, A., Linley, L., Sands, G., Bourjolly, J., & Stanhope, V. (2012). Training mental health providers in cultural competence: A transformative learning process. *American Journal of Psychiatric Rehabilitation, 15*, 334–356. doi:10.1080/15487768.2012.73387

Salter, D., & Salter, B. (2012). Competence with diverse populations. In S. Knapp, M. Gottlieb, M. Handelsman, & L. VandeCreek (Eds.), *APA handbook of ethics in psychology, Vol. 1: Moral foundations and common themes* (pp. 217–239). Washington, DC: American Psychological Association.

San Francisco State University, The Disability Programs and Resource Center. (2015). *A chronology of the Disability Rights Movement.* Retrieved from http://www.sfsu.edu/~dprc/chronology/index.html

Shapiro, J. P. (2015). The new civil rights: The Americans with Disabilities Act has unlocked the door; now it's time to open it. Retrieved from http://www.disabilityculture.org/course/article3.htm

Sherry, M. (2009). Barden-LaFollette Act. In S. Burch (Ed.), *Encyclopedia of American disability history* (p. 89). Retrieved from http://lib.myilibrary.com/Open.aspx?id=244003

State of Michigan, Department of Human Services. (2015). Events in the Development of Disability Policy. Retrieved from http://www.michigan.gov/dhs/0,4562,7-124-5453_25392_40237_42064-12436--,00.html

Stiers, W., Hanson, S., Turner, A., Stucky, K., Barisa, M., Brownsberger, M., . . . Ashman, T. (2012). Guidelines for postdoctoral training in rehabilitation psychology. *Rehabilitation Psychology, 57*, 267–279. doi:10.1037/a0030774

Sue, D. W., Arredondo, P., & McDavis, R. J. (1992). Multicultural counseling competencies and standards: A call to the profession. *Journal of Counseling & Development of a Conceptual Framework, 70*, 477–486.

Sue, D. W., & Sue, D. (2008). *Counseling the culturally diverse: Theory and practice* (5th ed.). Hoboken, NJ: John Wiley & Sons.

Sutton v. United Airlines, Inc., 527 U.S. 471 (1999).

Temple University. (2015). *Disability history timeline.* Retrieved from http://isc.temple.edu/neighbor/ds/disabilityrightstimeline.htm

Tilley, E., Fredricks, S., & Hornett, A. (2012). Kinship, culture and ethics in organizations: Exploring implications for internal communication. *Journal of Communication Management, 16*, 162–184.

Tummala-Narra, P., Singer, R., Li, Z., Esposito, J., & Ash, S. (2012). Individual and systemic factors in clinicians' self-perceived cultural competence. *Professional Psychology: Research and Practice, 43*, 165–174. doi:10.1037/a0025783

U.S. Department of Labor, Office of Disability Employment Policy. (2009, January). Disability history: An important part of America's heritage: Defining the next generation. Retrieved from http://www.dol.gov/odep/documents/Disability%20History_508%20compliant_links.pdf

U.S. Department of Transportation. (2015). Rehabilitation Act of 1973—Public Law (PL) 93-112 93rd Congress, H.R. 8070, September 26, 1973. Retrieved from https://www.civilrights.dot.gov/pl-93-112-rehabilitation-act-1973

U.S. Department of Transportation, Federal Transit Administration. (2015). *Disability rights movement timeline*. Retrieved from http://www.fta.dot.gov/12325_4064.html

U.S. Equal Employment Opportunity Commission. (1990). Titles I and V of the Americans with Disabilities Act of 1990 (ADA). Retrieved from http://www.eeoc.gov/laws/statutes/ada.cfm

Welch, P., & Palames, C. (1995). A brief history of disability rights legislation in the United States. In P. Welch (Ed.), *Strategies for teaching universal design* (pp. 5–12). Boston, MA: Adaptive Environments. Retrieved from http://www.udeducation.org/resources/61.html

Woidneck, M., Pratt, K., Gundy, J., Nelson, C., & Twohig, M. (2012). Exploring cultural competence in Acceptance and Commitment Therapy outcomes. *Professional Psychology: Research and Practice, 43,* 227–233. doi:10.1037/a0026235

World Bank. (2011). Main report. Vol. 1 of *World Report on Disability*. Washington, DC: The Worldbank. Retrieved from http://documents.worldbank.org/curated/en/2011/01/14440066/world-report-disability

World Health Organization. (2011). *World Report on Disability*. Retrieved from www.who.int/disabilities/world_report/2011

Wright, B. (1983). Impressions of people with disabilities. In B. A. Wright (Ed.), *Physical disability—a psychosocial approach* (2nd ed., pp. 52–77). New York, NY: HarperCollins Publishers.

CHAPTER EIGHT

THE EFFECTIVE USE OF CERTIFIED MEDICAL INTERPRETERS IN THE NEUROREHABILITATION SETTING

Julie Alberty and Jay M. Uomoto

The neurorehabilitation setting and the process of neurorehabilitation are likely novel experiences to most patients who receive services after a neurological disorder or event. The rehabilitation environment has its own culture. It requires the patient and those who support the patient to orient, accommodate, and assimilate to the way neurorehabilitation is delivered, all the while being challenged to adjust to a newly acquired neurological disability. This in and of itself can be a challenging situation for patients and their loved ones.

Now imagine what it is like to be in the hospital and meeting with a doctor who is speaking a language you do not understand and feeling quite overwhelmed by this experience. You are probably frightened and attempting to grasp what the doctor is saying and perhaps wondering if you as a patient or as a family member are missing information that might make a difference regarding your care and outcome. You try to explain to the doctor that you do not understand what is being said and ask if someone who speaks your language is available to help you understand what the doctor is saying. A certified medical interpreter is unavailable, so you ask your child to interpret what your doctor is saying. The doctor uses many terms the child does not know how to interpret. The child becomes anxious as he listens and tries to understand. The doctor is using medical jargon and the confused child does the best he can to interpret what he *thinks* the doctor is saying. The child does what he can because he wants to be helpful and does not want to be scolded for doing a bad job. This leads to a patient who remains confused and still does not fully grasp what is going on with her current state of health and does not understand the consequences of her neurological condition and prognosis.

How many vital things are communicated between you and your doctor when you are in the hospital? How many personal questions does the doctor ask you? Would you feel comfortable revealing all of those details in front of a child or a family member so they can interpret this for you? Language is one of the essential ways we communicate with one another. When in a doctor's office, let alone in the very busy and fast-paced clinical environment of neurorehabilitation, the patient is in a vulnerable situation and is asked to share private details of his life, not knowing why or how this information makes a difference in his outcome. This can be even more difficult when the patient has no choice but to use family members for his voice. Even under these circumstances, this assumes that there is a trusted and reliable family member available who is bilingual and who has enough health literacy to understand what must be translated. Most important, when a patient sees a doctor, key items are discussed, including diagnosis, prognosis, and follow-up treatment. How would you feel if suddenly you could not understand what was being told to you about your current state of health?

THE NEED FOR CERTIFIED INTERPRETERS

The United States is home to many immigrants and many different languages. According to the 2000 U.S. Census (see also Flores, 2005), 47 million Americans speak a language other than English at home. In fact, between 1990 and 2000, the number of people in the United States who spoke a language other than English at home rose from approximately 31.8 million to 47 million. According to the U.S. Census Bureau (2007), 21.4 million Americans are limited in their ability to speak English. These statistics were from the 2007 U.S. Census, but this number has continued to increase since then. Avery (2001) reported that over 300 languages are spoken in the United States. Moreover, Karliner, Jacobs, Chen, and Mutha (2007) reported that over 100 languages are commonly spoken in the United States, which only further magnifies the importance and necessity of certified medical interpreters. We live in a country that welcomes all ethnicities, cultures, religions, and languages, which leads to an immense amount of diversity. All patients have the right to get information from their health care providers in a language they can understand so they can make informed decisions about their treatment.

The U.S. Department of Health and Human Services interprets Title VI of the Civil Rights Act of 1964 as requiring that health care facilities provide trained, competent interpreters for limited-English-speaking persons. Studies have shown a need in the United States for certified medical interpreters to always be available during health care services. A recent literature review conducted by Ribera, Hausmann-Muela, Grietens, and Toomer (2008) demonstrated that multiple studies have shown that individuals with limited to no English proficiency (LEP) received a poorer quality of service, were prescribed less medication, had fewer tests done, and spent less time in the emergency department when compared to LEP patients who were assisted by an interpreter or English-proficient (EP) patients. In general, LEP patients demonstrated less comprehension of the diagnosis and prognosis compared to patients who were EP. This leads to less follow-through by LEP patients who do not necessarily understand what they are supposed to do or how they are supposed to follow up. Studies have also shown that this can lead to costly complications of disease processes (Ribera et al., 2008). This study also found that the literature clearly shows that LEP patients who were assisted by a professional/certified medical interpreter generally received the same quality of care and shared a comparable level of satisfaction as EP patients. Ribera et al. state, "Professional interpreters increase comprehension of medical recommendations, reduce risk of medical errors related to incorrect translations, increase trust and motivation (and therefore can increase adherence), and are the best option to maximize comprehension of informed consent and to ensure confidentiality of LEP patients" (p. 7). These findings are clearly alarming, showing that significant disparities resulting in lowered health outcomes and can eventually lead to longer-term lowered quality of life, can be solely attributed to being LEP.

Karliner et al. (2007), who also conducted a review of the literature, found that the quality of medical care is improved when certified medical interpreters are used or when the patient's health care provider is bilingual in the same language as the patient. This review demonstrated that the use of trained professional interpreters was associated with decreased disparities between LEP patients and EP patients or patients receiving care from health care providers who speak the patients' language. Both reviews concluded that the use of professional/certified interpreters is associated with an improved quality of health care for LEP patients. Professional interpreters appear to decrease errors in communication between the patient and the physician, increase patient comprehension, allow LEP patients to seek out health care on a more regular basis and at the same rate as EP patients, improve clinical outcomes, and increase satisfaction with communication and clinical services for LEP patients.

These findings are compelling in that they point out the importance for all patients in medical, or more specifically neurorehabilitation, settings to be afforded the opportunity to receive health care in their primary language. When sick, individuals want to be heard and be able to express their concerns and therefore participate in their health care. This chapter explains the importance of using a certified medical interpreter and how to appropriately use this service in a hospital setting. It also discusses the importance of patient perception on follow-through of treatment, the idea of cultural competence, and how to appropriately communicate and use interpreter services; it provides some case examples of successful and unsuccessful interpretation.

THE ROLE OF THE MEDICAL INTERPRETER

Avery (2001) discussed the role of the professional interpreter, which, at its most basic definition, is to allow for and provide communication between patients and health care providers who do not speak the same language. However, the role of the interpreter is more complicated than simply communicating oral information between two different languages. An interpreter needs to understand cultural beliefs and be able to effectively communicate the information between two individuals who are likely from different cultures. Many times an interpreter may need to communicate oral information in the form of a metaphor or a common expression that may not have a direct interpretation. In such cases, the interpreter must create a "linguistic conversion" (Avery, 2001), in which the main idea is still conveyed and communicated accurately. To the best of their ability, interpreters should be able to identify, understand, and respect the values and beliefs of the individuals for whom they are interpreting. Culture defines how health information is received, understood, and acted upon (Anderson et al., 2003). This is something that is too often ignored in the medical setting. How information is delivered—from verbiage, to eye contact, to the amount of physical space between the health care provider and the patient—involves the many ways that culture can impact what would allow a patient to feel heard and comforted versus ignored, rushed, or unimportant.

For example, one of the most important factors in the Latino culture is the concept of personal space, which is vastly different from mainstream American culture's beliefs. Although the American culture expects a certain amount of personal space in interactions with others (i.e., friends or professionals), Latinos have less of a barrier when it comes to personal space when interacting with others. For example, in the Latino culture, when a person meets a friend of a friend for the first time, they will greet each other with a hug and a kiss on the cheek. In contrast, in American cultures, it is customary to offer a handshake. In some cultures, a handshake is considered pushy, impolite, or even insulting. In many cultures, a hug is considered very personal and reserved for individuals who have a defined close relationship, such as family members. Latinos, on the other hand, believe that embracing one another is a sign of respect and is therefore expected. This is not to say that all providers should hug their Latino patients, but it demonstrates how cultural differences can lead to very different expectations. Many Latino patients will hug providers or will use some form of physical touch, such as a pat on the shoulder. An American provider or patient may be surprised by this and possibly put off by the invasion of personal space. Some disciplines in a neurorehabilitation setting have explicit professional ethics guidelines and cautions around the issue of touching patients. In the American culture, a hug can be seen as a patient blurring the boundaries between the patient and health care providers' professional boundaries, whereas for the patient it may simply be an acceptable way of saying, "Thank you for all your help during this difficult time." Not allowing that hug could be taken as an insult or as being disrespectful. If a Latino patient gave a provider or an interpreter a pat on the shoulder, the interpreter could explain the cultural importance and appropriateness of this action. If the provider pulled away, the interpreter could explain this to the patient as well. The trained and culturally sensitive medical interpreter can communicate verbal information and serve as a cultural bridge between two individuals who could have very different beliefs about everyday interactions with others. Culturally competent medical translators pay close attention to both the verbal nuances of language and the nonverbal norms and customs that may be significant in a health care interaction.

Because nonverbal expressions can differ among ethnic groups, it becomes an important part of the interpreter's role to be able to understand major themes in nonverbal communication and to be able to verbalize this communication to the physician or health care provider. Different cultures have different ideas about what is appropriate to discuss with health care providers. From handshakes to eye contact, each can represent a very different meaning to different cultures. Americans believe good eye contact is a sign of respect, and in the neurorehabilitation setting it may be an important "mental status" variable and a part of assessing such aspects as social cognition in the patient with a brain injury. However, in many Asian cultures, respect is shown by *not* maintaining consistent eye contact because it is considered rude. A health care provider could interpret a lack of eye contact as a patient being flippant or choosing to ignore the information the physician is discussing. This would be a good example of when an interpreter could explain the cultural differences that occur between physician and patient, allowing the interpreter to be the bridge of communication between the two.

If a health care provider of another culture reacts abruptly or chooses to decline the patient's gesture, the patient may not understand the meaning behind the health care provider's reaction, and the provider risks alienating the patient. If a patient feels alienated, disrespected, or misunderstood, the patient may not seek further medical care, including preventive care. Many cultural values are learned in childhood and become beliefs and expectations of how one is supposed to act in certain situations. In a country that has cultures within cultures (first-generation immigrants, American-born immigrants with monolingual parents, bilingual/bicultural immigrants, multicultural individuals, etc.), this can lead to many unnecessary misunderstandings. Professional certified interpreters are usually bilingual and understand the main components of the cultures that are tied to the languages they are interpreting. In essence, as noted earlier, the role of the certified professional interpreter is not only to communicate oral information but also to serve as a cultural bridge between two individuals to ensure both feel that adequate and respectful communication has taken place.

TYPES OF INTERPRETERS

The three types of interpreters are professional/certified interpreters, informal/ad hoc interpreters, and bilingual health practitioners. A professional or certified interpreter is a person with a formal background or certification in interpretation as well as cultural and medical competences. Although proving competency varies by site, these individuals have had to prove their competency in both languages by completing a class and then taking an oral and/or a written exam. In some facilities, interpreters are required to do all three (class, oral exam, written exam) before they can become certified. Different institutions may have different scoring or passing criteria because medical interpretation is not yet a universally licensed or credentialed field. Many institutions also offer medical language and interpretation courses, and these interpreters are required to undergo ongoing education and testing. In fact, in 2004, a *National Code of Ethics for Interpreters in Health Care* was published by the National Council on Interpreting in Health Care (NCIHC; see Ruschke et al., 2005). This document offers information on the standards of practice and the expected duties of certified medical interpreters. It also discusses ethical principles and how certified interpreters should respond to situations ethically, some of which are discussed later in this chapter.

There are different kinds of certified interpreters that vary by institution and what that institution has available. Many institutions have certified interpreters on staff to allow for an in-person interpretation during the appointment, with the physician, patient, and interpreter present in the same room. Some institutions use a telephone service that can be contracted by a monthly plan or paid by the minute (Fontes, 2008). The physician contacts the interpreter service via telephone, and the physician either puts the interpreter on speakerphone or the physician and the patient each have a handset. However, interpretation over the phone does not allow the interpreter to see the patient and be able to observe nonverbal communication or body language. The interpreter may miss a confused look or other nonverbal communication that the patient displays.

Some research has shown that patients who required the use of telephone interpreters reported identical overall visit satisfaction with patients who had language concordant physicians (Lee, Batal, Maselli, & Kutner, 2002). Finally, another option is when an interpreter communicates via video, such as Skype. This method has not been widely used. Most hospitals either have interpreters on staff or use the telephone service for professional interpreters.

Ad Hoc Interpreters

Ad hoc interpreters consist of anyone in the hospital setting, including family members (e.g., children), friends, nonmedical hospital staff, and even other patients who act as interpreters but have no formal training or testing of fluency. Avery (2001) reported that using ad hoc interpreters presented a "high risk of inadequate communication resulting in misdiagnosis and inappropriate treatment that could, in a worst case scenario, result in the death of the patient" (p. 2). These individuals often have little or no understanding of medical concepts or terminology. They can easily and possibly accidentally communicate oral information incorrectly, which can negatively impact the accuracy of the message that a physician or patient may be trying to convey. In general, research has shown that patients report significantly less satisfaction when an ad hoc interpreter is used. According to Lee et al. (2002), patient satisfaction was significantly less for provider listening, discussion of sensitive issues, manner, support, explanations, and answers when ad hoc interpreters were used.

Cultural factors are another important aspect that must be taken into account. Certain cultures and those from different ethnic backgrounds do not believe in discussing private matters (e.g., sexual concerns, family difficulties) with health providers. Often a family member may add information, change the emphasis of what may be concerning, or simply not include the information the patient is complaining about because she is too embarrassed to repeat the information. Fontes (2008) also reported that untrained interpreters are likely to omit and/or embellish information on behalf of the patient. In regard to children, Fontes reported that often patients will minimize or completely omit their true level of distress in front of their children, which can be highly problematic when discussing health issues with the physician. Fontes also stated that some information should never be conveyed by children. Undue pressure may be placed on the child who feels "responsible for the outcome of the interview and might be blamed by the family if the outcome was not to their liking. The child might not have adequate vocabulary or understanding to convey sexual detail or legal or medical information" (p. 150).

Older family members may believe they are protecting the patient by omitting or overly emphasizing certain symptoms. Overall, research has shown that ad hoc interpreters often add new information, omit information, and end up changing the nature of the original message, which can lead to critical and life-threatening errors (Avery, 2001; Fontes, 2008). Individuals who do not have training in interpretation often blur the lines between communicating oral information by reporting what is told to them and discussing what they believe are only the most important aspects of the patient and health care provider conversation. Moreover, what is most concerning is that individuals who have no medical interpretation training may not understand the terminology or medical jargon that the mental health provider is discussing.

Bilingual Health Providers

Bilingual health practitioners are those who are bilingual but may or may not have gone through a formal certification process. It is important for bilingual health practitioners to know their limits when doing interpretation. For languages that may have different dialects or slang (i.e., Spanish or many indigenous tribal languages), the interpreter or bilingual provider should be comfortable asking for further elaboration if unfamiliar with a slang term or admitting that he does not understand a certain dialect. In the Flores (2005) review, it was stated that LEP patients tend to ask more questions, have better information recall, are more comfortable discussing sensitive or embarrassing issues, have less pain and better physical functioning, and have higher patient satisfaction when they have a bilingual health provider. According to Romero (2004), patients report that they receive a better quality of care when it is delivered by a person of their own culture or someone who understands their culture.

The importance of cultural understanding is frequently discussed in the literature. One of the most important aspects of the health care provider and patient relationship is that the patient feels understood and heard by the health care provider. This is yet another example of how professional interpreters and bilingual health providers can be helpful. A patient who feels understood is more willing to ask follow-up questions and more likely to have a better understanding of the diagnosis and the next steps for treatment.

When possible, the use of a professional interpreter or bilingual health care provider is the gold standard with individuals who have limited English proficiency. Professional interpreters increase the patient's understanding, they interpret all the questions the patient may have, and they use the same tone as both the physician and patient when interpreting. In general, research has shown that this leads to the patient having a greater understanding of medical instructions, reduces the risk of medical errors related to mistranslation, increases trust and motivation, and increases the patient's adherence to medical recommendations. Interpreters are able to maximize understanding of informed consent and ensure patient confidentiality (Ribera et al., 2008). In fact, patients with limited English proficiency who were assisted by an interpreter were more willing to return to the same emergency department if more medical problems arose in the future compared to LEP patients who were not assisted by an interpreter.

When patients do not have an accurate understanding of how to appropriately follow up with medical recommendations or if they feel uncomfortable interacting with their health care providers due to language barriers, then the overall cost of care will increase significantly. Patients will not seek medical health care until the patient believes it is necessary. For individuals who may have chronic diseases such as diabetes, that may mean avoiding preventive care or routine follow-ups until the complications require acute hospitalization. Once a patient is hospitalized, the cost of medical care and the burden of payment significantly increase. Review of the literature demonstrates that using professional interpreters increases the use of preventive care for patients with limited English proficiency, improves patients' ability to report symptoms, improves patients' ability to comprehend physician recommendations, decreases the risk of dangerous misunderstanding due to inefficient or incorrect translations, and increases LEP patients' access to basic health care (Ribera et al., 2008).

Moreover, interpreters have the added advantage of being able to communicate with patients at their level of understanding and meaning. If patients do not understand medical terminology, the interpreter can explain with a combination of medical terms and lay terms that is appropriate to the patients' educational levels. An interpreter opens the door for both the patient and the health provider to ask questions and, more important, provides the bridge of communication. This bridge allows these individuals to understand one another clearly and effectively.

HOW TO WORK WITH AN INTERPRETER

When first working with a certified interpreter, it is ideal to meet with the interpreter before meeting with the patient. This is particularly important if the content that will be discussed is of a particularly sensitive nature (e.g., sexuality or sexually related information, a bad prognosis) or frightening or could be perceived or accepted differently by certain cultures. If discussing information of a sexual nature (as occurs frequently on neuro-rehabilitation services), it is important to ask the interpreter about any cultural issues related to the patient, especially if this is a population you have not worked with in the past. It is also good to give the interpreter some basic demographic information about the patient before the meeting, such as age, ethnicity, and what other family members or significant others may be present. This becomes particularly important when discussing information of a sexual nature. In certain cultures, such as Latino cultures, it can be embarrassing to receive information concerning sexuality or sexual intercourse from an older female figure rather than from a male figure. This is important to note if the interpreter happens to be an older female.

It can also be uncomfortable for interpreters at first and something they may have to prepare themselves for prior to entering the room. For example, when working with patients who have experienced a spinal cord injury, the topics of sexual intercourse and sexual education are important to discuss. This conversation usually includes a review of the patient's injury and how spinal cord injury can affect future sexual functioning. This is a particularly important topic to review when talking to a young couple who may be interested in having a family in the future. If you have an older female interpreter and a young Mexican couple, for example, it will likely be an awkward conversation. In Latino cultures, discussing information about one's own sexual life can be seen as taboo in general, even with a health care provider. Most interpreters should be able to participate in such a conversation without any difficulty, but it is important to inform them in advance that they will be interpreting this topic. Because standards and education differ per site, it may be important to review limits of confidentiality with the interpreters to ensure they have been exposed to this concept and understand both their and your responsibilities in regard to confidentiality.

Interpreters should repeat *exactly* what is said to both the patient and the provider. The interpreter should first introduce himself or herself in the patient's language and describe the reason for the meeting. Usually, the introduction goes something like this:

> My name is Jane Doe, and I am a certified interpreter. I am here so I can interpret what the provider says to you and any information or questions you may have for the provider. I wanted to ask you if you would be comfortable with this?

After the patient consents, the interpreter can tell the provider that the patient is agreeable to the conversation. It is important that the interpreter let the provider know that she will communicate all spoken information, including any side conversations the provider may have with anyone else in the room, so everyone knows what information is being discussed during the session. This ensures that most of the social interactions can be captured in the room as if all were speaking the same language. This also builds trust within the patient and alleviates suspicions of physicians or staff speaking "behind the patient's back" or "speaking badly about the patient."

In general, the interpreter usually sits slightly behind the provider so the provider can maintain eye contact with the patient. The rapport is meant to be between the patient and the provider, and it is essential that the interpreter allow for this by not standing or sitting between the two. It is too easy for the patient to lapse into a conversation with the interpreter, thus degrading the patient–provider relationship. The provider should maintain eye contact with the patient and not look at the interpreter when speaking to the patient about the patient's health. If more than one provider is present during the session, the interpreter should communicate to the patient any side conversations the providers may have. This is to ensure that the patient does not feel alienated during the session.

A major purpose of interpretation is to allow the patient to feel as comfortable as possible despite the language barriers. When interpreting, the interpreter should always communicate using the same person of speech as the patient uses. If the patient reports, "I feel lightheaded," then the verbatim interpretation should use first-person language as opposed to third-person speech.

An interpreter's tone of voice should always match the tone of the provider during the session. Speech prosody can be difficult to track and translate, especially if the interaction is fairly rapid. Further, this can be particularly difficult during emotional sessions that include delivering devastating news. A family member or ad hoc interpreter may communicate oral information incorrectly merely because it is devastating, whereas a certified medical interpreter should be able to match the tone and communicate what the provider is telling the patient as close to verbatim as possible. For example, a provider may tell a patient who recently suffered a spinal cord injury that the patient will most likely never walk again and must learn to use a wheelchair. An ad hoc interpreter, however, might say, "The doctor said it will be difficult for you to learn to walk again, but with faith and hard work, you can do it." This requires immediate intervention because the patient is being given false information and false hope. The patient may become depressed, angry, or frustrated because he was led to believe he would be able to walk by the time of discharge and blame himself for not trying hard enough. The provider may not even know the interpreter gave the patient this erroneous information.

Professional interpreters are trained in medical terminology and know they should avoid religious terms such as "faith." Also, errors in interpretation are much less likely with professional interpreters, and when they do occur, they are usually slight and do not significantly alter the provider's meaning (Karliner et al., 2007). Ad hoc interpreters also may sound excited or apathetic, which can make the patient feel anxious or uncomfortable.

At times, providers can attempt to listen to the interpreter's fluency. If while communicating oral information the interpreter appears to have halting speech or does not seem to be as fluid, the provider can check in with the interpreter to ensure that the interpreter feels capable of correctly interpreting the information. This is a good time to attend to the patient's nonverbal cues as well. If the patient looks confused, a provider can ask the patient, through the interpreter, if the patient understands all the information she is receiving or if she has any questions.

In general, providers should use short sentences so the interpreter can remember everything that is said. Some interpreters prefer to communicate oral information while the provider is speaking. It is usually better if the interpreter waits for the provider to stop speaking and then communicates oral information. Patients can get confused if they have to listen to two people speaking at the same time. Simultaneous translation can also be complicated by the level of cognitive impairment (e.g., processing speed deficits, memory deficits) that the patient experiences. The provider should speak directly to the patient, always using the first person. The interpreter is a tool to help you communicate with the patient, but the provider is speaking to the patient about his health care. The provider should make eye contact with the patient and ask all questions in the first person—for example, "How are you feeling today?" Suggestions for working with a certified interpreter appear at the end of the chapter.

When a Family Member Is a Certified Interpreter

In an ideal world, it is best for a staff member who is a certified interpreter to ask patients whether they would be more comfortable with the staff interpreter or a family member who is a certified interpreter. In most cases, patients are comfortable with having a family member interpret for them, but they should always be given the choice. To maintain a therapeutic alliance and respectful and productive patient–family–provider relationships, patients' preferences should be confirmed at the beginning of each translated interaction. If a patient consents to having a family member interpret in one situation, that may not be the case another time. It is important to respect a patient's right to choose what information is shared with whom.

ETHICAL GUIDELINES FOR INTERPRETERS

The *National Standards of Practice for Interpreters in Health Care* (Ruschke et al., 2005) were created to be used as a guideline for health care interpreters and to define ethical and best forms of practice for interpreters. This allows health care interpreters to provide accurate and complete communication between two people—provider and patient—who speak different languages, while still supporting and maintaining the patient–provider therapeutic relationship. More important, professional interpreters must abide by these standards, whereas ad hoc interpreters have no restrictions. Some facilities require that interpreters undergo an ethics training course before becoming a certified interpreter.

The standards require interpreters to be accurate by "striving to render the message accurately, conveying the content and spirit of the original message, taking into consideration the cultural context" (p. 5). This means interpreters must communicate *all oral information*, even if it is a highly sensitive topic, and maintain transparency. An interpreter should *respect the patient's confidentiality* and *provide impartiality.* Interpreters should *not allow their own personal or cultural values to interfere* with what or how they communicate oral information. Interpreters will *display respect for all parties involved*, have *cultural awareness*, and *understand their professional boundaries and roles* as interpreters. It is of upmost importance that interpreters refrain from personal involvement with patients and maintain their professional role as interpreters.

Interpreters should encourage *direct communication* between the provider and the patient, including directing the individuals to address each other rather than the interpreter in the conversation. The interpreter should be seen as someone who is merely allowing for clear communication between two parties. Interpreters should display professionalism, maintain professional development, and *provide advocacy*, if needed. As part of professionalism, interpreters should be able to *acknowledge their limitations.* For example, if a highly technical medical term is used that the interpreter is not familiar with, the interpreter should ask for an explanation from the provider so she can accurately communicate the information to the patient. In regard to professional development, interpreters should request feedback on their services and try to stay current on medical terminology and slang in the languages they interpret. *Advocacy* refers to interpreters speaking out to protect individuals from serious harm, whether it is a patient who has a life-threatening allergy or to report a pattern of disrespect toward patients.

THE COST OF USING A CERTIFIED INTERPRETER

The literature shows that using interpreters leads to lower costs of health care over time. Some research has shown that LEP patients who used professional interpreters and were provided with a similar level of service as EP patients accrued fewer costs than their EP counterparts (Ribera et al., 2008). This same review of the literature also pointed out that the LEP patients were more likely to receive unnecessary diagnostic tests and therapeutic interventions to exclude erroneous diagnoses. It was posited that this is mostly likely due to poor communication and the need for the physician to order more tests to rule out a wide spectrum of differential diagnoses. A review of the literature demonstrated that LEP patients who were assisted by a professional interpreter or bilingual practitioner showed almost no difference in test costs compared with EP patients. LEP patients were more likely to be admitted and have longer lengths of stay in the hospital compared to the EP cohort, which can lead to a tremendous difference in overall cost, especially if a longer length of stay is due to poor communication.

Ribera et al. (2008) reviewed a study conducted in Belgium that demonstrated that the use of professional interpreters leads to increased quality of care and preventive measures, especially in patients who have diabetes. In Europe, according to this study, it was estimated that 72% of diabetic patients will have at least one complication, and between 3% and 8% of diabetic patients will have a diabetic foot. Up to 20% of total costs in diabetes are attributed to diabetic foot, with over 70% of these costs occurring after an amputation. This study demonstrated that language difficulties were associated with less than optimal monitoring of diabetes among diabetics, which can lead to costly consequences. If the use of an interpreter can prevent one case of diabetic foot with gangrene, the interpreter's annual salary will be fully recovered in avoided medical costs. It also would be interesting to calculate the costs and benefits of the regular use of an array of certified medical interpreters in the delivery of neurorehabilitation services.

Ribera et al. (2008) also reported that the literature shows that linguistic barriers across different countries tend to negatively affect access to medical resources, preventive care, quality of care, nondominant-language-proficient patient satisfaction, and health personnel satisfaction. Many other studies have demonstrated similar results (Flores, 2005; Karliner et al., 2007). Overall, the literature showed decreased disparities between patients with a language barrier as compared with patients receiving care from language-concordant clinicians (Karliner et al., 2007). The findings of this review suggest that professional interpreters are associated with an overall improvement of care for LEP patients. They appear to decrease communication errors, increase patient comprehension, equalize health care utilization, improve clinical outcomes, and increase satisfaction with communication and clinical services for LEP patients. Professional interpreters improve clinical care more than ad hoc interpreters do, and they can raise the quality of clinical care for LEP patients to match or approach that for patients without a language barrier (Flores, 2005; Karliner et al., 2007; Ribera et al., 2008). It is likely that what is spent on interpreters is made up for with improvements in quality of care, fewer unnecessary diagnostic tests, fewer emergency department visits, better preventive care, and more follow-up. Over time, using professional interpreters is cost-efficient compared to the use of an ad hoc or no interpreter (Flores, 2005).

CASE EXAMPLES BY DR. ALBERTY

As a bilingual provider, I have often had the opportunity to sit with interpreters while they provided services to patients in my second language. At one institution, I could not provide interpreter services without first being a certified medical interpreter and passing all of the requirements needed to do so. The following are some personal experiences and interactions I have had with professional interpreters.

Case Vignette #1: Earlier in the chapter, it was explained how important it is to debrief the interpreter before the session if the conversation involves culturally sensitive or taboo information. I learned this from personal experience. At that session, I had assumed, without fully debriefing the interpreter, that she would be comfortable in the scenario. We were going to be discussing sex and sexuality after incurring a spinal cord injury. Having worked with this interpreter before, I immediately asked her if she was comfortable with this topic. She said she was, and we began the session. This interpreter was a Latina woman in her 60s. The patient was a Latino male in his early 30s, whose wife was present at the session. At a previous appointment, I had obtained the patient's consent to discuss sexuality after spinal cord injury.

As always, the interpreter first introduced herself to the couple. After receiving consent from the patient and his wife to proceed, we began providing psychoeducation on sexuality after spinal cord injury. It quickly became apparent to me that the interpreter was uncomfortable with this topic. She did not know how to communicate words like *lover* and *sex*. A few times, she asked me how to say something. I was taken aback because she was a very skilled interpreter and usually had no difficulty. The patient and his wife were receptive to the information, but their discomfort was obvious. It was particularly important that I help the interpreter feel comfortable, as well as the patient and his wife. At the same time, I wanted to make sure the interpreter did not feel I was overstepping her authority or that the patient and his wife did not sense my confusion. As we continued discussing the patient's future, he asked whether his paralysis would be permanent. I responded that most likely it would be permanent due to the severity and location of the injury. The interpreter relayed this as "Well, it may be permanent due to the nature of your injury, but with faith, you may be able to walk again." I quickly interrupted and explained that from a medical standpoint, it was very unlikely that he would ever be able to walk again. This is a common mistake that occurs even with professional interpreters. The interpreter does not want to deliver bad news or tries to couch it in a positive way and, in doing so, alters the meaning of the provider's words. I quickly clarified that I did not use the word *faith*, and from a purely medical perspective, the patient would probably never walk again. The patient had already been given this news by his primary physician, but he did not want to accept it. I followed up with the patient a few days later to see if he had any further questions about the psychoeducation that was provided or any concerns. He stated that he was grateful to have been provided the information and felt the session was helpful to his future lifestyle.

I was lucky enough to understand what was being said in this scenario and able to interrupt and tactfully correct certain parts of the interpretation that I was not comfortable with. What I learned most from this session was that it is always important to debrief the interpreter prior to beginning a session that will have taboo or emotionally salient information. If I could do it again, I would have set aside 10 minutes before the meeting to discuss the patient's prognosis and topic of sexuality with the interpreter. I would have confirmed with the interpreter that she was comfortable with the topic and asked if she had any questions. Often, no other interpreter is available, and even if she is uncomfortable with the topic, she has to provide the service. However, discussing key points in advance can put the interpreter at ease and help the provider form an alliance prior to going in with the patient. This may seem like a lot of extra work, but once you have used the same interpreter a few times, meeting with the patient will be easier and quicker. The most important thing is that the patient feels heard and is able to understand the information provided.

Case Vignette #2: Here is an another example of where using a professional interpreter can be extremely helpful. In this case, I had a young Latino patient who had recently suffered a spinal cord injury. The interpreter who was available was experienced in spinal cord injury and had assisted in sessions like this many times before. Prior to meeting with the patient, I met with the interpreter and explained the purpose of session, the patient's diagnosis, and his age. I asked the interpreter if he had any questions before meeting with the patient, and he said he was ready to proceed. As soon as the conversation began, the patient became very upset and started to cry. He said he had finally begun to accept that his life would never be the same. We discussed the importance of grieving the changes that had occurred and the parts of oneself that were lost. The interpreter was able to match my tone of voice, consistently sat slightly behind me, and allowed me to maintain good eye contact and rapport with the patient. Despite using short sentences and pauses so the interpreter could communicate oral information, the session flowed along without interruption. The patient was able to be fully vulnerable and open with me despite having a third party present. His vulnerability was rather astounding because he was a Latino male, and, culturally, it was unusual for him to cry, especially in front of another male (the interpreter). The interpreter was able to match my tone of voice as well as the patient's. In emotional moments like this, it is important that the interpreter be able to match the patient's tone without overly exaggerating emotions.

Case Vignette #3: It is important to note that sometimes just being from a similar culture and speaking the same language as your patient can make him or her feel more confident in you as a provider. Research has shown that, in general, patients who were seen by providers who spoke the same language as they did were more satisfied with their interactions with their providers (Flores, 2005; Green et al., 2005; Lee et al., 2002). I once had a young Latino patient in his early teens who had suffered a severe traumatic brain injury. He was nonverbal, unable to walk, and was barely able to move his extremities. When my supervisor and I first met with him and his parents, it was apparent that his parents were at varying levels of distress. His father had a flat affect and was obviously trying to be strong. He appeared to be filling the *machismo* role of Latino men. He was the head of the family, and he was not going to show any emotion. His wife was very tearful and distressed. At this time, I had already become a certified medical interpreter. I introduced myself to the parents in Spanish. The father stated that he was comfortable speaking in English, and the mother stated that she preferred to speak in Spanish.

I decided to talk to the mother, and my supervisor spoke with the patient's father. The mother was visibly distraught. She told me the patient's brother was also involved in the accident and sustained injuries as well, but did not sustain a traumatic brain injury. She was confused about what to do about her other son. He refused to visit his brother in the hospital. We discussed the details of the accident and the different emotions her other son might be feeling. After processing these ideas, the mother stated that she had not cried before this session. She said she had been trying to be strong for both of her sons and would not allow herself to break down. We discussed the importance of grieving and the difference between mourning a death and mourning a change that has occurred, such as the changes her son now had to deal with. She told me she could not talk to her husband about what was going on and that she just knew she needed to be strong for her family.

If I had not been able to speak Spanish, I would not have learned all of this information. I would not have known that she was holding back her emotions and felt that she did not have anyone to confide in. Through our conversation, I was able to form an alliance as a confidant and provide a safe place for her to release a month's worth of emotional turmoil. She did not feel comfortable speaking English, and her husband felt an interpreter was not necessary. We were able to address significant topics and come up with different times that she could allow herself to break down and other people she could do so with. Sometimes, just being from the same culture and speaking the same language make it possible to be vulnerable and open with a provider. With time, the wife was able to speak more openly with her husband, and the husband was also more open to talking to me about the patient.

Case Vignette #4: In another case, I had a patient who had suffered a severe stroke during a neurosurgery. After his stroke, he was unable to walk and was mostly nonverbal. The patient was Latino, in his late 60s, and had a military background. It was very important to the family that the patient be addressed by his military position because that was how he was addressed in everyday life prior to his stroke. It is important to note that certain cultures demand a level of respect for elders that may not be as apparent in other cultures.

For example, in the American culture, you can call any adult "Mr.," "Ms.," or "Mrs.," which are all considered respectful ways to address an individual. In the Latino cultures, there is a familial form of "tu" and respectful form of "ud." One uses the "ud." form whenever speaking to anyone who is older or may have higher authority. This is an important fact to take into consideration. I always use the respectful form of "ud." when interacting with Latino patients until I have been given permission by the patient to use the familial "tu" form. This allows me to show my patients that from a cultural perspective, I respect that they are my elders, and despite my position as a doctor, I still consider it appropriate to address them using the formal "ud." format. Most patients will quickly tell me that I can switch to the familial "tu" format, but this simple act allows us to quickly build a rapport and shows my patient that I understand certain cultural values that they may hold dear.

With this patient I made sure to announce to the rehabilitation team that he would like to be addressed by his military rank or by "Señor," the Spanish form of "Sir." The patient was not to be addressed by his first name because that was too informal for someone of his prestige. Although this may sound slightly narcissistic or odd to a reader who may not be as familiar with Latino cultures, this is considered showing earned respect within the Latino culture. I spent many sessions providing psychoeducation and support to the patient's wife and family. When it was my time to leave the rehabilitation setting, the patient's wife hugged me and thanked me for my help. She wished me well on my educational journey. It may seem odd to some individuals that a patient's family member would embrace a provider, but in the Latino culture, hugging is an acceptable form of gratitude among Latinos. The patient's wife knew my background. She had asked me in an earlier session how I learned Spanish, and she knew that I was also Latina. She felt comfortable expressing her gratitude with an embrace, and I felt comfortable accepting it, knowing the cultural norms. Had she not been Latina, or even had she been a male Latino, this may have been a different interaction or response. Within each culture, we automatically learn things that are expected and acceptable, which is why having a professional interpreter can be invaluable. Sometimes you may not know something truly important about cultural expectations that could explain a patient's behavior. It is not necessary for a provider to feel the need to return the embrace because the provider should always do what is most comfortable for them; however, it is important to know where the gesture is coming from and have an understanding of why it may not be inappropriate for this particular patient.

CONCLUSIONS

The literature has shown that the immigrant and minority populations will continue to grow in the United States. It is expected that by 2050, certain minority groups will have a greater population in the United States than the White majority. The United States is a country full of immigrants and continues to expand its immigrant population. Professional interpreters are becoming a necessity, especially in a medical setting. The research has shown that the use of interpreters over time actually ends up saving money and cutting costs of expensive surgeries that could have been avoided with better preventive care, better follow-up, and better adherence with treatment. Language is the essential tool we use to communicate our concerns and needs. When language is a barrier, individuals do not feel heard or understood. When using an interpreter, the patient does feel heard and is more likely to follow through with treatment because she has a better understanding of why treatment is necessary and how to appropriately follow up. Professional interpreters and bilingual providers are invaluable because not only do they allow for fluid communication between the patient and the provider, but they also understand cultural values and how they can impact a patient's perspective or expectations within the medical setting. Professional interpreters provide an invaluable service that allows patients who are not proficient in the dominant language to have their voices heard.

ADDITIONAL RESOURCES

Partners for Applied Social Sciences (www.pass-international.org)
Diversity Rx (www.diversityrx.org)

Cross-cultural health care program (www.xculture.org)

Information about caring for patients with limited English proficiency (www.lep.gov)

American Translators Association (www.atanet.org)

National Hispanic Medical Associates (www.nhmamd.org)

Spanish-speaking neuropsychologist directory (http://hnps.org/find-a-spanish-speaking-neuropsychologist)

If you are looking for a board-certified neuropsychologist who speaks another language, see www.theaacn.org/findboardcertifiedcn.aspx

SYNOPSIS: WORKING WITH A PROFESSIONAL INTERPRETER IN A MEDICAL SETTING

The following is a synopsis of some considerations when working with a professional interpreter:

- If this is your first time working with a specific interpreter, review the limits of confidentiality.
- Debrief the interpreter about the patient's basic demographics and the topic if it is one that is emotionally salient or taboo, such as a bad prognosis, or if sexuality will be addressed in this session.
- Ask the interpreter about cultural issues or factors if you think they may be relevant to your patient.
- Have the interpreter stand slightly to the side or behind the provider, allowing the provider and patient to maintain direct eye contact. This also makes it possible for the patient to look directly at both of you and not have to turn his or her head.
- Have the interpreter introduce himself and explain why he is there before the session begins. Make sure the interpreter asks the patient if she would like an interpreter. Do not assume that all patients will.
- Speak to the patient using first-person language as you would with any of your patients.
- Maintain eye contact with your patient, and address the patient. Do not address the interpreter.
- Speak in your normal tone of voice. Use short sentences, and pause frequently to allow the interpreter to be able to communicate oral information accurately.

- Attend to your patient's nonverbal cues, and ask your patient through-out the session if he or she has any questions.
- Attend to the interpreter's tone of voice, and if it does not match yours or the patient's, ask the interpreter to ensure his tone matches each person he is interpreting for.
- When the session is completed and you have left the patient, ask the interpreter if he has any questions or needs to debrief what occurred in the session.

REFERENCES

Anderson, L. M., Scrimshaw, S. C., Fullilove, M. T., Fielding, J. E., Normand, J., & the Task Force on Community Preventive Services. (2003). Culturally com-petent healthcare systems. *American Journal of Preventative Medicine, 24*(3S), 68–79.

Avery, M. B. (2001). The role of the health care interpreter: An evolving dia-logue. *The National Council on Interpreting in Health Care Working Papers Series.* Retrieved from www.ncihc.org/index.php?option=com_content&view=arti cle&id=103

Flores, G. (2005). The impact of medical interpreter services on the quality of health care: A systematic review. *Medical Care Research and Review, 62*(3), 255–299.

Flores, G., Laws, B. M., Mayo, S. J., Zuckerman, B., Abreu, M., Meidna, L., & Hardt, E. (2003). Errors in medical interpretation and their potential clinical consequences in pediatric encounters. *Pediatrics, 111*(1), 6–14.

Fontes, L. A. (2008). *Interviewing clients across cultures: A practitioner's guide.* New York, NY: Guilford Press.

Green, A. R., Ngo-Metzger, Q., Legedza, A. T. R., Massagli, M. P., Phillips, R. S., & Lezzoni, L. I. (2005). Interpreter service, language concordance, and health care quality: Experiences of Asian Americans with limited English proficiency. *Journal of General Internal Medicine, 20*, 1050–1056.

Karliner, L. S., Jacobs, E. A., Chen, A. H., & Mutha, S. (2007). Do professional inter-preters improve clinical care for patients with limited English proficiency? A systematic review of the literature. *Health Services Research, 42*(2), 727–754.

Lee, L. J., Batal, H. A., Maselli, J. H., & Kutner, J. S. (2002). Effect of Spanish inter-pretation method on patient satisfaction in an urban walk-in clinic. *Journal of General Internal Medicine, 17*, 641–646.

Ribera, J. M., Hausmann-Muela, S., Grietens, K. P., & Toomer, E. (2008). Is the use of interpreters in medical consultations justified? A critical review of the literature. Retrieved from http://www.tvgent.be/downloads/interpreters inmedicalconsulations.acriticalrev.pdf

Romero, C. M. (2004). Curbside consultation: Using medical interpreters. *American Family Physician, 69*(11), 2720–2723.

Ruschke, K., Bidar-Sielaff, S., Avery, M. B., Downing, B., Green, C. E., & Haffner, L. (2005). *National standards of practice for interpreters in health care*. Retrieved from http://www.ncihc.org/assets/documents/publications/National_ Standards_5-09-11.pdf

U.S. Census Bureau. (2007). *Facts for features: Hispanic heritage month 2007: Sept 15–Oct 15*. Press release CB07–FF.14. Issued July 16, 2007.

RECOMMENDED READING

Andres-Hyman, R. C., Ortiz, J., Anez, L. M., Paris, M., & Davidson, L. (2006). Culture and clinical practice: Recommendations for working with Puerto Ricans and other Latinas(os) in the United States. *Professional Psychology: Research and Practice, 37*(6), 694–701.

Casas, R., Guzman-Velez, E., Cardona-Rodriguez, J., Rodriguez, N., Quinones, G., Juan, S., . . . Tranel, D. (2012). Interpreter mediated neuropsychological testing of monolingual Spanish speakers. *Clinical Neuropsychology, 26*(1), 88–101.

Derose, K. P., & Baker, D. W. (2000). Limited English proficiency and Latinos' use of physician services. *Medical Care Research and Review, 57*(1), 76–91.

Fagan, M. J., Diaz, J. A., Reinert, S. E., Sciamanna, C. N., & Fagan, D. M. (2003). Impact of interpretation method on clinical visit length. *Journal of General Internal Medicine, 18*, 634–638.

Gany, F., Leng, J., Shapiro, E., Abramson, D., Motola, I., Shield, D. C., & Changrani, J. (2007). Patient satisfaction with different interpreting methods: A randomized controlled trial. *Journal of General Internal Medicine, 22*(Suppl. 2), 312–318.

Garcia, E. A., Roy, L. C., Okada, P. J., Perkins, S. D., & Wiebe, R. A. (2004). A comparison of the influence of hospital trained, ad hoc, and telephone interpreters on perceived satisfaction of limited English proficient parents presenting to a pediatric emergency department. *Pediatric Emergency Care, 20*(6), 373–378.

Gerrish, K., Chau, R., Sobowale, A., & Birks, E. (2004). Bridging the language barrier: The use of interpreters in primary care nursing. *Health and Social Care in the Community, 12*(5), 407–413.

Hampers, L. C., & McNulty, J. E. (2002). Professional interpreters and bilingual physicians in a pediatric emergency department. *Archives of Pediatric Adolescent Medicine, 156*, 1108–1113.

Howard, S. (2006). Use of interpreters in palliative care. *End of Life/Palliative Education Resource Center Medical College of Wisconsin*. Retrieved from https://drive .google.com/file/d/0By/FEWCSwGsUWWtLeEluX0FZVzg/view?pli=1

Hudelson, P. (2005). Improving patient-provider communication: Insights from interpreters. *Family Practice, 22,* 311–316.

Jacobs, E. A., Sadowski, L. S., & Rahouz, P. J. (2007). The impact of an enhanced interpreter service intervention on hospital costs and patient satisfaction. *Journal of General Internal Medicine, 22*(Suppl. 2), 306–311.

Jacobs, E. A., Shepard, D. S., Suaya, J. A., & Stone, E. L. (2004). Overcoming language barriers in health care: Costs and benefits of interpreter services. *American Journal of Public Health, 94*(5), 866–869.

Karliner, L. S., Perez-Stable, E., & Gildengorin, G. (2004). The language divide: The importance of training in the use of interpreters for outpatient practice. *Journal of General Internal Medicine, 19,* 175–183.

Laws, M. B., Heckscher, R., Mayo, S. J., Li, W., Wilson, I. B. (2004). A new method for evaluating the quality of medical interpretation. *Medical Care, 42*(1), 71–80.

Mindt, M. R., Arentoft, A., Germano, K. K., D'Aquila, E., Scheiner, D., Pizzirusso, M., . . . Gollan, T. H. (2008). Neuropsychological, cognitive, and theoretical considerations for evaluation of bilingual individuals. *Neuropsychological Review, 18,* 255–268.

Mindt, M. R., Byrd, D., Saez, P., & Manly, J. (2010). Increasing culturally competent neuropsychological services for ethnic minority populations: A call to action. *Clinical Neuropsychology, 24*(3), 429–453.

Ramirez, D., Engel, K. G., & Tang, T. S. (2008). Language interpreter utilization in the emergency department setting: A clinical review. *Journal of Health Care for the Poor and Underserved, 19*(2), 352–362.

CHAPTER NINE

REHABILITATION IN MILITARY AND VETERAN POPULATIONS: THE IMPACT OF MILITARY CULTURE

Alison N. Cernich, Heather G. Belanger, Michael Pramuka, and William L. Brim

The United States has a strong history of military service, with individuals serving in various declared wars, conflicts, and operations through the decades. Currently, approximately 21,973,000 U.S. citizens are military veterans (National Center for Veterans Analysis and Statistics, 2014). With approximately 2.65 million deployments in support of Operation Enduring Freedom/Operation Iraqi Freedom/Operation New Dawn (OEF/OIF/OND) through June 2014 (OSD Press Office, personal communication, 2014), a significant portion of the population is placed at high risk for incurring an injury that might require rehabilitation. In addition, approximately 1.2 million individuals have had more than one deployment, increasing their risk for incurring a deployment-related injury (OSD Press Office, personal communication, 2014). Many individuals who have served in combat present with complex conditions, multiple comorbidities, polytrauma, and mental health disorders. This may also be the case for those individuals who have not deployed but who have suffered injuries or illnesses as a result of training exercises or routine military tasks.

Rehabilitation providers who work with service members and veterans face significant cultural challenges that may impact the rehabilitation process. Part of this challenge is maintaining an awareness that any individual engaged in rehabilitation could have had prior military service that could impact rehabilitation care. This chapter provides an overview of military culture, including specific aspects of this culture that may affect the rehabilitation process, the various co-occurring disorders that are common in military/veteran populations, and resources and programs that are particularly useful when working with service members and veterans.

UNDERSTANDING MILITARY CULTURE

A provider who works with service members or veterans can benefit from developing a cultural competency with all aspects of military life. Understanding the individual's service characteristics (active duty, Reserve, National Guard), branch of service (e.g., Army, Navy, Marines, Air Force), era of service (e.g., Vietnam, Korea, Gulf War, OEF/OIF/OND, humanitarian missions), and occupational classification helps the provider to understand the context in which the individual served. Asking about deployments and the nature of those deployments gives the provider further understanding of the context in which the individual served and may provide valuable information related to the potential physical, psychological, or environmental risks to which the service member or veteran was exposed. Finally, understanding military culture provides the framework needed for the individual to serve with dignity and honor.

Identification of the military ethos requires an understanding of both the overt and subtle characteristics of military life. Most apparent to a provider would be designation of an individual by uniform, medals, specification of rank, and outward signs of military participation (e.g., service paraphernalia, clothing, tattoos). At a more subtle level, service members and veterans live by a creed, oath, and set of core values that are specific to their branch or even to their unit. Specific underlying attributes that are part of the military culture may require more understanding and exploration by the provider to discover how it may impact rehabilitation, including the individual's commitments to discipline, teamwork, loyalty to team, self-sacrifice, fighting spirit, and warrior values and beliefs. Each branch of the service has a unique set of core beliefs that sets it apart, and it is important to understand the individual's commitment to those beliefs and how those beliefs shape his or her behavior. Even within each branch of service, different units deploy with different missions, including as combatants, support to other units, or protectors of other people or territories. Understanding that these roles can change over time and can affect the way service members views themselves is another aspect of the role of military culture.

The military ethos is often greater than just the role of the service branch. Underlying all branches is a set of values that is instilled and emphasized, and designed to make the individual service member better able to function in the military environment. Teamwork is a major emphasis in the military, and it is taught as part of initial training and reemphasized throughout service because it is the key to successful military operations. The values of selflessness, honesty, and loyalty in service to the unit, the military, and the nation are constantly reinforced. The service member is infused with a moral focus and trained to make quick ethical decisions in situations that are morally ambiguous. Finally, the service member is encouraged to develop a sense of loyalty and commitment to fellow service members to enable strong team functioning. Understanding how service members see themselves and their experiences in the context of this ethos may help a provider to understand the roles of loss, shame, or guilt in the presentation of clinical symptoms. Also, an overdeveloped sense that an individual can rely on himself and his unit can interfere with seeking help from health care providers or assist in ignoring problems in service of other goals.

Accepting the warrior ethos as part of one's self-concept plays several protective roles for the service member. Living by the military ethos gives the service member the strength to persevere in periods of great danger and deprivation of resources. One powerful reason for living according to a warrior ethos or code is that it may protect the service member herself from serious psychological damage. In wartime, service members must do things that are not always pleasant, and the combination of their own disgust at what they see on the battlefield and the uncivilized nature of what they do could cause feelings of severe self-loathing if they have not accepted the higher moral calling of a warrior. What a warrior does is not for his own pleasure but out of a sense of duty and a respect of his country's values. By adhering to these higher standards, service members can create a lifeline that will help them assimilate their role into a healthy view of themselves and to reintegrate into society after war.

The military ethos and the standards infused in those who have served at times make the individual vulnerable to "moral injury," which comes from witnessing, doing, or not doing something that violates the individual's moral values. For those who perceive their actions as contrary to their values or who feel they have failed to live up to their standards, there may be a great deal of shame or guilt. There may be feelings of inadequacy or incompetence that reflect a failure to live up to military standards. If they view others as not living up to those ideals, anger may be the primary reaction.

The military ethos, although protective in some scenarios, can also create challenges for service members, especially when it comes to seeking health care. For example, the value of selflessness—putting the well-being of others above one's own needs—is an important tenet of military culture, but it may also mean that service members will not seek medical help because they feel their own needs are not a priority. The ability to display toughness and to stoically endure hardship without complaint is a bedrock of military culture, but it might also mean that it is anathema to the service member to acknowledge his or her own pain and suffering. For service members who have been trained and have accepted that they must show excellence in all they do, physical or emotional injuries are a reason for shame.

The military culture and the health care culture are in many ways so diametrically opposed that what is perceived as a strength in one is a weakness or even pathological in the other. Whereas the warrior culture values self-sacrifice, the health care culture values self-care. The warrior values group achievement, and health care focuses on self-determination. The service member values increased pain tolerance and emotional suppression, and health care focuses on pain reduction and values emotional expression.

The provider who incorporates strength-based conceptualizations and uses an active skills training approach focused on functional outcomes that are valuable to the service member will make a bigger impact on that member's life. The provider who is always aware of these deeply held culture differences and tries to understand them and work with the member's self-view will be significantly more effective at treating the service member.

As in other cultures, there are degrees of acculturation, and it varies among individuals. Before assuming the warrior ethos and values are standard, the provider should ask the patient about personal experiences and determine the degree to which the patient embraces the military culture and ethos. This may vary due to particular experiences during the time of service, the length of service, the quality of the experience in the military, and/or demographic or social characteristics. Further, the military may not be the primary culture with which the person identifies, in which case other aspects of culture still need to be explored to provide culturally competent care (e.g., family of origin, religion, culture of origin).

Conveying an awareness and understanding of the military culture and a willingness to work with service members within their view of their illness or injury begins with the questions that are asked in the initial interview. With a heightened sense of the heterogeneity of the military culture, the culturally aware provider understands that it is no longer sufficient to just ask, "Are you a veteran or currently serving in the military?" Table 9.1 lists some questions that can help you compile the military history portion of your assessment. The culturally sensitive provider will recognize that not all of these questions will be relevant in every interview, but they are

Table 9.1 *Interview Questions Relevant to Military Service*

Question	Clinical Implication
What branch of service are/were you in?	Recognizing which service the patient is/was in can provide insight into the types of missions in which the service member may have participated.
Were you ever in the Guard or Reserve?	Following up a positive response to this question with the next questions about duties and deployments is important.
What years did you serve?	This question gives you a time frame of their service and lets you know how long they were in the military. You can use this information to inform later questions— for example, if service dates were between 1965 and 1973, they may have served in Vietnam, or if between 1969 and 1972, they may have been drafted.
What was your rank?	Be aware of the rank structure. A basic understanding of the potential responsibilities associated with ranks is helpful.
What is/was your occupation(s) in the military?	The career field tells what a person does in the military and can include fields such as Armor, Infantry, Aviation, Hospital Corpsman, or Dental Technician.
How many duty assignments did you have, and where were they?	Often people are surprised with the number of moves that military members may have had over the course of their time in service. It might also be relevant if they had only a few assignments over the course of a 20-year career. In general, military members can expect to have a move (called a permanent change of station, or PCS) every 3 to 4 years, but many will have more or fewer.

(continued)

Table 9.1 *Interview Questions Relevant to Military Service (continued)*

Question	Clinical Implication
What were some of the reasons you decided to join the military originally? Were they different than the reasons you stayed in the military (if they served more than 1 to 4 years).	
What were the major milestones in your career?	The answers may be related to promotions, selection for leadership positions, or the earning of awards. This information may also be valuable as a part of your conceptualization and treatment planning because it will give you some insight into the types of things they value.
What was the impact of military service on your family?	Military members clearly indicate that family concerns are a top stressor. Understanding the member's perspective of how military service in general affected the family is an important acknowledgment of their whole military service.
Were you ever deployed?	*Deployed* is a relatively new term in the general public. You may also ask if they ever served in combat, "went to war," or served during a war or conflict.
What was most rewarding part of deployment?	It is also not good to assume that deployment did not have rewarding aspects or was even a growth experience. Members and veterans will report learning about strengths that they were not aware of, quitting smoking, starting a healthier lifestyle, and forming bonds with others as examples of rewarding aspects of being deployed.
What was most difficult part of deployment?	Never assume that the answer to this question will be seeing combat or other war-related trauma.
When did you deploy? Where?	Understanding where and when members were deployed may give significant insights into what their experiences may have been.
How many times did you deploy, and how long were the deployments?	In Operation Iraqi Freedom/New Dawn/Operation Enduring Freedom, members and veterans experienced multiple deployments. You may have to inquire about the experience of each deployment separately.

(continued)

Table 9.1 *Interview Questions Relevant to Military Service (continued)*

Question	Clinical Implication
What were your duties in theater?	Many times the duties assigned to members in the deployed environment are different from what they do as a regular duty when in garrison.
Did you see combat? / How often were you "outside the wire"?	Members will not necessarily have been "combatants" to have seen combat or to be exposed directly and intimately with combat-related experiences.
Did you deploy with your unit, or were you an individual augmentee?	Members who deploy as an augmentee to a larger, already intact, unit often report more psychological health issues and report they felt less unit cohesiveness and support.
If Guard or Reserve, how did being deployed impact your life compared to coming home and returning to civilian life?	Guard and Reserve members are at higher risk for psychological health issues.
Did you feel supported by the unit?	Several recent studies and surveys have indicated that unit cohesion and the impression of unit leadership can have an impact on psychological health.
Were you exposed to blasts while deployed?	This is an opportunity for you to assess the possible presence of traumatic brain injury and add to your differential diagnosis, and it may lead to referral for neurological evaluation.
What was your exposure to the deaths of unit members, enemy combatants, or civilians?	This can be a difficult topic to broach with a new client and should be addressed carefully.
Do you feel like there are any lasting physical or psychological effects of your exposure to these potentially traumatic events?	This is a way to transition from discussing an event to a person's reaction to the event.
What is the possibility that you will get deployed again?	Military member may report that they wish to deploy again as soon as possible. Often the deployed setting is one that is more compatible for their "new normal." They may be reluctant to deploy again.

(continued)

Table 9.1 *Interview Questions Relevant to Military Service (continued)*

Question	Clinical Implication
How was coming home from deployment? Was it different than you expected?	Often members come home with high expectations for the homecoming. There are many stressors associated with homecoming. Members often report feeling overwhelmed by the number of people who want to see them or have some of their time.
What was impact of deployment on your family?	Many members will report that the deployment was hardest on the spouse or family members. Often you will hear from family members that they learned they had strengths and capabilities they did not know they had when the member was deployed.

Source: Adapted from and published with kind permission from the Center for Deployment Psychology at the Uniformed Services University of the Health Sciences. For more information regarding culturally sensitive interviewing with service members and veterans, or for online training in military culture, please visit www.deploymentpsych.org

meant to be an extensive, though not exhaustive, guide and a potential starting point for understanding the member's worldview. The member's responses may generate more inquiry along a particular topic or may indicate that this is not a relevant area.

UNIQUE STRESSORS IN MILITARY AND VETERAN POPULATIONS

Service members and veterans face unique challenges and stressors that are over and above some of the routine sources of stress that others face in the workplace. Service members are considered 24/7 employees—that is, they are essentially on call all the time. During times of conflict and deployment to theaters of operations or peacekeeping missions, training requirements and operational demands may lengthen workdays and increase stress levels. Stress can come from participating in combat, including exposure to traumatic events, risk of injury, and fears about deployment. Further, operational stressors may be involved that include exposure to extreme environments, prolonged separation from support systems, and exposure to significant injuries or traumas over multiple missions, including the death of colleagues.

Even in nondeployed or noncombat settings, service members face routine stressors as part of their everyday jobs. They are required to make a PCS move to new posts every 2 to 3 years, and they have no say in where they are sent. They must participate in drills, hazardous training activities, natural disaster exercises, and other mandatory training in addition to their jobs. Finally, they are required to maintain a high level of physical fitness throughout their time of service.

Deployment is a separate and unique stressor requiring service members to serve at a location other than their permanent duty station, without family, for periods of up to 2 years. Deployment is often with the individual's unit, but a service member can be assigned to another unit as needed by the mission as an individual augmentee. In the most recent conflicts, service members experienced multiple deployments, some of which lasted for periods greater than a year and with time between deployments less than the Department of Defense's benchmark of 5 years.

Certain components of the military, including the National Guard and Reserve Components, face unique stressors because of the manner in which they serve. Reserve Component members are federal service members who serve as augmentees to the active duty force. National Guard components are state-level service members who can also be called to augment the active duty force. Both groups, when activated, receive benefits commensurate with their active duty counterparts and face similar deployment stressors. Although these roles have some good benefits, including base privileges and retirement pay, these members also have unique stressors in that they maintain other employment in the civilian sector when they are not on active duty, which may be interrupted by a deployment. Also, often, they are located away from military installations and communities where their families can receive support. If Reserve or Guard members are deployed, they return more quickly to their communities, often away from military facilities and their deployment cohort.

IMPACT OF MILITARY CULTURE ON REHABILITATION

It is important to understand certain unique aspects of military life when working in military/veteran rehabilitation settings. Adjustment to injury is a key part of the rehabilitation process for any patient. With postdeployed service members and veterans, adjustment is multiplicative—that is, besides having to adjust to an injury and resulting disability, members also face separation from their unit or base and possibly from the United States and their families.

Characteristics of military life vary by service and rank. As already mentioned, each branch has a unique tradition and set of missions that will shape the individual's service. However, some global aspects of military culture can interact with the treatment setting. Often, military service members and veterans are accustomed to early-morning activities and meetings. In addition, punctuality and preparedness are key aspects of military life. Tardiness and lack of preparation are often considered signs of incompetence. Providers should be aware that structure and clear definitions of tasks are inherent to most military tasks and operations. As such, it is helpful for providers to ensure that rehabilitation groups or interventions address a very specific and delineated goal or a specific challenge. The process of defining the goal is useful to set expectations and limits and is culturally consistent with the way jobs or tasks are assigned in military settings.

Service members who have chosen a military career often have an attraction to physically active or high-risk tasks and environments. Their expectations for recovery and their choice of leisure or vocational activities after injury often continue to reflect this preference. Rehabilitation providers need to be aware that service members and veterans will continue to expect a lot of themselves, which poses both opportunities and challenges. Veterans and service members may engage in functional activities or mobility tasks prematurely (i.e., before cleared by their clinician) and immediately return to walking, running, weight lifting, or engaging in demanding cognitive tasks. Although it may seem to be evidence of their determination to recover fully, this may hamper or impede rehabilitation progress at times. Service members or veterans may demonstrate a desire to engage in high-risk activities (water sports, skydiving, driving), which clinicians may see as contraindicated given their level of recovery. This requires a delicate balance between understanding the contribution of these activities to the individual's quality of life and encouraging awareness of the risks involved and the possible setbacks that could occur. Moreover, because of the complex nature of many of the injuries in the current and past cohort, clinicians often have to understand the potentially different requirements for mobility devices (prosthetics, wheelchairs, ankle–foot orthoses) to support this population in strenuous physical activity, recreational activity in rugged environments, and team sports.

Not only do service members often retain a commitment to physical performance as they engage in rehabilitation, but the organizational structure of the military may affect the individual's choice of providers and interaction with rehabilitation interventions as well. For example, service members and veterans may express a preference for providers who are in uniform or are themselves veterans. Sometimes the military hierarchy may create uncomfortable situations in rehabilitation. For example, a high-ranking officer may be uncomfortable disclosing personal information to a lower-ranking junior medical officer, or vice versa. Junior ranking officers may be more inclined to see a civilian provider because of perceived risks to their career. Service branch and rank may be salient in group-based interventions (recreation therapy, group counseling) and may inhibit lower-ranking individuals from providing feedback to higher-ranking individuals in the group or interfere with group dynamics.

The dynamic of the individual who has a history of or is currently serving in the military is also strongly tied to his interaction not only with the military but with the family system. As with other cultures, military families have specific characteristics that may affect the individual's inability to interact with a rehabilitation program. Military families specifically have frequent deployments or moves from one duty station to another over the course of the service members' careers. Different families choose either to move frequently or to allow for separation of the service member if a tour or operation will be brief. These frequent moves, especially if they are in small military communities that do not have a large military post, may affect the individual's connection with the larger community and social supports. In addition, there are particular challenges to individuals in the National Guard and Reserve Components who may deploy with a unit but do not return to a military post or base and become disconnected from the unit with which they deployed. These separations from the military family and their nuclear family or family of origin may cause additional stressors that will impact the rehabilitation process due to lack of social support or ongoing family conflicts that began during deployment or were sustained through multiple permanent changes of stations. It is important to understand the effects of military service on the family so they can be considered in the overall rehabilitation plan. It is also possible that during the individual's rehabilitation stay, she is receiving treatment far away from the family and thus has no regular social support.

Finally, as a provider working with service members and veterans, one needs to understand one's own biases and beliefs related to those who served in the military that may affect practice patterns or interactions with the patient. This can include the providers' beliefs about individuals who serve in the military, beliefs related to war and national security, views on social or political issues that are tied to military service, and providers' willingness to welcome veterans and service members in the community and into the practice. As a provider working with this population, it is important to try to remain neutral in the expression of beliefs or attitudes that might interfere in offering the best possible treatment. In addition, one needs to understand the context in which one is working with this population. If the provider is engaged in diagnostic or assessment work as part of a medical evaluation for separation or compensation, the context of the interaction is different than if one is engaged in work that is aimed at symptomatic recovery and/or rehabilitation. Understanding one's role with the patient and ensuring cultural competence with the population are integral to providing care to this population. Training opportunities are available for those who have not worked with this population. Veterans Affairs (VA) and the Department of Defense jointly host a training program through the Center for Deployment Psychology that provides a beginning point for those who are interested in working with this population (www.deploymentpsych.org/military-culture-course-modules).

CO-OCCURRING DISORDERS THAT MAY IMPACT REHABILITATION

Perhaps even more than in other populations, co-occurring disorders and comorbidities are particularly relevant in the military/veteran rehabilitation setting (Cernich, Chandler, Scherdell, & Kurtz, 2012; Friedemann-Sanchez, Sayer, & Pickett, 2008; Lew et al., 2009). Lew et al. (2009) found that in veterans presenting to outpatient clinics, nearly 82% had more than one diagnosis, and 42% had three. In contrast, civilian traumatic brain injury (TBI) is typically associated with fewer comorbidities when compared to other rehabilitation populations (such as stroke and orthopedic injury; Holcomb, Millis, & Hanks, 2012). Due to the nature of war-induced injury, other (i.e., non-TBI) physical and psychological injuries are common. Combat presents some unique psychological experiences, as well as physical injuries. In the psychological realm, posttraumatic stress disorder (PTSD), readjustment issues (i.e., readjustment to home life, adjustment to injury), and grieving for fallen colleagues are common issues that may impact the rehabilitation process. In the physical realm, due to the ubiquity of explosive devices used in modern combat, blast injuries are prevalent and can create a host of challenges.

Indeed, in the postdeployment realm, much attention, both in the popular press and in the medical literature, has been directed at "blast injuries" that result from exposure to high-energy explosions. *Blast injury* as a general term refers to the biophysical and pathophysiological events and the clinical syndromes that occur when the human body is exposed to a blast or explosion. Blast injuries most typically come from improvised explosive devices (IEDs), rocket-propelled grenades (RPGs), and land mines, and they account for approximately 50% to 78% of injuries sustained in combat (Coupland & Meddings, 1999; Owens et al., 2008; Ritenour et al., 2010). Ritenour et al. (2010) found that from 2003 to 2006, incidence of primary blast injury increased, whereas return-to-duty rates decreased, suggesting increasing injury survival and severity associated with these types of events.

Blast injuries typically are divided into four categories: primary, secondary, tertiary, and quaternary injuries. Individuals may be injured via high-force blast waves (primary blast injuries) or by the mechanical aftermath of the explosion, such as expelled missile fragments, being forcefully thrown, or being crushed by collapsing objects (secondary, tertiary, or quaternary blast injuries, respectively; DePalma et al., 2005; Taber et al., 2006). As such, exposure to blast-level forces can cause a multitude of injuries, including damage to internal organs, multiple fractures, amputations, burns (both on the skin and through inhalation), and ruptured tympanic membranes. Table 9.2 lists some common blast injuries. Sayer et al. (2008), in an inpatient VA rehabilitation sample, found that blasts produced a unique constellation of comorbidities but did not differentially affect outcomes.

From a psychological perspective, PTSD is obviously something about which rehabilitation specialists should be aware when working with military and veteran patients. Controversy has existed regarding whether PTSD and TBI can co-occur following a traumatic event. The issue at hand is whether it is possible to be psychologically traumatized by an event when one is unconscious. As such, the controversy applies more to moderate to severe than to mild TBI because the diagnostic criteria for the former but not the latter require loss of consciousness. PTSD is more common in the postdeployed population in milder TBI groups (Belanger, Kretzmer, Vanderploeg, & French, 2010; Jamora, Young, & Ruff,

Table 9.2 *Common Blast Injuries*

System/Organ	Injury or Condition
Auditory/ vestibular	Tympanic membrane rupture, ossicular disruption, cochlear damage, foreign body, hearing loss, distorted hearing, tinnitus, earache, dizziness, sensitivity to noise
Eye, orbit, face	Perforated globe, foreign body, air embolism, fractures
Respiratory	Blast lung, hemothorax, pneumothorax, pulmonary contusion and hemorrhage, atrioventricular fistula (source of air embolism), airway epithelial damage, aspiration pneumonitis, sepsis
Digestive	Bowel perforation, hemorrhage, ruptured liver or spleen, mesenteric ischemia from air embolism, sepsis, peritoneal irritation, rectal bleeding
Circulatory	Cardiac contusion, myocardial infarction from air embolism, shock, vasovagal hypotension, peripheral vascular injury, air embolism–induced injury
Central nervous system	Concussion, closed or open brain injury, petechial hemorrhage, edema, stroke, small blood vessel rupture, spinal cord injury, air embolism–induced injury, hypoxia or anoxia, diffuse axonal injury
Renal/urinary tract	Renal contusion, laceration, acute renal failure due to rhabdomyolysis, hypotension, hypovolemia
Extremity	Traumatic amputation, fractures, crush injuries, burns, cuts, lacerations, infections, acute arterial occlusion, air embolism–induced injury
Soft tissue	Crush injuries, burns, infections, slow healing wounds
Emotional/ psychological	Acute stress reactions, posttraumatic stress disorder, survivor guilt, postconcussion syndrome, depression, generalized anxiety disorder
Pain	Acute pain from wounds, crush injuries, or traumatic amputations; chronic pain syndromes

Source: Reprinted with kind permission of the author and publisher from Scott, S. G., Vanderploeg, R. D., Belanger, H. G., & Scholten, J. (2005). Blast injuries: Evaluating and treating the postacute sequelae. *The Federal Practitioner, 22,* 67–75.

2012). A recent review of the controversy suggests that varying methodologies (i.e., self-report versus structured interview) used in research studies has led to contradictory findings (Sbordone & Ruff, 2010) in more severely injured groups.

Regardless, when both TBI and PTSD are present, King (2008) purports that they can be "mutually exacerbating" (p. 3). Longitudinal study suggests that PTSD symptoms reported in theater more strongly predict postdeployment symptoms and outcomes than does a history of mild TBI (Polusny et al., 2011). Furthermore, PTSD symptom severity has been found to mediate the relationship between war zone exposure and postdeployment symptoms (Wachen et al., 2013).

In one study, sustaining a TBI nearly doubled the PTSD rates for participants with less severe predeployment PTSD symptoms (Yurgil et al., 2014). An important thing to remember in the context of milder forms of TBI and enduring symptoms is that two or more different etiologies may be present simultaneously. Within the psychological realm, there could be normal reactions to abnormal levels of stress and readjustment, as well as potentially abnormal responses that include clinical disorders defined by the *Diagnostic and Statistical Manual of Mental Disorders,* Fifth Edition (e.g., anxiety syndromes, adjustment disorders, conversion syndromes, depressive disorders, psychotic reactions), as well as malingering (American Psychiatric Association, 2013). Within the physiological injury realm, direct injury to the brain could be involved, as well as other physical injuries. Also underappreciated is that these two independent processes (physiological and psychological) could potentially interact and compound the effects of each other (Vanderploeg, Belanger, & Brenner, 2013).

Another common comorbidity in military populations is alcohol abuse. Psychiatric epidemiology studies have repeatedly found higher rates of substance-related disorders among veterans compared to the general population (Eisen et al., 2004; Thomas et al., 2010). Clearly, substance use and abuse raise the risks for injury. However, although it has been reported that acute alcohol intoxication exerts both detrimental and beneficial effects on TBI severity and outcome, the data are often contradictory, and mechanisms have not been clearly elucidated (Andelic et al., 2010). Substance abuse is associated with the presence of other neuropsychiatric disorders (Castano-Monsalve, Bernabeu-Guitart, Lopez, Bulbena-Vilarrasa, & Quemada, 2013).

Sleep difficulties are common in postdeployed individuals and therefore constitute an important consideration in military rehabilitation settings. To begin with, individuals with TBI report significantly more difficulty with sleep than the general population (Fogelberg, Hoffman, Dikmen, Temkin, & Bell, 2012). Further, Fogelberg et al. found that participants with one or more conditions (i.e., depression, anxiety, pain) had significantly worse sleep than those without these comorbidities. Added to that, deployment heightens the likelihood of poor sleep, particularly when

PTSD is present. Indeed, disturbed sleep is a prominent feature of PTSD. It is important to consider these factors because poor sleep is associated with worse outcomes and poorer quality of life (Cantor et al., 2012; Duclos et al., 2013; Fogelberg et al., 2012; Nakase-Richardson et al., 2013b) in TBI patients. Obviously, poor sleep can adversely impact participation in rehabilitation therapies, cognitive performance (Brownlow, Hall Brown, & Mellman, 2014), and overall motivation. There is some suggestion that individuals recovering from TBI need more sleep than normal during the acute recovery phase (Sommerauer, Valko, Werth, & Baumann, 2013).

Given the prevalence of comorbidities in the postcombat patient population, then, what are the practical implications of the aforementioned physical and psychological comorbidities for the rehabilitation specialist? One consideration is that medical concerns often are necessarily more of a focus in patients with comorbidities than is typical in the rehabilitation setting. When numerous physical injuries are present, medical complexity increases, and medical staff may need a greater presence on the rehabilitation service, beyond the physiatrist (Friedemann-Sanchez et al., 2008). Patients who have sustained crush injuries in war may require fasciotomies due to impending compartment syndrome. Many patients who have sustained severe head trauma will require partial craniectomy to control for edema. Infections and pain are also common in postcombat rehabilitation patients (Nakase-Richardson et al., 2013a; Sayer et al., 2008). Multiple revisions of amputated limbs may be required, as well as multiple interventions for burned patients, such as repeated skin grafting. These types of medical issues require medical monitoring and oversight. In addition, multiple medications may be prescribed, which can interact and have unintended consequences.

Another consideration is the need to possibly alter or modify prognosis, based on the type and number of comorbidities present. Data from the private sector suggest that comorbid injuries may interact with TBI severity to adversely impact outcome (Leitgeb, Mauritz, Brazinova, Majdan, & Wilbacher, 2013). Also, consideration should be given to the extent to which any comorbidities are "treatable." So, for example, a broken leg may impede physical recovery to some extent but eventually will heal, and typically TBI-specific rehabilitation would not necessarily be delayed. In contrast, severe cases of PTSD may impede the rehabilitation process without additional specialized treatment, which can be time-consuming. Although empirically supported treatments for PTSD exist, the patient must be motivated to participate in psychological treatment, and the duration of treatment may extend beyond the rehabilitation services. Similarly, drug and alcohol dependence may also prolong recovery if not properly treated.

A final practical consideration presented by comorbidities is that equipment and procedures may need to be modified. A patient with severe PTSD may not be able, at least initially, to participate in community outings with recreational therapy. Similarly, a patient who is not sleeping (possibly due to PTSD) will have trouble fully participating in rehabilitation. Working with mental health providers to modify activities can be helpful in adapting rehabilitation activities accordingly and to address the underlying mental health disorder. Cotreatment across disciplines is probably more common in rehabilitation settings with greater prevalence of comorbidities (Friedemann-Sanchez et al., 2008), due to the need to rely on others' specialized knowledge about disorders affecting the foci of one's rehabilitation efforts. Finally, equipment may need modification in any number of ways, depending on comorbidities. For example, the VA's Polytrauma Centers have treated many TBI patients who are blind. The communication boards, typically used by speech therapists to facilitate communication, had to be redesigned in Braille. Creative problem solving, along with greater reliance on other disciplines' knowledge, are paramount when working with complex, postdeployed patients.

RESOURCES AND PROGRAMS

Stateside, the rehabilitation process for those returning from combat theaters begins at acute medical settings such as military treatment facilities (MTF) with the initiation of individual physical, occupational, and speech therapies. Collaboration via video teleconferences has allowed earlier physiatric input into the care of these complex patients and helped to coordinate a smooth transition from acute care facilities to rehabilitation units.

In response to the complexity inherent in those returning from war for rehabilitation, and in recognition of many of the issues related to comorbidities just mentioned, the VA began describing these injuries as "polytrauma injuries" to reflect the importance of the comorbidities. *Polytrauma* means injuries to multiple parts of the body secondary to trauma. The VA set up a Polytrauma System of Care at its existing TBI centers. Because injuring multiple body parts or systems most typically includes TBI, polytrauma can be defined in practice as injury to the brain in addition to other body parts or systems, resulting in physical, cognitive, psychological, or psychosocial impairments, and functional disability (Scott et al., 2008). Injury to the brain is the impairment that typically guides the course of rehabilitation.

Belanger, Uomoto, and Vanderploeg (2009) and Sigford (2008) describe the system in greater detail, but, briefly, the five polytrauma rehabilitation centers (PRC; Tampa, Florida; Minneapolis, Minnesota; Palo Alto, California; Richmond, Virginia; San Antonio, Texas) are the first component of the Veteran's Health Administration (VHA) Polytrauma System of Care. These centers provide acute medical and rehabilitation care, research, and education related to polytrauma and TBI within the context of accreditation by the Commission on Accreditation of Rehabilitation Facilities (CARF) for both TBI and comprehensive rehabilitation. Clinical care is provided by a dedicated interdisciplinary staff of rehabilitation specialists and medical consultants with expertise in the treatment of the comorbidities that accompany TBI.

The polytrauma network sites (PNS), one located in each of the VHA's 22 regional Veterans Integrated Service Networks (VISN), comprise the second component of care within the Polytrauma System. These PNS programs may provide postacute rehabilitation care for individuals with polytrauma/TBI, including inpatient and outpatient rehabilitation and vocational rehabilitation programs. They are responsible for coordinating access to services to meet the needs of patients recovering from polytrauma. The PNS consults with and collaborates with PRCs in transitioning care from the acute rehabilitation setting to the community.

In addition, the Polytrauma System of Care network includes polytrauma support clinic teams (PSCT). With their geographical distribution across the VHA, the PSCT facilitate access to specialized rehabilitation services close to the veterans' and active duty service members' home communities. These interdisciplinary teams of rehabilitation specialists are responsible for managing the care of patients by providing treatment plans, regular follow-up, and any further care needs as they arise. The PSCT consults with the affiliated PNS or PRC when more specialized services are required. Finally, the remaining VHA medical centers have an identified Polytrauma Point of Contact who is responsible for managing consultations for patients with polytrauma and referring these patients to appropriate programs.

CONCLUSIONS

Service members and veterans have unique and culturally specific experiences that shape both their personal values and their beliefs, as well as their everyday lives. Their training and values may be a critical part of the rehabilitation process, depending on their degree of acculturation and identification with military service or veteran status. The culturally aware rehabilitation provider should be armed with the requisite awareness of military culture and begin with at least a basic understanding of the individual's service branch, occupation, and deployment history. Simply beginning with the knowledge that the individual is or was a member of the armed services is a major first step in understanding how that individual will approach the rehabilitation process. Multiple resources are available to begin this conversation through the Department of Defense Center for Deployment Psychology (deploymentpsychology.org) and the Department of Veterans Affairs Mental Health Service (mentalhealth.va .gov/communityproviders/screening).

After beginning the conversation, the provider with an understanding of military and veteran culture may begin to see the effect of the unique stressors with which service members are faced and the potential comorbid conditions that may impact rehabilitation and recovery. This will facilitate anticipation of needed referrals, proactive identification of services, and additional discussion with the service member or veteran about his or her recovery. Understanding unique stressors and comorbidities also tends to allow for more specialized care and coordination with specific programs or supports that may not be available in the general community.

Service members and veterans do not often raise the subject of their service independently; in fact, many may never mention it. It is up to the provider, absent overt signs of military service, to ask the questions and convey the recognition that this is an important part of these individuals' lives. Following that recognition, identification of the potential impacts of their status as service members or veterans on their rehabilitation process and the potential benefits to which they may have access can be an important part of the rehabilitation planning process. If the rehabilitation provider is engaged with these populations, the time spent learning about the culture, traditions, missions, values, and benefits afforded to those who have served in the military will be well spent.

REFERENCES

American Psychiatric Association. (2013). *Diagnostic and statistical manual of mental disorders* (5th ed.). Washington, DC: Author.

Andelic, N., Jerstad, T., Sigurdardottir, S., Schanke, A. K., Sandvik, L., & Roe, C. (2010). Effects of acute substance use and pre-injury substance abuse on traumatic brain injury severity in adults admitted to a trauma centre. *Journal of Trauma Management Outcomes, 4*, 6.

Belanger, H. G., Kretzmer, T., Vanderploeg, R., & French, L. M. (2010). Symptom complaints following combat-related TBI: Relationship to TBI severity and PTSD. *Journal of the International Neuropsychological Society, 16*(1), 194–199.

Belanger, H. G., Uomoto, J. M., & Vanderploeg, R. D. (2009). The Veterans Health Administration's (VHA's) Polytrauma System of Care for mild traumatic brain injury: Costs, benefits, and controversies. *Journal of Head Trauma Rehabilitation, 24*(1), 4–13.

Brownlow, J. A., Hall Brown, T. S., & Mellman, T. A. (2014). Relationships of posttraumatic stress symptoms and sleep measures to cognitive performance in young-adult African Americans. *Journal of Traumatic Stress, 27*(2), 217–223.

Cantor, J. B., Bushnik, T., Cicerone, K., Dijkers, M. P., Gordon, W., Hammond, F. M., . . . Spielman, L. A. (2012). Insomnia, fatigue, and sleepiness in the first 2 years after traumatic brain injury: An NIDRR TBI model system module study. *Journal of Head Trauma Rehabilitation, 27*(6), E1–E14.

Castano-Monsalve, B., Bernabeu-Guitart, M., Lopez, R., Bulbena-Vilarrasa, A., & Quemada, J. I. (2013). Alcohol and drug use disorders in patients with traumatic brain injury: Neurobehavioral consequences and caregiver burden. *Revista de Neurologia, 56*(7), 363–369.

Cernich, A. N., Chandler, L., Scherdell, T., & Kurtz, S. (2012). Assessment of co-occurring disorders in veterans diagnosed with traumatic brain injury. *Journal of Head Trauma Rehabilitation, 27*(4), 253–260.

Coupland, R. M., & Meddings, D. R. (1999). Mortality associated with use of weapons in armed conflicts, wartime atrocities, and civilian mass shootings: Literature review. *British Medical Journal, 319*(7207), 407–410.

DePalma, R. G., Burris, D. G., Champion, H. R., & Hodgson, M. J. (2005). Blast injuries. *New England Journal of Medicine, 352*, 1335–1342.

Duclos, C., Dumont, M., Blais, H., Paquet, J., Laflamme, E., de Beaumont, L., . . . Gosselin, N. (2013). Rest-activity cycle disturbances in the acute phase of moderate to severe traumatic brain injury. *Neurorehabilitation and Neural Repair, 28*, 472–482.

Eisen, S. A., Griffith, K. H., Xian, H., Scherrer, J. F., Fischer, I. D., Chantarujikapong, S., . . . Tsuang, M. T. (2004). Lifetime and 12-month prevalence of psychiatric disorders in 8,169 male Vietnam War era veterans. *Military Medicine, 169*(11), 896–902.

Fogelberg, D. J., Hoffman, J. M., Dikmen, S., Temkin, N. R., & Bell, K. R. (2012). Association of sleep and co-occurring psychological conditions at 1 year after traumatic brain injury. *Archives of Physical Medicine & Rehabilitation*, *93*(8), 1313–1318.

Friedemann-Sanchez, G., Sayer, N. A., & Pickett, T. (2008). Provider perspectives on rehabilitation of patients with polytrauma. *Archives of Physical Medicine & Rehabilitation*, *89*(1), 171–178.

Holcomb, E. M., Millis, S. R., & Hanks, R. A. (2012). Comorbid disease in persons with traumatic brain injury: Descriptive findings using the modified cumulative illness rating scale. *Archives of Physical Medicine & Rehabilitation*, *93*(8), 1338–1342.

Jamora, C. W., Young, A., & Ruff, R. M. (2012). Comparison of subjective cognitive complaints with neuropsychological tests in individuals with mild vs. more severe traumatic brain injuries. *Brain Injury*, *26*(1), 36–47.

King, N. S. (2008). PTSD and traumatic brain injury: Folklore and fact? *Brain Injury*, *22*(1), 1–5.

Leitgeb, J., Mauritz, W., Brazinova, A., Majdan, M., & Wilbacher, I. (2013). Impact of concomitant injuries on outcomes after traumatic brain injury. *Archives of Orthopaedic and Trauma Surgery*, *133*(5), 659–668.

Lew, H. L., Otis, J. D., Tun, C., Kerns, R. D., Clark, M. E., & Cifu, D. X. (2009). Prevalence of chronic pain, posttraumatic stress disorder, and persistent postconcussive symptoms in OIF/OEF veterans: Polytrauma clinical triad. *Journal of Rehabilitation Research and Development*, *46*(6), 697–702.

Nakase-Richardson, R., McNamee, S., Howe, L. L., Massengale, J., Peterson, M., Barnett, S. D., . . . Cifu, D. X. (2013a). Descriptive characteristics and rehabilitation outcomes in active duty military personnel and veterans with disorders of consciousness with combat- and noncombat-related brain injury. *Archives of Physical Medicine & Rehabilitation*, *94*(10), 1861–1869.

Nakase-Richardson, R., Sherer, M., Barnett, S. D., Yablon, S. A., Evans, C. C., Kretzmer, T., . . . Modarres, M. (2013b). Prospective evaluation of the nature, course, and impact of acute sleep abnormality after traumatic brain injury. *Archives of Physical Medicine & Rehabilitation*, *94*(5), 875–882.

National Center for Veterans Analysis and Statistics. (2014). *Projected Veteran population 2013 to 2043*. U.S. Department of Veterans Affairs. Retrieved from http://www.va.gov/vetdata/Veteran_Population.asp

Owens, B. D., Kragh, J. F., Jr., Wenke, J. C., Macaitis, J., Wade, C. E., & Holcomb, J. B. (2008). Combat wounds in Operation Iraqi Freedom and Operation Enduring Freedom. *Journal of Trauma*, *64*(2), 295–299.

Polusny, M. A., Kehle, S. M., Nelson, N. W., Erbes, C. R., Arbisi, P. A., & Thuras, P. (2011). Longitudinal effects of mild traumatic brain injury and posttraumatic stress disorder comorbidity on postdeployment outcomes in national guard soldiers deployed to Iraq. *Archives of General Psychiatry*, *68*(1), 79–89.

Ritenour, A. E., Blackbourne, L. H., Kelly, J. F., McLaughlin, D. F., Pearse, L. A., Holcomb, J. B., & Wade, C. E. (2010). Incidence of primary blast injury in U.S. military overseas contingency operations: A retrospective study. *Annals of Surgergy, 251*(6), 1140–1144.

Sayer, N. A., Chiros, C. E., Sigford, B., Scott, S., Clothier, B., Pickett, T., & Lew, H. L. (2008). Characteristics and rehabilitation outcomes among patients with blast and other injuries sustained during the Global War on Terror. *Archives of Physical Medicine & Rehabilitation, 89*(1), 163–170.

Sbordone, R. J., & Ruff, R. M. (2010). Re-examination of the controversial coexistence of traumatic brain injury and posttraumatic stress disorder: Misdiagnosis and self-report measures. *Psychological Injury and Law, 3*(1), 63–76.

Scott, S. G., Scolten, J. D., Latlief, G. A., Humayun, F., Belanger, H. G., & Vanderploeg, R. D. (Eds.). (2008). *Polytrauma rehabilitation* (2nd ed.). Philadelphia, PA: Elsevier.

Sigford, B. J. (2008). "To care for him who shall have borne the battle and for his widow and his orphan" (Abraham Lincoln): The Department of Veterans Affairs polytrauma system of care. *Archives of Physical Medicine and Rehabilitation, 89*(1), 160–162.

Sommerauer, M., Valko, P. O., Werth, E., & Baumann, C. R. (2013). Excessive sleep need following traumatic brain injury: A case-control study of 36 patients. *Journal of Sleep Research, 22*(6), 634–639.

Taber, K. H., Warden, D. L., & Hurley, R. A. (2006). Blast-related brain injury: What is known? *Journal of Neuropsychiatry and Clinical Neuroscience, 18*, 141–145.

Thomas, J. L., Wilk, J. E., Riviere, L. A., McGurk, D., Castro, C. A., & Hoge, C. W. (2010). Prevalence of mental health problems and functional impairment among active component and National Guard soldiers 3 and 12 months following combat in Iraq. *Archives of General Psychiatry, 67*(6), 614–623.

Vanderploeg, R. D., Belanger, H. G., & Brenner, L. A. (2013). Blast injuries and PTSD: Lessons learned from the Iraqi and Afghanistan conflicts. In S. P. Koffler, J. E. Morgan, I. S. Baron, & M. F. Greiffenstein (Eds.), *Neuropsychology science and practice* (pp. 114–148). New York, NY: Oxford University Press.

Wachen, J. S., Shipherd, J. C., Suvak, M., Vogt, D., King, L. A., & King, D. W. (2013). Posttraumatic stress symptomatology as a mediator of the relationship between warzone exposure and physical health symptoms in men and women. *Journal of Trauma Stress, 26*(3), 319–328.

Yurgil, K. A., Barkauskas, D. A., Vasterling, J. J., Nievergelt, C. M., Larson, G. E., Schork, N. J., . . . Baker, D. G. (2014). Association between traumatic brain injury and risk of posttraumatic stress disorder in active-duty marines. *JAMA Psychiatry, 71*(2), 149–157.

CHAPTER TEN

RACIAL AND ETHNIC MICROAGGRESSIONS IN THE NEUROREHABILITATION SETTING

Fred Loya and Jay M. Uomoto

Over the course of the past few decades, neurorehabilitation has emerged as an empirically supported method of treatment for neurological injury. The science and practice of neurorehabilitation have benefited from many noteworthy innovations in rehabilitation tools and clinical methodologies to address myriad forms of cognitive dysfunction and functional impairment resulting from brain injury. As a result of these rapid developments, neurorehabilitation has gained wider acceptance within health care and academic settings as a viable treatment option (Haskins, Cicerone, & Trexler, 2012). These advances have also helped neurorehabilitation mature as a discipline, allowing researchers and practitioners to consider potential mechanisms underlying treatment response as well as additional factors that might impact the process of neurorehabilitation more generally.

One area of critical importance to all helping professionals that has received comparably little attention within neurorehabilitation is the establishment and maintenance of a quality working alliance between providers and their clients. Decades of counseling and psychotherapy research have identified the working alliance as one of the most robust and consistent predictors of treatment outcomes, regardless of the type of therapy provided (Horvath & Symonds, 1991; Martin, Garske, & Davis, 2000). For any therapeutic relationship to be maximally effective, the working alliance requires routine monitoring so that any potential sources of strain or disruption can be addressed in a timely and therapeutically helpful manner. This requires, in part, that providers acknowledge and understand how aspects of their own behavior and ways of interacting with their clients may contribute to tension and fissures within the relationship (Safran & Muran, 2000). This is particularly relevant to cross-cultural therapy dyads (Vasquez, 2007), given that ethnic minorities report frequently experiencing discrimination and race-related stress at the hands of helping professionals (Constantine, 2007; Constantine & Sue, 2007; Owen, Tao, Imel, Wampold, & Rodolfa, 2014; Sue et al., 2007).

However, within the field of neurorehabilitation, there has been minimal discussion of the complex interpersonal dynamics that develop between cross-cultural dyads or recognition of its potential impact on the rehabilitation process. At present, there is little professional guidance available to help neurorehabilitation providers understand the specific relevance of cultural factors to neurorehabilitation settings or how cultural differences between providers and their clients may impact the rehabilitation process. In the allied disciplines of clinical and counseling psychology, there is increasing recognition, however, that one particularly virulent way providers negatively impact the working alliance is when they convey prejudicial attitudes or discriminatory behaviors to their clients in the form of *racial and ethnic microaggressions*[1]—that is, as Solórzano, Ceja, and Yosso (2000) explain, through "subtle insults (verbal, nonverbal, and/or visual) directed toward people of color, often automatically or unconsciously"(p. 60). According to Sue (2005), helping professionals, like all people, are cultural beings that are not immune from the sociocultural developmental processes that shape racial and ethnic prejudices, some of which undoubtedly impact how clients are viewed and treated. If providers interact with their ethnic minority clients in ways that mirror broader negative societal attitudes, they may risk reinforcing these messages, which can be counterproductive to treatment goals. Indeed, mounting evidence suggests that microaggressions play a critical and detrimental role in the lives of ethnic minorities (Wong, Derthick, David, Saw, & Okazaki, 2014) and that ignoring these transgressions in clinical settings damages the working alliance and detracts from therapeutic progress (e.g., Owen et al., 2014).

This chapter explores the concept of microaggressions in neurorehabilitation settings, describes their potential impact on the rehabilitation process, and offers recommendations on how to address and potentially mitigate infractions when they do occur. Consider, for example, the following brief illustrations of different types of microaggressions that might transpire in neurorehabilitation settings.

[1]Subsequently, "microaggressions" is used to refer to this concept.

Case Vignette #1: A 22-year-old Native American woman was admitted to a neurobehavioral unit after acute hospitalization for viral encephalitis. The woman was displaying substantial behavioral outbursts, including significant verbal anger directed toward any nursing or rehabilitation staff that took care of her. She also had struck out at nursing staff while on the acute medicine unit. Behavioral outbursts were very sudden, interspersed with poor initiation of actions and minimal verbal interaction. The neurobehavioral unit at the time of this woman's hospitalization was staffed by female nurses and one male nurse. One of the occupational therapists had discovered through talking with the patient's family that she liked to dance and sing, and she had been taking dance coursework while in college. The patient could be engaged therapeutically if music and dance were incorporated into the rehabilitation therapy. The male nurse started calling her "Pocahontas" as a joke, eliciting uncomfortable smiles on behalf of other rehabilitation and nursing staff. He persisted calling her "Pocahontas" despite admonitions by the psychology staff to stop. His rationale was that it helped to relieve the stress of some of the nursing staff who had close contact with the patient in light of her behavioral outbursts and physical striking-out behaviors.

Case Vignette #2: A Chinese American neuropsychologist was leading a training focused on strengthening attention regulation skills and goal management strategies for a group of military combat veterans with chronic mild to moderate traumatic brain injury and symptoms of posttraumatic stress. Group members consisted of a Caucasian Vietnam War veteran and two younger veterans of the recent wars in the Middle East, one a Caucasian male who served in the Iraq war and the other a Palestine American male veteran of the war in Afghanistan. Early in the treatment, when the group was still in its initial forming stage, the veterans exchanged brief "war stories" as a means of establishing trust and highlighting their common experiences. Although they reflected on the horrors of war, they all lamented the fact that nothing in civilian life compared to the "thrill" and "excitement" of direct combat. The Iraq war veteran stated, "There's nothing more exciting than knocking down a door and punching *Haji* in the face." He then looked at the Vietnam War veteran and added, "Well, in your case, punching *Charlie* in the face." These statements were not intended to offend, but were made without acknowledgment that they could possibly be construed as hostile and derogatory to the Chinese American neuropsychologist or the Palestine American veteran. These epithets were stated matter-of-factly, as if these ethnic minority persons were simply not present in the room.

These vignettes highlight the potentially complex ways that micro-aggressions might manifest in neurorehabilitation settings and raise important questions about their impact on the rehabilitation process. For instance, in Vignette #1, how might a racial indignity perpetrated by one member of a larger rehabilitation treatment team affect the client's relationships with other team members? Could this negative interaction limit the effectiveness of neurorehabilitation as a whole? In what way does the behavior of one staff member become an accepted norm on a neurorehabilitation unit? What steps should be taken to resolve the potential rupture to the working alliance resulting from the nurse's actions, both at the level of the individual provider and the treatment team as a whole? Vignette #2 raises a different set of questions that are less frequently considered in discussions on microaggressions but are nevertheless important. For instance, how should the clinician handle microaggressions that occur between two group members? Further, how might microaggressions directed toward a treatment provider impact the care he or she is able to provide? These questions are not necessarily unique to neurorehabilitation but may require special consideration in this treatment setting, given the neurocognitive vulnerabilities and common comorbidities (e.g., posttraumatic stress, chronic pain) that characterize this population. How do these factors contribute to the management of microaggressions, and what training and resources are required to help providers successfully navigate infractions when they do occur? These are complex questions without clear and straightforward answers.

We begin our discussion with a brief and selective review of the theoretical and empirical literatures on microaggressions, with the understanding that its study is still in its relative infancy and has not yet been examined within the context of neurorehabilitation. Consequently, our focus is on the small body of research that has been conducted in other clinical settings that might bear direct relevance on neurorehabilitation. We also highlight features unique to neurorehabilitation settings that may be important to consider for microaggressions, underscoring the need for future study in this area. We conclude with a discussion of training needs in the field to help raise awareness for the clinical impact of microaggressions, as well as strategies for their clinical management when they do occur. We offer rational, clinical suggestions based upon theory and the available evidence and raise important questions the field would benefit from investigating.

MICROAGGRESSIONS: THEORETICAL BACKGROUND AND EMPIRICAL FINDINGS

As larger societal attitudes began to shift in the wake of the Civil Rights Movement, overt forms of bigotry, hatred, and racial condemnation started to fall out of practice. Traditional beliefs regarding the rights of Whites to castigate, abuse, deny services to, or subject ethnic minorities to ridicule based simply upon their race or ethnic background stood in direct opposition to newly forged democratic ideals of racial equality, meritocracy, and the hopes of creating an inclusive, "color-blind" society. An unintended consequence of these progressive strides was the creation of a virtual racial vacuum, where deeply engrained and conditioned racial discriminatory attitudes and beliefs could no longer be so openly expressed despite their continued persistence. Within this climate, new, subtler forms of racism emerged, often characterized by an ambiguous and subtle nature.

Chester Pierce (1995), in his psychiatric practice with African American clients in the 1970s, was the first to identify and define this new breed of racism. He coined the term *microaggressions* to describe a process of "subtle, innocuous, preconscious, or unconscious degradations, or putdowns" (p. 281) directed at people of color. He explained that the power of these "putdowns" lay in their commonplace and often unintended nature, which allow them to hide in plain sight, virtually unnoticed and rarely addressed. As a mainstay of the everyday experiences of ethnic minorities, Pierce further stressed that the cumulative effects of microaggressions over the lifetime were likely significant, particularly regarding their impact on ethnic minority health, self-confidence, and well-being. While any particular microaggression, in and of itself, may appear small to an outsider or may even be experienced as inconsequential by the recipient, their ubiquity in the daily lived experiences of ethnic minorities communicates a clear message of devaluation and otherness.

Since its inception, the concept of microaggressions has been explored from a variety of different academic perspectives, each conceptualizing it in slightly different terms and operating via unique mechanisms (e.g., as "symbolic racism" [Kinder & Sears, 1981], "modern racism" [McConahay, 1986], or "aversive racism" [Gaertner & Dovidio, 1986]). Although each approach emphasizes different facets of this phenomenon, they all hold the common view that racism continues to plague modern society but is now more likely to be expressed and perpetuated through covert means that are difficult to detect and nearly impossible to "prove." Take, for example, an employer who unwittingly asks fewer questions of a minority job applicant during an interview due to unconsciously held stereotypical views of the applicant as being intellectually inferior and incompetent. In this scenario, the reduced number of questions posed to the applicant is subtle and the motivation for these actions is unclear (perhaps not even to the interviewer). The minority applicant may leave the interview feeling that something was awry but not sure if she or he was in fact a victim of discrimination (as compared to more traditional, explicit forms of racism such as refusal to provide an ethnic minority entrance into a business establishment). These feelings of unease and uncertainty are common among ethnic minorities who have experienced microaggressions (Sue et al., 2007). But in the absence of direct proof, ethnic minorities often do not directly combat these transgressions in a manner that may help preserve their self-esteem and well-being.

As a topic of scholarly inquiry, the study of microaggressions is complicated by the subtle ways they frequently manifest, rending them difficult to operationalize and observe. Further, because the behaviors, attitudes, and stereotypes that comprise microaggressions reflect deeply ingrained societal values, they occur with alarming regularity and are often perpetuated by individuals who otherwise espouse egalitarian worldviews. Most people consider themselves to be upstanding, moral, and well intentioned, and they have difficulty acknowledging (particularly on self-report questionnaires) that certain of their behaviors may be motivated by more implicit forms of prejudice and bias (Greenwald, Poehlman, Uhlmann, & Banaji, 2009). This reluctance to consider the potential for acting in a racially biased manner may be even more pronounced among the highly educated and those with increased economic and social capital, individuals who likely consider themselves to be among the more progressive segments of society. Taken together, these dynamics enable microaggressions to persist largely unchallenged as a normal part of majority–minority social exchange.

A major advance in the study of microaggressions occurred with the publication of a taxonomy by Sue et al. (2007). Their classification system provided a framework that allowed clinicians and researchers to approach the study of microaggressions in a more systematic, hypothesis-driven fashion. Sue et al. (2007) defined microaggressions as "brief and commonplace daily verbal, behavioral, and environmental indignities, whether intentional or unintentional, that communicate hostile, derogatory, or negative racial slights and insults to the target person or group" (p. 273). They also delineated three separate categories of offense. The first is microassaults, or consciously held and explicitly expressed racist communications or behaviors, committed with the intent to harm or demean persons of color. Within this categorization are behaviors such as discriminatory acts, referring to ethnic minorities through the use of racial epithets, or blatantly displaying racially offensive messages or imagery (e.g., the Confederate flag). Sue et al. likened these acts to more traditional forms of racism, but noted they typically occur in private, thus providing the perpetrator with a degree of protection and anonymity. Within neurorehabilitation settings, these forms of explicit racism are possible but unlikely given professional standards and the strong legal and ethical prohibitions against racial discrimination in health care settings. Sue et al.'s (2007) second category is microinsults, or communications and behaviors that demean a person's racial heritage or identity and often occur outside conscious awareness of the perpetrator. Examples of this type of microaggression include treating minorities in accordance with ethnic stereotypes, such as African Americans as criminals or Asian Americans as good at math. Within neurorehabilitation settings, microinsults may manifest via reduced expectations for the recoveries of minority clients (i.e., an ethnic minority's assumed baseline inferiority places limits on what providers consider as realistic rehabilitation goals), less time and less intensive work provided to minority clients, or expressions of surprise for demonstrated competence in areas assumed to be deficient. The third category is microinvalidations, or communications and behaviors that deny, minimize, or negate the psychological and experiential reality of ethnic minorities. These include acts such as minimizing the impact of racism on the lives of ethnic minorities, treating ethnic minorities as second-class citizens (i.e., as foreigners), or otherwise marginalizing ethnic minorities' cultural identity. A rehabilitation psychologist who dismisses an ethnic minority client's fears of finding a job after undergoing rehabilitation might be committing this type of microaggression. Sue et al. (2007) further identified nine common themes of microaggressions: Ethnic minorities are treated as intellectually inferior, second-class citizens, aliens in their own land, criminals, or holding pathological cultural values, whereas White individuals deny the existence of individual racism, espouse a color-blind worldview, promote myths of meritocracy, and contribute to environmental invalidations.

Sue et al.'s (2007) proposed taxonomy and research agenda helped usher in a new era of research on microaggressions. With stronger theoretical underpinnings in place, researchers were able to develop measurement tools that allowed for microaggressions to be quantified (e.g., Nadal, 2011) and investigated within various ethnic minority groups and across different life settings. Within a very short period of time, the study of microaggression has grown exponentially, and researchers have accumulated mounting evidence demonstrating that microaggressions are associated with substantial psychological distress for ethnic minorities (Ong, Burrow, Fuller-Rowell, Ja, & Sue, 2013; Owen, Imel, Tao, Wampold, Smith, & Rodolfa, 2011; Schoulte, Schultz, & Altmaier, 2011; Torres, Driscoll, & Burrow, 2010; Torres-Harding & Turner, 2014; Wang, Leu, & Shoda, 2011). There is also some suggestion that the distress associated with experiencing microaggressions may lead to negative behavioral consequences, such as binge drinking (Blume, Lovato, Thyken, & Denny, 2012) or decreased work productivity (Hunter, as cited in Wong et al., 2013). Furthermore, and consistent with theoretical accounts regarding the impact that the attributional ambiguity (Major & Crocker, 1993) of microaggressions may have on ethnic minorities (Sue et al., 2007), research has also shown that ethnic minorities dedicate a great deal of time and internal resources determining whether perceived slights are racially motivated (Watkins, LaBarrie, & Appio, 2010), resulting in considerable additional stress and increased negative affect (Wang et al., 2011). As initially discussed by Sue et al. (2007), the lack of certainty regarding whether a microaggression occurred often prevents ethnic minorities from adequately processing and responding to these instances in a manner that helps resolve the psychological distress these situations engender.

One particularly damaging instance of microaggressions identified by Sue et al. (2007) occurs in the context of clinical practice settings. Clinical and counseling research has demonstrated that ethnic minority clients experience microaggressions frequently in their interactions with providers and that, if left unresolved, they have the potential to negatively impact the course of therapy. In one of the earliest studies of this process, Constantine (2007) conducted focus groups with African American college students regarding their experience of microaggressions with White counselors. Counseling clients identified 12 different categories of microaggressions they had experienced, ranging from therapists espousing a color-blind worldview, to accusing minority clients that they were overly sensitive to issues of race and ethnicity, to frank endorsement of racial and ethnic stereotypes. Furthermore, minority clients' perceptions of microaggressions committed during therapy were negatively associated with ratings of the working alliance, which, in turn, predicted lower ratings of counselors overall and cultural competence. Direct associations were also found between perceived microaggressions and treatment satisfaction (Constantine, 2007). Similarly, Owen et al. (2011, 2014) found that college counseling clients frequently perceived their White therapists as committing microaggressions during treatment and that these instances negatively impacted the working alliance and clients' overall well-being. Moreover, the vast majority (74%) of counseling clients that reported experiencing a microaggression never discussed it with their therapist. Failure to discuss these transgressions negatively impacted the working alliance, whereas addressing them resulted in alliance ratings that were comparable to those who had never experienced a microaggression (Owen et al., 2014). Finally, Morton (2000, as cited in Wong et al., 2014) reported that White therapists' endorsement of color-blind ideology predicted the occurrence of microaggressions in cross-racial therapy dyads, most frequently involving avoiding discussing race and culture and minimizing racial and culture experiences of the counseling client.

For health care providers, these findings highlight the critically important role that microaggressions play in the delivery and receipt of care and suggest that the helping relationship be continually monitored and assessed for breaches of this nature. As discussed by Sue et al. (2007) and Constantine (2007), microaggressions perpetuated by helping professionals may potentially be more damaging than those committed by the public at large. They caution that in clinical settings, microaggressions may retraumatize clients in particularly powerful ways, given that the therapeutic environment is presumed to be safe and encouraging of personal growth, honesty, and self-reflection. If ethnic minorities view their health care providers as being guilty of treating them in an insensitive, disrespectful, and demeaning manner, even if such slights are unintended, positive treatment outcomes are less likely. Most importantly, addressing microaggressions in a clinically sensitive manner may offset some of their ill effects (Owen et al., 2014), reflecting the importance of resolving ruptures in therapy more broadly (Safran & Muran, 2000). However, if providers fail to address microaggressions, ethnic minority clients may withdraw from their treatment and end therapy prematurely. Indeed, unresolved transgressions of this kind have been postulated as one factor that may account for some of the ethnic disparities in help-seeking behaviors (U.S. Department of Health and Human Services, 2001).

Taken together, available research indicates that microaggressions are a common indignity experienced by many ethnic minorities and are associated with psychological distress that can be quite profound, even reaching levels associated with more direct forms of abuse and injury (Schoulte et al., 2011). The power of microaggressions lay in the subtle and ambiguous nature in which they occur, making them difficult to recognize and especially challenging to address. They can be perpetrated within any interracial relationship but may be particularly damaging when committed by a person in a position of authority, such as within a health care setting. Unfortunately, addressing transgressions within the helping professions appears to be the exception rather than the general rule and may likely reflect providers' reluctance to acknowledge their own racial biases or discomfort associated with discussing matters of race and ethnicity (Sue et al., 2007).

MICROAGGRESSIONS IN THE NEUROREHABILITATION SETTING

This section examines several unique features of neurorehabilitation settings that may contribute to the occurrence of microaggressions and impact the rehabilitation process. In highlighting these aspects, we aim to raise the self-awareness of rehabilitation specialists so they can better identify situations that may lend themselves to microaggressions in their workplaces. Each of the areas also represents an important avenue for future investigation.

One of the first aspects to consider is that neurorehabilitation services are frequently delivered by multiple providers working together as a larger treatment team. One patient's care may be coordinated among several different specialists, involving contributions from neurology; neuropsychology; social work; and speech, recreation, occupation, and physical therapy, among others. This treatment milieu differs in important ways from individualized forms of care (e.g., counselor–client relationship), which likely influences how microaggressions function in this environment. For example, the treatment team may magnify the power differential between the client and the providers, potentially increasing the likelihood of providers committing microaggressions but also imposing barriers on acknowledging and appropriately attending to them when they occur (Link & Phelan, 2001; Sue, 2010a, 2010b; Sue, Capodilupo, Nadal, & Torino, 2008). From the perspective of the patient undergoing neurorehabilitation, confronting microaggressions among a team of professionals may be intimidating and fraught with anxieties about the potential negative repercussions on other areas of clinical care. Some patients may fear reprisals for blowing the whistle on a team member, particularly given that these infractions can be denied with relative ease. For the providers, the treatment team may make it more difficult to acknowledge personal bias out of concern for being perceived negatively or as culturally incompetent by peers. In addition, given that most microaggressions are unintended and difficult to recognize, the professional group dynamic may encourage alternative explanations for ambiguous behaviors over critical self-reflection and taking personal responsibility. Finally, in the situation of a patient who asserts some form of microaggression toward a rehabilitation staff member, as in the second vignette, the net stress experienced by staff in a complex health care environment may increase. Such staff members may feel obligated not to disclose these encounters to fellow colleagues or supervisors for fear of being seen as "overly sensitive" or intolerant of those patients whose neurobehavioral disposition or long-term interpersonal style may reveal a history of prejudgment of certain staff of a particular cultural background.

In addition to power differentials between neurorehabilitation clients and the treatment team, providers within the team may also be considered to occupy different positions of power and influence. A treatment team's hierarchical structure is likely to reflect the professional credentials of team members, as well as how members' individual contributions are collectively valued. This power dynamic may also make it difficult to address microaggressions within the team setting. For instance, team members of lower status may find it difficult to question or confront a senior team member regarding actions they consider possibly reflective of a microaggression. This is further complicated due to the relative invisibility of microaggressions (Sue et al., 2007), meaning that levying a criticism of this nature to a colleague in the absence of definitive proof may carry significant professional risk. Consider, for example, the potential consequences of a speech pathologist questioning the behaviors of a neurologist on her standing within the team or with her own professional ambitions. Without direct evidence, raising concerns of this sensitive nature might be interpreted more as accusations than as constructive and professional criticism. Establishing safe environments where self-reflection and honesty are encouraged are needed in order for this form of self-policing and critical dialogue to occur.

Finally, as illustrated in Vignette #1, how might microaggressions perpetrated by one team member affect the client's relationship with the team as a whole? If transgressions are not addressed, could this lead to the establishment of team norms condoning microaggressive behavior? Although many different factors contribute to this dynamic, the best safeguard against the generalization of negative feelings toward the team is likely through explicitly addressing instances of microaggressions in a timely and thoughtful manner. Owen et al. (2014) demonstrated that therapeutic dyads that could successfully discuss clinical experiences of microaggressions were able to generally preserve the working alliance and recover from the therapeutic rupture. Developing a better understanding for ways to redress microaggressions that occur as part of a treatment team is an important area for future investigations.

A second factor that is important to consider in neurorehabilitation settings is the intensity of the treatment environment itself. As just mentioned, neurorehabilitation clients typically receive a variety of therapies simultaneously to address their varied treatment needs. For many clients, this experience can be confusing and result in substantial fatigue. It may be difficult for persons with cognitive vulnerabilities to track and remember their various providers and the therapies they are engaged with, further contributing to a sense of frustration and confusion. In addition, the neurobehavioral sequelae of brain injuries themselves are often difficult to manage and introduce substantial stress to the treatment setting. For instance, many persons with brain injuries have limited awareness of their deficits, act impulsively, have difficulty regulating their emotions, and may behave in a socially inappropriate manner. These factors can lead to interpersonal strain between providers and clients, as well as pose specific complications with treatment compliance and working toward rehabilitation goals. In addition, many clients in neurorehabilitation settings experience ongoing struggles with accepting the profound changes in their physical and cognitive abilities that result from brain injuries. The process of coming to terms with new limitations is often associated with significant psychological distress, frustration, desperation, sadness, anger, or despair.

Within this intense treatment context, providers may be at increased risk for committing microaggressions. Racial stereotypes represent efficient means of organizing and categorizing information about social groups (Major & O'Brien, 2005), which might be relied upon to a greater extent under conditions when cognitive resources are scarce (Macrae & Bodenhausen, 2000). That is, providers in neurorehabilitation settings, experiencing the impact of an intense work environment and significant mental fatigue, may utilize cultural stereotypes more frequently because they require fewer cognitive resources to process. Further, providers under considerable stress and pressure may be less capable of engaging their own self-regulatory capacities to override deeply ingrained social stereotypes (Payne, 2005). In a similar vein, the intensity of the neurorehabilitation setting combined with a reduced capacity to self-regulate on the part of neurorehabilitation clients and providers alike may result in more intense and volatile reactions to microaggressions when they do occur. This may contribute to a downward spiral of escalation and greater challenge to resolve situations to be of most help to patients.

Another important feature to consider with respect to microaggressions in neurorehabilitation settings is the close relationship between certain neurobehavioral deficits on the one hand and common racial stereotypes on the other. For instance, consider the example of an African American male who sustained significant damage to the frontal lobes from a car accident and has been acting aggressively in a neurorehabilitation setting. How might this individual be treated differently from his Caucasian counterpart, given widespread stereotypes of African American males as violent and aggressive? In such situations, there are at least two possible responses that may reflect different manifestations of microaggressions. First, behaviors may be misattributed to racial stereotypes rather than as a result of injury or underlying neurological dysfunction. This may lead to providers responding more punitively and less compassionately (e.g., through administrating sedatives), potentially missing opportunities to work with clients on the exact deficits they are in treatment to address. Second, neurobehavioral symptoms that conform to racial stereotypes may be experienced as more intense, extreme, debilitating, or threatening. If providers hold negative stereotypes of their clients, they may be more prone to selectively seek out and latch onto behaviors that confirm their perspective. Interpreting symptoms and behaviors in this manner may result in lower expectations for treatment and recovery or elicit disproportionate responses. For instance, activation of stereotypes regarding the intellectual inferiority of ethnic minorities may limit expectations for cognitive rehabilitation.

Finally, special consideration needs to be given to microaggressions that may occur around setting rehabilitation goals. This is not necessarily unique to neurorehabilitation, but it may be more pronounced in these settings. Providers may differ considerably from patients and their families with respect to therapeutic targets, potentially reflecting Eurocentric views of independence. For instance, providers may place greater value on promoting independent living skills than persons of certain ethnic backgrounds that hold strong communal values. Here, microaggressions do not necessarily always occur in verbal form but may manifest in the behavior of the rehabilitation setting, such as the way one is encouraged in establishing rehabilitation goals that do not conform to their cultural background. Take, for example, the case of an older Native American male who sustained a left cerebral artery stroke and whose rehabilitation team prioritizes gait training due to his right hemiparesis with slowly returning sensation in his right leg. Gait training becomes an interdisciplinary goal, but the patient and his family are seen as "resisting" or being "noncompliant" with treatment when he and his family refuse gait training in both physical and occupational therapy. Rather, they believe it is more important for the staff to have the patient undergo speech therapy and worry about him learning to walk later. When questioned about this, the family explains that their home community will provide for the patient's mobility needs, but it cannot assist with the return of language. In this scenario, the act of identifying return of right-sided mobility as a priority goal, in a somewhat paternalistic fashion, and the negative nonverbal behaviors conveyed to the patient and family can be seen as a behavioral manifestation of microaggression centered on goal setting. Overriding a patient and family's autonomy and preferences can be a very difficult rehabilitation dilemma, raising the potential of communicating microaggressions through nonverbal means of disapproval. This may fall into Sue et al.'s (2007) category of microinvalidation, although how "micro" that may be is a somewhat subjective determination. It is also important for providers to acknowledge that certain rehabilitation goals might be more difficult to identify properly to align with the goals of ethnic minority patients. For instance, racial disparities in employment may present different obstacles and be associated with unique anxieties for ethnic minority clients. Failing to recognize this aspect of their experience risks invalidating certain ethnic minorities experiential reality.

The potential disruption of clinical care resulting from microaggressions, such as via stress on the therapeutic relationship, likely shares many commonalities across clinical settings. However, for neurorehabilitation providers, it is important to recognize and acknowledge how certain features of the neurorehabilitation setting may increase the likelihood of providers committing microaggressions; make microaggressions more difficult to recognize, manage, or address when they do occur; or result in unique manifestations. Increasing awareness and understanding for how microaggressions may function in this environment can help providers addressing these issues in a clinically appropriate way that preserves the integrity of the professional relationship.

EDUCATION AND TRAINING FOR THE CLINICAL MANAGEMENT OF MICROAGGRESSIONS

The preceding discussion provided some ways to educate and train neurorehabilitation staff to be aware of how microaggressions can lead to poorer rehabilitation outcomes for those with neurological disorders. As Sue (2005) noted, microaggressions derive their power by their subtle and invisible nature as transmitted by the perpetrator and as registered by the recipient. Given the sometimes elusive nature of microaggressions in the neurorehabilitation setting, more explicit training and education may be needed. The following are some general recommendations to serve as a starting point.

Neurorehabilitation settings are usually fast-paced and stressful and require a significant degree of organization and collaboration. That said, under such conditions, one's self-awareness of interpersonal communications that may convey certain prejudices and biases may not be at its best. Microaggressions could arise as a means of coping, similar to that of "gallows humor" that sometimes appears during times of significant stress in a health care environment. Katie Watson (2011) discussed the function of such humor in the treatment setting, including facilitating clinical decision making (such as might be expected in brainstorming), dismantling aggressive stances made by a clinician, and helping clinicians to cope with difficult situations. As such, it seems that the challenge is balancing what may be helpful and needed in a situation versus what may be deemed as unprofessional. Regarding dark humor, Tomlinson (2012) adds, "The joke doesn't obscure the seriousness of the situation. It relies on it, and for that reason, once the laughter subsides, attention can quickly return to the patient's needs" (p. 9). When dark humor might be considered a microaggression, microinsult, or microinvalidation, one must consider that an ethical and clinically practical line has been crossed. In the case of the nurse who called the patient "Pocahontas," it seems that although this might be considered gallows humor (i.e., the patient's neurobehavioral problems were partially remedied by capitalizing upon her background of dance), at the same time it reflects a negative stereotype of Native American culture in terms of being adept at dance.

Using microaggressions as a means to cope with one's duties should be eradicated from the neurorehabilitation setting. In the same manner that the increase of sexual harassment in the workplace fostered training programs, so too should education and training be made available for the broad area of microaggressions. This may need to be an ongoing activity, perhaps a yearly requirement to remind rehabilitation staff of the pernicious nature of microaggressions affecting the neurorehabilitation environment as a whole, affecting patients and families in their trust of the health care system, and affecting functional outcomes.

In addition to training, it may be helpful to have regular debriefing sessions on difficult patient care situations. A debriefing session might allow for making explicit what may be implicit with respect to microaggressions that may have occurred in the rehabilitation process of the patient. Consider, for example, a World War II veteran who presents with a neurodegenerative condition and is receiving acute neurorehabilitation for a recent stroke. This patient refers to a Korean neuropsychologist staff member as an "Oriental doctor" in a somewhat demeaning tone of voice. Although the neuropsychologist may be accustomed to people using that term or being mistaken for someone of a different Asian culture, his coworkers may also resent the veteran's comments in support of their colleague. Without discussing this more openly, therapeutic alliances could easily be eroded, perhaps subtly (e.g., responding to the call light a bit later than for another patient). Coping with microaggressions on the part of the provider may be welcomed as a part of routine neurorehabilitation team care. As in the clinical vignette of a Chinese American neuropsychologist and her veteran patients, she may have been aided by discussing and processing the impact of his comments with colleagues so she would not risk developing negative countertransference that could undermine her work.

The preceding two issues raise an administrative policy dilemma. Much in the same way that sexual harassment and violence in the workplace are taken seriously, some consideration of a "no-tolerance" policy regarding microaggressions may need to be debated. A conversation between key stakeholders from hospital administration/agency administration with managers and clinicians would be beneficial to educate individuals about the issue, integrate training on microaggressions within curriculum on diversity, and develop a strategic plan around sustaining and dynamically responding to cultural differences in that specific setting. For example, in Vignette #1, cultural competency training might include specific issues of racial/ethnic disparities in neurorehabilitation in Native American populations and discussion of potential microaggressions that can occur in that setting if it served a proportionally high number of patients from Native American cultures. Jones and Galliher (2015) reported on the use of the Daily Racial Microaggressions Scale in a Native American young adult population. A high percentage (98%) of participants experienced at least one type of microaggression, and females showed a higher degree of upset from microinvalidations compared to male Native Americans in this study. Studies such as these underscore the specificity by which individuals of different cultures experience microaggressions.

In recent times, Muslim Americans have been the target of prejudice and discrimination. Not surprisingly, once marginalized, what follows are unique microaggressions that are used in public conversations, political venues, media, and also likely within health care settings. Research in this population is sparse, though emerging, and is consistent with research on other ethnic minorities. Nadal et al. (2012), in conducting qualitative interviews with ten Muslim college students, found that several of them had experienced microaggressions around six major themes: stereotypes of

Muslims as terrorists; the Muslim religion as pathological; the assumption that all Muslims share the same homogeneous experience in terms of their religious practices; microaggresions related to viewing and commenting on the Muslim religion as being an "exotic" or "trendy" religion; microaggressions that use "lslamophobic" and spiteful language when discussing the Muslim faith; and comments that connote being a foreigner despite a strong identification of the United States as their home country or even being born in the United States. Sadly, this post-9/11 era has also introduced a new arena of racial/ethnic and religious microaggressions. This type of information can be most enlightening when embarking upon cultural competency training. It also provides caution against overgeneralizing across cultures for findings on racial/ethnic microaggressions. Training must be aware of key populations to educate staff on some unique features of the experience of microaggressions in different cultures.

Education and training in cultural competency and management of incidences of microaggressions span many different cultures, many of which intersect. Microaggressions may also interact with other often marginalized individuals who identify with, for example, the lesbian, gay, bisexual, and transgender (LGBT) culture (e.g., see Platt & Lenzen, 2013). In this regard, Balsam, Molina, Beadnell, Simoni, and Walters (2011) developed a measure of what they call "multiple minority stress," called the LGBT People of Color Microaggressions Scale, which emphasizes these interacting cultures. Although this is a research instrument, the item development and factor structure can alert clinicians of some of the key constructs and experiences of microaggressions that are unique to this population of individuals.

In the neurorehabiliation setting, it may be assumed that individuals with brain injury, stroke, brain tumor, and other neurological disorders are in the "majority" culture because their disability is acquired. However, those who experience disability also experience other forms of microaggressions—for example, when a rehabilitation staff member talks louder to a person with an expressive aphasia (talking louder does not affect that person's ability to express language any better than if a comment were whispered). Another example is when nursing staff feel free to say whatever they want when caring for someone with a severe traumatic brain injury who is in a minimally conscious state because "they won't hear or remember it anyway." Keller and Galgay (2010) provide many other examples in one of the few published works to date that highlight the subtle (and perhaps not so subtle) means that microaggressions are expressed toward people with disabilities. Based on what they note as an "able-centric worldview" (p. 242), microaggressions can occur when there is a perception of the person as deviating from the norm of being able-bodied, and in brain injury, also deviating from an expectation of having normal thinking abilities. Clearly, such findings must be used in clinical practice and administrative policy when caring for individuals from diverse and intersecting cultures who may be vulnerable targets of microaggressive behavior.

CONCLUSIONS

The neurorehabilitation setting is not immune from microaggressions and, in fact, likely contains several unique facets that affect the manner in which these types of microaggressions manifest, are experienced by the patient, and require addressing. In this chapter, we highlight the aspects of neurorehabilitation settings and the practice of neurorehabilitation more broadly so providers might consider them when working with ethnic minority patients. Providers in these settings may benefit from cultural competency training to develop a greater appreciation for how microaggressions may impact the quality of their work with ethnic minorities, detract from the working alliance, and limit therapeutic success. Increased familiarity with factors (structural as well as interpersonal and intrapersonal) that might contribute to microaggressions may help providers better identify them and intervene in a timely and therapeutically helpful manner. However, given that a defining feature of microaggressions is their unintended nature, neurorehabilitation and other clinical settings would be well advised to establish policies that encourage critical self-examination and dialogue regarding specific issues of race, ethnicity, and culture without fear of harsh reprimand. Such policies should not only function as a means of examining potential microaggressions but also as an opportunity to provide ongoing training and support in a fast-paced health care setting marked by challenging patients. Establishing specific institutional guidelines and expectations regarding how to educate, train, and manage microaggressions may assist with promoting a safer and more inclusive clinical environment for neurorehabilitation to occur.

REFERENCES

Balsam, K. F., Molina, Y., Beadnell, B., Simoni, J., & Walters, K. (2011). Measuring multiple minority stress: The LGBT People of Color Microaggressions Scale. *Cultural Diversity and Ethnic Minority Psychology, 17,* 163–174.

Blume, A. W., Lovato, L. V., Thyken, B. N., & Denny, N. (2012). The relationship of microaggressions with alcohol use and anxiety among ethnic minority college students in a historically White institution. *Cultural Diversity and Ethnic Minority Psychology, 18,* 45–54.

Constantine, M. G. (2007). Racial microaggressions against African American clients in cross-racial counseling relationships. *Journal of Counseling Psychology, 54,* 1–16.

Constantine, M. G., & Sue, D. W. (2007). Perceptions of racial microaggressions among black supervisees in cross-racial dyads. *Journal of Counseling Psychology, 54,* 142–153.

Gaertner, S. L., & Dovidio, J. F. (1986). The aversive form of racism. In J. F. Dovidio & S. L. Gaertner (Eds.), *Prejudice, discrimination, and racism* (pp. 61–89). San Diego, CA: Academic Press.

Greenwald, A. G., Poehlman, T. A., Uhlmann, E. L., & Banaji, M. R. (2009). Understanding and using the Implicit Association Test: III. Meta-analysis of predictive validity. *Journal of Personality and Social Psychology, 97,* 17–41.

Haskins, E., Cicerone, K., & Trexler, L. (2012). *Cognitive rehabilitation manual: Translating evidence-based recommendations into practice.* Reston, VA: American Congress of Rehabilitation Medicine.

Horvath, A. O., & Symonds, B. D. (1991). Relation between working alliance and outcome in psychotherapy: A meta-analysis. *Journal of Counseling Psychology, 38,* 139–149.

Jones, M. L., & Galliher, R. V. (2015). Daily racial microaggressions and ethnic identification among Native American young adults. *Cultural Diversity and Ethnic Minority Psychology, 21,* 1–9.

Keller, R. M., & Galgay, C. E. (2010). Microaggressive experiences of people with disabilities. In D. W. Sue (Ed.), *Microaggressions and marginality: Manifestation, dynamics, and impact* (pp. 241–268). Hoboken, NJ: John Wiley & Sons, Inc.

Kinder, D. R., & Sears, D. O. (1981). Prejudice and politics: Symbolic racism versus racial threats to the good life. *Journal of Personality and Social Psychology, 40,* 414–431.

Link, B. G., & Phelan, J. C. (2001). Conceptualizing stigma. *Annual Review of Sociology, 27,* 363–385.

Macrae, C. N., & Bodenhausen, G. V. (2000). Social cognition: Thinking categorically about others. *Annual Review of Psychology, 51,* 93–120.

Major, B., & Crocker, J. (1993). Social stigma: The consequences of attributional ambiguity. In D. M. Mackie & D. L. Hamilton (Eds.), *Affect, cognition, and stereotyping: Interactive processes in group perception* (pp. 345–370). San Diego, CA: Academic Press, Inc.

Major, B., & O'Brien, L. T. (2005). The social psychology of stigma. *Annual Review of Psychology, 56,* 393–421.

Martin, D. J., Garske, J. P., & Davis, M. K. (2000). Relation of the therapeutic alliance with outcome and other variables: A meta-analytic review. *Journal of Consulting and Clinical Psychology, 68,* 438–450.

McConahay, J. B. (1986). Modern racism, ambivalence, and the Modern Racism scale. In J. F. Dovidio & S. L. Gaertner (Eds.), *Prejudice, discrimination, and racism* (pp. 91–125). San Diego, CA: Academic Press, Inc.

Nadal, K. L. (2011). The Racial and Ethnic Microaggressions Scale (REMS): Construction, reliability, and validity. *Journal of Counseling Psychology, 58,* 470–480.

Nadal, K. L., Griffin, K. E., Hamit, S., Leon, J., Tobio, M., & Rivera, D. P. (2012). Subtle and overt forms of Islamophobia: Microaggressions toward Muslim Americans. *Journal of Muslim Mental Health, 6,* 15–37.

Ong, A. D., Burrow, A. L., Fuller-Rowell, T. E., Ja, N. M., & Sue, D. W. (2013). Racial microaggressions and daily well-being among Asian Americans. *Journal of Counseling Psychology, 60,* 188–199.

Owen, J., Imel, Z., Tao, K. W., Wampold, B., Smith, A., & Rodolfa, E. (2011). Cultural ruptures in short-term therapy: Working alliance as a mediator between clients' perceptions of microaggressions and therapy outcomes. *Counselling and Psychotherapy Research, 11,* 204–212.

Owen, J., Tao, K. W., Imel, Z. E., Wampold, B. E., & Rodolfa, E. (2014). Addressing racial and ethnic microaggressions in therapy. *Professional Psychology: Research and Practice, 45,* 283–290.

Payne, B. K. (2005). Conceptualizing control in social cognition: How executive functioning modulates the expression of automatic stereotyping. *Journal of Personality and Social Psychology, 89,* 488–503.

Pierce, C. (1995). Stress analogs of racism and sexism: Terrorism, torture, and disaster. In C. Willie, P. Rieker, B. Kramer, & B. Brown (Eds.), *Mental health, racism, and sexism* (pp. 277–293). Pittsburgh, PA: University of Pittsburgh Press.

Platt, L. F., & Lenzen, A. L. (2013). Sexual orientation microaggressions and the experience of sexual minorities. *Journal of Homosexuality, 60,* 1011–1034.

Safran, J. D., & Muran, J. C. (2000). *Negotiating the therapeutic alliance: A relational treatment guide.* New York, NY: Guilford Press.

Schoulte, J. C., Schultz, J. M., & Altmaier, E. M. (2011). Forgiveness in response to cultural microaggressions. *Counselling Psychology Quarterly, 24,* 291–300.

Solórzano, D., Ceja, M., & Yosso, T. (2000). Critical race theory, racial microaggressions, and campus racial climate: The experiences of African American college students. *Journal of Negro Education,* 60–73.

Sue, D. W. (2005). Racism and the conspiracy of silence: Presidential Address. *The Counseling Psychologist,* 100–114.

Sue, D. W. (2010a). *Microaggressions in everyday life: Race, gender, and sexual orientation.* Hoboken, NJ: John Wiley & Sons.

Sue, D. W. (Ed.). (2010b). *Microaggressions and marginality: Manifestation, dynamics, and impact.* Hoboken, NJ: John Wiley & Sons.

Sue, D. W., Capodilupo, C. M., Nadal, K. L., & Torino, G. C. (2008). Racial microaggressions and the power to define reality. *American Psychologist, 63,* 277–279.

Sue, D. W., Capodilupo, C. M., Torino, G. C., Bucceri, J. M., Holder, A., Nadal, K. L., & Esquilin, M. (2007). Racial microaggressions in everyday life: Implications for clinical practice. *American Psychologist, 62,* 271–286.

Tomlinson, T. (2012). Uncomfortable humor. *Hastings Center Report, 42,* 9.

Torres, L., Driscoll, M. W., & Burrow, A. L. (2010). Racial microaggressions and psychological functioning among highly achieving African-Americans: A mixed-methods approach. *Journal of Social and Clinical Psychology, 29,* 1074–1099.

Torres-Harding, S., & Turner, T. (2014, September). Assessing racial microaggression distress in a diverse sample. *Evaluation and the Health Professions,* 1–27.

U.S. Department of Health and Human Services. (2001). *Mental health: Culture, race, and ethnicity—A supplement to Mental Health: A Report of the Surgeon General.* Washington, DC: U.S. Department of Health and Human Services.

Vasquez, M. J. (2007). Cultural difference and the therapeutic alliance: An evidence-based analysis. *American Psychologist, 62,* 878–885.

Wang, J., Leu, J., & Shoda, Y. (2011). When the seemingly innocuous "stings": Racial microaggressions and their emotional consequences. *Personality and Social Psychology Bulletin, 37,* 1666–1678.

Watkins, N. L., LaBarrie, T. L., & Appio, L. M. (2010). Black undergraduates' experience with perceived racial microaggressions in predominantly White colleges and universities. In D. W. Sue (Ed.), *Microaggressions and marginality: Manifestation, dynamics, and impact* (pp. 25–58). Hoboken, NJ: John Wiley & Sons.

Watson, K. (2011). Gallows humor in medicine. *Hastings Center Report, 41,* 37–45.

Wong, G., Derthick, A. O., David, E. J. R., Saw, A., & Okazaki, S. (2014). The what, the why, and the how: A review of racial microaggressions research in psychology. *Race and Social Problems, 6,* 181–200.

CHAPTER ELEVEN

SPIRITUALITY, RELIGIOUSNESS, AND CULTURE IN NEUROREHABILITATION

Vicky T. Lomay and Brick Johnstone

*T*he neurorehabilitation process can be a time of significant adjustment for patients with chronic disabling conditions and their families, given the many impairments and issues that can impact multiple facets of their lives. As individuals recover and adjust to their disabilities, they rely on their medical team, family members, friends, and community for assistance, encouragement, and help. In addition to these resources, they also frequently rely on spiritual or religious practices and beliefs as a source of support. Spiritual resources can provide people with the necessary comfort and strength needed to successfully navigate through challenging periods of life (Kerferi & Riemer-Ross, 2007).

People often rely on religious beliefs to help them cope during stressful life circumstances, such as after the loss of health and independence, indicating that religious practices give them a sense of control and help them to adapt (Koenig, 2008). As a result, rehabilitation psychologists must be aware of the manner in which individuals use spiritual and religious resources in a neurorehabilitation setting.

RELIGION AND SPIRITUALITY IN THE UNITED STATES AND THE WORLD

The vast majority of individuals, from all cultures and from around the world, have specific spiritual beliefs and religious practices. According to one survey, 92% of Americans believe in God or a universal spirit (Pew Forum, 2008). Seventy-six percent to 78% of Americans identified themselves as Christians (Kosman & Keysar, 2009; Pew Forum, 2008), and 4% to 5% self-affiliated with other religions. Fifty-four percent reported that they attend religious services fairly regularly (i.e., once or twice a month; Pew Forum, 2008). On a global level, more than 8 in 10 people identified with a religious group, including 32% Christians, 23% Islamists, 15% Hindu, 7% Buddhists, and 0.2% Jews. Furthermore, 6% of individuals practice folk or traditional/indigenous religious belief systems (Pew Forum, 2012). It is clear that the majority of U.S. citizens use religion to help them cope with life's struggles, so it is important that psychologists become aware of such spiritual beliefs and religious practices and how individuals use them to cope with chronic health disorders and disabling conditions.

DEFINITIONS

This chapter discusses spirituality, religiousness, and indigenous/folk belief systems in a multicultural context. The terms *spirituality* and *religiosity* are often used interchangeably, and it is difficult to have a consensus of definitions. Therefore, the following are meant to be general descriptors.

Religion

Religion has many definitions, but it usually refers to adherence or allegiance to a set of institutionalized beliefs or doctrines (Keferl & Riemer-Ross, 2007). Koenig (2008) defines it as "a system of beliefs and practices observed by a community, supported by rituals that acknowledge, worship, communicate with, or approach the Sacred, the Divine, God or Ultimate Truth" (p. 10). Stated simply, religion involves the behavioral practice of culturally based rituals associated with specific worldviews about humankind's place in the cosmos.

Spirituality

Spirituality also has multiple definitions and often refers to anything that is subjectively experienced and considered to be transcendent, sacred, holy, or divine (Miller & Thoresen, 2003). It is also defined as the way through which humans recognize the exalted meaning and value of their lives (Rahnama, Khoshknab, Maddah, & Ahmadi, 2012). Whereas religion is conceptualized as being primarily based in cultural practices, spirituality can be conceptualized as being primarily based in neuropsychological processes (e.g., feeling of emotional connectedness with a higher power, however one conceives such).

RESEARCH ON RELIGION, SPIRITUALITY, AND NEUROREHABILITATION

There is growing interest in determining the mechanisms that exist among religion, spirituality, and health, with general conclusions that increased religiosity/spirituality is associated with better health and decreased mortality (e.g., Hummer, Rogers, Nam, & Ellison, 1999; Koenig, 2008; Koenig, King, & Carson, 2012; McCullough, Larson, & Koenig, 2001; Pargament, Koenig Tarakeshwar, & Hahn, 2004; Shatenstein & Ghadirian, 1998; Strawbridge, Shema, Cohen, & Kaplan, 2001). The majority of religion and health research to date has primarily focused on persons with life-threatening diseases and conditions (e.g., cancer), as persons facing death may use religion to help them accept their condition, come to terms with unresolved life issues, and prepare for death. In contrast, rehabilitation patients who suffer acute injuries or chronic progressive disorders may live for decades after the onset of their condition and use religious and spiritual resources to help them cope with their disability, give new meaning to their lives based on their newly acquired disabilities, and help them to establish new goals (Johnstone, Glass, & Oliver, 2007). As such, it is important for rehabilitation psychologists to be aware of general religious practices and spiritual beliefs, as well as how they can accommodate such coping skills appropriately into their practices.

General Rehabilitation Populations

Several studies have investigated the relationships among religious, spiritual, and health variables for heterogeneous rehabilitation populations, although the type of disabilities assessed and measures of religion and spirituality used have varied considerably. For example, Campbell,

Yoon, and Johnstone (2010) investigated relationships among religious/ spiritual variables and physical health in a heterogeneous sample of individuals with traumatic brain injury (TBI), spinal cord injury (SCI), cerebral vascular accidents (CVA), and cancer. They reported that increased positive spiritual beliefs and increased religious attendance were associated with better physical health. In contrast, Cohen, Yoon, and Johnstone (2009), using the same sample, indicated that both positive spirituality and positive congregational support were associated with better mental health. Investigating just those individuals in this sample from a rehabilitation center, Johnstone and Yoon (2009) indicated that positive spirituality and increased willingness to forgive were associated with better physical health and that increased negative spirituality was associated with both worse physical and mental health. Results from these studies suggest that spiritual beliefs, both positive and negative, and congregational support were more closely associated with health outcomes than religious variables. It was suggested that this is because individuals with more severe disabilities pray more regardless of their condition (e.g., pray more for recovery, pray more in supplication in declining health), thus negating any statistically identifiable relationships.

Although most studies on religion, spirituality, and health have been cross-sectional, several longitudinal studies have been completed that suggest possible causal relationships. For example, a 4-month longitudinal study of a general rehabilitation population indicated that religion did not promote better recovery or adjustment, although it may have been a source of consolation for some patients with limited recovery (Fitchett, Rybarczyk, DeMarco, & Nicholas, 1999). In addition, negative religious coping and anger with God were found to be risk factors for poor recovery. Kim, Heinemann, Bode, Sliwa, and King (2000) completed a longitudinal study of medical rehabilitation patients and indicated that spiritual well-being did not change over time (i.e., admission until 3 months after discharge), although 37% of the sample experienced gains of at least 2 standard deviations in spiritual well-being over time, and 32% reported experiencing declines of at least 2 standard deviations in spiritual well-being. These results indicated that some individuals with disabilities may turn to religious and spiritual resources to help them cope in times of crisis, whereas others may feel spiritually abandoned or that their disability is punishment from God.

Specific to populations with TBIs and SCIs, McColl et al. (2000) conducted a qualitative study to explore expressions of spirituality at the onset of injury. They identified five themes—awareness, closeness, trust, purpose, vulnerability—and three relationships—intrapersonal, interpersonal, and transpersonal—that appear to be important to these populations.

Traumatic Brain Injury

Several studies have investigated relationships among religion, spirituality, and health for specific rehabilitation populations. This is important because individuals with different types of injuries/disorders may use different religious and spiritual resources to help them cope. This may be particularly true for individuals with cognitive versus physical disabilities or a combination of both.

One study of individuals with TBI indicated that persons who experienced a stronger sense of meaning in their lives and who possessed stronger values/beliefs were more likely to have better perceived physical health, and those who received more support from their religious congregations were more likely to have better mental health (Johnstone, Yoon, Rupright, & Reid-Arndt, 2009). Another study of individuals with nonacute TBI indicated that increased spirituality was associated with positive psychological coping strategies (e.g., cognitive restructuring, information seeking), but not with negative psychological coping strategies (e.g., self-blame, wish fulfilling fantasy; Mahalik, Johnstone, Glass, & Yoon, 2007).

In a study of Canadian Aboriginal clients recovering from a brain injury, Keightly et al. (2009) identified culturally sensitive care and traditional healing methods as a challenge in providing specialized needs for Aboriginal clients. They also found health practitioners' clinical experiences with brain injury as well as working specifically with Aboriginal clients influenced the perceived challenges.

Stroke

Other studies have investigated these relationships for persons with stroke, which by nature is typically a group of older individuals. In general, Giaquinto, Spiridigliozzi, and Caracciolo (2007) suggested that religious beliefs may be a potential protective factor against emotional distress for persons with stroke. Johnstone, Franklin, Yoon, Burris, and Shigaki (2008) indicated that those individuals with stroke who reported stronger religious and spiritual coping skills were more likely to have better mental health. However, no religious or spiritual variables were significantly associated with physical health, likely related to the severity of physical impairments associated with the strokes (i.e., prayer and spiritual belief can assist individuals in coping with their disability but cannot improve significant physical conditions). Increased attendance at religious services has been shown to be associated with reduced incidence of stroke (Colantonio, Kasl, & Ostfeld, 1992; Colantonio, Kasl, Ostfeld, & Berkman, 1993), which is likely related to the better health habits of persons who regularly attend church. Similarly, increased attendance at religious services has been shown to be associated with better overall physical health for individuals who sustained a first-time stroke (Berges, Kuo, Markides, & Ottenbacher, 2007). This may be because individuals with better physical functioning are better able to attend religious services, and not that attendance at religious services leads to better physical functioning.

Spinal Cord Injury

Additional studies have focused on individuals with SCI. Matheis, Tulsky, and Matheis (2006) interviewed participants with SCI and reported that "existential spirituality" was significantly related to general health but that "religious spirituality" was not predictive of any outcomes. These results suggest that nonreligious beliefs (i.e., existential worldview) may be more important in relating to health than religious beliefs for persons with SCI. Another study indicated that individuals with SCI who reported receiving greater congregational support were more likely to report better mental health (Franklin, Yoon, Acuff, & Johnstone, 2008). This is consistent with other studies that stress the importance of social support for persons with SCI who may have limited socialization due to difficulties with transportation and mobility.

Chronic Pain

Rippentrop, Altmaier, Chen, Found, and Keffala (2005) investigated relationships among health and religious, spiritual, and congregational support variables for individuals with chronic pain. Hierarchical multiple regressions indicated that forgiveness, negative spiritual coping, positive spiritual coping, and congregational support all predicted mental health. They noted that "lack of forgiveness and engaging in negative religious coping seem to contribute to poor mental health and higher pain intensity" (p. 319). This result is consistent with other studies that suggest that negative beliefs such as a punishing or abandoning God is related to worse health outcomes (e.g., Fitchett et al., 1999; Kim et al., 2000).

SPIRITUAL/RELIGIOUS INTERVENTIONS

Most of the research on individuals with disabilities has been correlational, with few interventional studies. Although health professionals traditionally have not been encouraged to provide religious or spiritually based interventions, it is important to be aware of those services that have been shown to be related to positive outcomes. For example, several meditation studies have been completed with persons with TBI, with variable results published. Brief mindfulness training has been shown to have variable results for attention difficulties (McMillan, Robertson, Brock, & Chorlton, 2002), whereas mindfulness-based stress reduction has been shown to have long-term benefits (Bedard et al., 2005). Mindfulness practices show promise in helping individuals to cope with disability, although further studies are needed—especially for individuals with and without brain dysfunction.

Forgiveness interventions are also showing promise as effective psychological interventions in rehabilitation. Many individuals in rehabilitation suffer injuries as the result of the actions of others (e.g., motor vehicle accidents, drunk driving, physical assault) and harbor intense, persisting feelings of anger toward perceived offenders. Such anger often impedes effective recovery, and for them to fully recover psychologically, it is sometimes beneficial to forgive offenders. Recent studies suggest that forgiveness interventions may be helpful for individuals with disabilities who are injured as the result of another person's actions (Gisi & D'Amato, 2000; Johnstone et al., 2014). The efficacy of such religious and spiritual interventions with rehabilitation populations clearly needs more study.

REHABILITATION AND FAITH TRADITIONS

A review of the literature did not reveal any studies regarding relationships among religion, spirituality, and health for persons with disabilities from different faith traditions. However, one study investigated the relationships among these variables for individuals from five different faith traditions, including Catholics, Protestants, Muslims, Jews, and Buddhists (Johnstone, Yoon et al., 2012). The results indicated that the different faith traditions differed in terms of personality and self-reported religiosity and spirituality but that faith tradition was not a significant predictor of better or worse health. Future research will need to address the role of different cultural practices and beliefs in the maintenance of health for different rehabilitation populations.

SPIRITUALITY AND RELIGIOUSNESS IN MULTICULTURAL POPULATIONS

Most rehabilitation psychologists come from traditional religious backgrounds (i.e., Christian) and are most familiar with the Christian religion. However, given the increased religious pluralism in the United States today, it is necessary to have at least introductory knowledge of different cultures and religions to best meet the needs of those individuals we serve. As stated earlier, 76% to 78% of the U.S. population identify with Christianity (Kosman & Keysar, 2009; Pew Forum, 2008) as their religious tradition. When the racial and ethnic compositions of other religious traditions were explored, the Pew Forum on Religious & Public Life (2008) found that 92% of congregants from historically Black churches were African American, followed by Hispanic at 4%. Eighty-eight percent of followers of Hinduism in the United States were identified as Asian American. Among those who practice Buddhism, 53% of followers are White (non-Hispanic), followed by Asian Americans at 32%. Of the Muslim faith tradition, the largest racial and ethnic group representations were White at 37%, African American at 24%, Asian American at 20%, and other/mixed groups at 15%. As such, beliefs and practices are as varied as the multiple faith traditions around the United States and the world. Following are some ways that individuals from particular faith traditions use religious coping strategies to assist them in their recovery from chronic illness and disability.

Koffman, Morgan, Edmonds, Speck, and Higginson (2008) explored how religion and spirituality influenced the experience of Black Caribbeans in coping with cancer. They found religious beliefs were important in helping these individuals conceptualize their cancer in the context of their existential well-being. They also found that the church community provided participants with social, practical support and that a small number believed the cancer experience was linked to their ultimate meaning and magnified their religiosity (Koffman et al., 2008).

Similarly, in their study of Iranian patients, Rahnama et al. (2012) explored the spiritual beliefs of a Muslim population dealing with cancer of different types and found three themes: God was perceived as the spiritual truth, moralities were seen as a spiritual sign, and spiritual resources were viewed as a source of hope. Many defined their spirituality as a relationship with God and the act of trusting Him. In addition, they reported that their own personal and interpersonal ethical considerations were an essential part of their spirituality. That is, being trustworthy, respecting others, and offering help or support to others were core components of their being. Examples of spiritual resources included worship activities such as engaging in prayer or visiting shrines or holy places. Rahnama et al. encouraged health care providers to allow patients the opportunity to perform spiritual activities, including those activities that incorporate a moral or ethical perspective.

Krause and Hayward (2013) conducted a study with a Mexican American population to determine if trust-based prayer expectancies (i.e., the belief that God answers prayers at the right time and in the best way) are associated with health. They found that this group used three spiritual practices: making *mandas* or requests of the Virgin Mary or a saint; leaving a *milagro* (a charm or offering) at a religious shrine or altar; and maintaining a home altar. They also found that older Mexican Americans who attend church more frequently are more likely to report they have a close relationship with God and that those who have a close relationship with God are more likely to endorse trust-based expectations. They found that a higher sense of self-esteem was associated with more favorable self-rated health. Further analysis found the indirect effect of trust-based expectations on health through self-esteem was statistically significant (Krause & Hayward, 2013).

In a review of research on religion, spirituality, and mental health from Western and Middle Eastern countries where Christianity and Muslim faiths predominate, Koenig, Al Zaben, and Khalifa (2012) found that both faith traditions overlap in many ways. Individuals from both faith traditions worshipped one God. In addition, the basic morals, values, and many rituals/practices were very comparable, and both Christians and Muslims reported a desire to live a life that emulates their respective prophets (i.e., Jesus and Mohammed; Koenig et al., 2012). The differences noted between the two faiths were mainly in belief rather than practice. The influence of these faith traditions on mental health suggests that greater religious involvement is associated with better mental health, regardless of the specific nature of the religion.

INDIGENOUS HEALING METHODS AND HEALTH

The World Health Organization (WHO; 2000) defines traditional indigenous healing as "the sum total of the knowledge, skills, and practices based on the theories, beliefs, and experiences indigenous to different cultures, whether explicable or not, used in the maintenance of health, as well as in the prevention, diagnosis, improvement, or treatment of physical and mental illness."

In American Indian tribal communities, traditional healing and ceremonies long predate biomedical care (Gurley et al., 2001). Traditional or indigenous healing practices were conducive to finding meaningful ways to live with the challenges of ill health or just everyday life (Hunter, Logan, Goulet, & Barton, 2006) and usually placed an emphasis on the spirit world, supernatural forces, and spirituality. Possible supernatural causes for health problems could include soul loss, possession by an evil spirit, the magical insertion of a foreign body, or the machinations of offended or malicious ancestral ghosts (Frank & Frank, 1993). Other causes could be violating taboos, offending spirits, or disrespecting natural elements. This in turn causes some kind of disequilibrium or disharmony, which can result in injury. That is, the actual physical injury may be quite natural, such as a fall resulting in a broken leg, but the fall may have been caused by supernatural means (i.e., an evil thought or sorcery; Frank & Frank, 1993).

Indigenous traditional healing rituals are typically used to provide a holistic approach to healing, and tribal people believe that traditional healing can help one on a path to general wellness (Struthers & Eschiti, 2005). In many indigenous populations, this holistic healing concept involved all aspects of the person's being (i.e., physical, emotional, spiritual, and social). Hunter et al. (2006) found in their study of Aboriginal healing that holistic healing is conceptualized as "following a cultural path," regaining balance, and sharing in the circle of life. Traditional healing is often used to address both the physical and spiritual needs of American Indian people, as well as the presumed causes of symptoms (Gurley et al., 2001).

The current service ecology for some tribal communities incorporates both traditional and biomedical forms (Gurley et al., 2001). Different systems of care are often seen to address different problems; for example, biomedicine may be utilized in the context of dental health, obstetrics, women's health, surgical intervention, emergency and trauma services, pediatrics, orthopedics, or general family medicine.

In their study of the Yup'ik in the Yukon-Kuskokwim Delta of Alaska, Wolsko, Lardon, Mohatt, and Orr (2007) found those who identified more with their traditional Yup'ik way of life reported greater happiness and used religion and spirituality to cope with stress. They further emphasized that the traditional (Yup'ik) values are a source of wellness and that connecting with the community and wilderness helps to both heal and sustain a sense of well-being (Wolsko et al., 2007). Clearly, adhering to one's cultural background and beliefs can be a source of comfort and strength.

In a study describing the use of biomedical services and traditional healing options for American Indians, Novins et al. (2004) found a higher prevalence of use of traditional healing methods than those reported for non-Indians using complementary or alternative methods of healing. This suggests traditional healing as an important source of care for tribal members. These researchers also found general differences in traditional healing practices between two tribes. One tribe featured traditional healing that is fairly informal, with a core set of ceremonies, any of which could be used for multiple forms or causes of distress. The other tribe had traditional healers who used very specialized and carefully scripted ceremonies that addressed specific symptoms to determine the spiritual cause of an individual's distress (Novins et al., 2004).

Buchwald, Beals, and Manson (2000) conducted a study to determine the extent to which traditional health practices were used by urban American Indian/Alaska Native patients. They found that 70% reported using traditional practice for health-related reasons during the past year, and

52% reported finding the practices helped quite a bit. Similarly, Bush and NiaNia (2012) described a traditional healing approach for a young man who was hearing disturbing voices and experiencing seizure-like events. He was treated with psychiatric medications. Over a 2-month period, the voices reduced in intensity and frequency, and the seizure-like episodes also decreased. The young man and his family also accepted a referral to a cultural practitioner because they suspected this may be more related to a traditional spiritual issue. After the consultation and at a later follow-up, the young man and his family reported that he was doing well, with a complete resolution of distressing symptoms and that he had stopped taking the psychiatric medication. Although many factors could account for this change in symptoms, the most important point is that the spiritual intervention provided the young man and his family with an explanation that fit with their cultural worldview, instilled hope, and encouraged him to take action (Bush & NiaNia, 2012).

Research on indigenous or traditional healing methods is scarce, probably due to fear of ridicule by the practitioner and user of traditional indigenous methods; concerns about misuse of the information divulged; or patients' belief that healing is a private matter and sacred. Also, healing practices are rarely recorded, and the scientific community may consider the lack of education and more metaphysical elements of indigenous healing methods to be unacceptable (Struthers, Eschiti, & Patchell, 2004). Rehabilitation psychologists must become familiar with the specific practices and beliefs of the individuals they work with so they can relate to their attitudes about disability and determine the best way to provide services.

CASE EXAMPLES

Following are some examples of the different ways rehabilitation psychologists can address religious and spiritual beliefs with individuals from different faith traditions. The first vignette illustrates how psychologists need to be aware of, and encourage and support, how the spiritual beliefs and cultural practices of American Indians can be used to promote their health, well-being, and recovery.

Case Vignette #1: Jim is a middle-aged American Indian man who sustained a TBI after a motor vehicle accident. He lives with his wife on his tribe's reservation in a remote area of the state. He has five adult children who are very supportive of him. During the course of his medical care, he is admitted to the inpatient neurorehabilitation unit for further care. He did not require any surgical intervention, but he is experiencing some cognitive deficits. The rehabilitation psychologist is consulted regarding his coping and adjustment, as well as about recommendations for discharge planning. He is agreeable to speaking with the therapist, and after several sessions, he and his family share their concerns about the cause of the accident being attributed to negative energy or spirits. He has been having a difficult time adjusting to the changes associated with his injuries, as well as changes in his mood and attitude that his family think are uncharacteristic of him. This is distressing to his family, and they would like to ask a tribal healer to intervene on a more supernatural, spiritual level. The rehabilitation psychologist recognizes how important and beneficial this healing ceremony could be for Jim, and the family arranges, with the help of the rehabilitation team, for a tribal healer of his choosing to visit Jim in the unit. The day after the private session with the healer, Jim exhibits a slightly more optimistic change in his motivation, energy, and effort. He says he believes the negative energy has been dispelled, and he feels he can concentrate now on participating fully with his therapies. He plans to have another healing ceremony at home after he is discharged. His family comments that his optimistic outlook and generally jovial mood are more like his preinjury personality.

The following vignette illustrates how faith practices are used positively by individuals in rehabilitation and presents issues that psychologists are likely to face in rehabilitation.

Case Vignette #2: Karen is a 32-year-old African American Baptist who incurred a C-2 SCI in a motor vehicle accident. She is now a quadriplegic, and she will not be able to return to her previous job as a corporate attorney, a position from which she developed her core identity. Her fiancé does not feel comfortable with the situation and tends to withdraw, although Karen's family and congregation are extremely supportive of her. She suffers from bouts of depression and concerns about what she is going to do with the rest of her life. She is followed by rehabilitation psychology primarily to deal with issues of depression, self-concept, and changes in her work, home, and relationships. The psychologist also provides forgiveness interventions for Karen's intense anger with the driver of the car in the accident in which she was injured, as well as with her fiancé, who she is anticipating is going to leave her. Karen relies on prayer as a coping mechanism and asks her health care providers to pray with her on occasion. She participates in religious rituals that involve the laying on of hands and asks her psychologist to participate in such ceremonies.

This next vignette illustrates how more common faith practices are used negatively by individuals in rehabilitation and presents issues that psychologists are likely to face in rehabilitation.

Case Vignette #3: Paul is a biracial man in his 20s who incurred a significant TBI in a fight with gang members. He suffered frontal lobe hemorrhages and demonstrates difficulties with cognition, impulsivity, and emotional lability, which were also preexisting to a lesser extent. Paul earned his GED but has never been able to hold steady employment. His family support is nonexistent, and his peer group generally ignores him because they do not seem to know how to deal with his cognitive, emotional, and behavioral changes. Paul is provided with psychological services for severe depression, behavioral impulsivity, and a lack of motivation to participate in therapies or get involved in the community. Paul attended a Fundamentalist church with his grandmother during his youth, but he quit attending when he became independent. He now views his injury as a sign of divine punishment for his previous wayward behavior and therefore finds little motivation to engage in therapies or life because "God has it in for him." He subsequently expressed the opinion that he therefore no longer needed psychological interventions.

SUMMARY

To summarize, research indicates that positive spiritual beliefs and congregational support are generally associated with better mental health for persons with disabilities, and for physical health to a lesser extent.

Religious practices appear to have minimal statistical relations to health outcomes, which is likely related to methodological issues (i.e., individuals pray more as their health both improves and worsens). Studies also consistently indicate that persons with negative spiritual beliefs have worse health outcomes. Spiritual, religious, and congregational support variables are differentially related to health outcomes for different rehabilitation populations (e.g., SCI, CVA, TBI, pain). Current research is focusing on the efficacy of different spiritual interventions (e.g., meditation, forgiveness interventions, mindfulness-based stress reduction) for persons with disabilities, with an acknowledged need to identify persons with positive versus negative beliefs.

RECOMMENDATIONS

It is well documented that spiritual beliefs and religious practices, in whatever context a patient chooses to believe, are a source of support and are often used in the coping process. The specific mechanism by which these belief systems assist the patient is relatively unimportant. In addition, spirituality is associated with both culture and religion, and all of these three factors influence our understanding of health and disease (Rahnama et al., 2012).

Rehabilitation psychologists, at a minimum, need to be aware of the cultural, religious, and spiritual backgrounds of their patients. In general, psychologists are not trained to engage in religious or spiritual practices, although more are becoming comfortable in doing so (Johnstone, Glass, & Oliver, 2008). This may include referring individuals back to their spiritual leaders, passively engaging in religious practices with their patients (e.g., prayer), or offering interventions that can be delivered in both religious and nonreligious contexts (e.g., forgiveness interventions, meditation). However, proselytizing is never acceptable in health care.

Following are several general recommendations for how rehabilitation psychologists can address the spiritual and religious needs of their patients based on cultural factors. During the rehabilitation process, it can be helpful to ask questions to facilitate a better understanding of how religious or spiritual beliefs may influence perceptions of health and illness (Koffman et al., 2008). Kerferi and Riemer-Ross (2007) recommended the following when working with patients in the rehabilitation setting:

1. Providers should acknowledge the importance of spirituality in their patients' lives.
2. Providers should be willing to accept and consult with other spiritual and/or religious leaders in their clients' lives.
3. Providers should parallel their clients' worldviews with congruent terminology and imagery in conceptualizing rehabilitation strengths and limitations.
4. Providers should address spiritual themes that are meaningful to their patients and encourage the presence of those themes in the therapeutic process.
5. Providers should be aware of their own limitations and provide the most ethical care.

In an article on prayer as a therapeutic tool, Farah and McColl (2008) suggested some guidelines to determine if prayer with the patient may be beneficial and helpful to coping with health issues. They recommended asking the following questions, and suggested that if the answer was yes, it might be helpful to incorporate prayer into the therapist–patient relationship:

Is there a spiritual component to the client's problems?
Is the therapist equipped to offer prayer? If so, would it be authentic?
Would the client be receptive to prayer?
Would the therapist's workplace support the use of prayer?

Neimeier and Arango-Lasprilla (2007) provided some general recommendations for rehabilitation providers working with ethnic/minority cultures. These recommendations include increased awareness of and knowledge of cultural beliefs, customs, and histories; increased self-knowledge regarding personal biases and specific prejudices; preservice education and mentoring; decreased rehabilitation health disparities; and increased advocacy and research regarding working minority cultures.

Lomay and Hinkebein (2006) also suggested a number of culturally sensitive considerations, particularly when working with those who identify as members of an indigenous, an Aboriginal, or a tribal group. Their recommendations include awareness of beliefs and possible stereotypes, knowledge of historical and contemporary information specific to that group, exploring basic value structures and how culture may influence those values, awareness of spiritual beliefs and implications for how illness and/or injury is understood and conceptualized, and understanding how spiritual beliefs may influence how disability is understood.

CONCLUSIONS

It is clear that spiritual and religious beliefs are an important source of support, comfort, and strength for individuals as they cope with the challenges of adjusting to a chronic disabling condition. This chapter discusses the diverse and multifaceted aspects of religion and spirituality, with the hope that practitioners will use this as an introduction to further explore how they can incorporate this knowledge into their clinical work.

REFERENCES

Bedard, M., Felteau, M., Gibbons, C., Klein, R., Mazmanian, D., Fedyk, K., & Mack, G. (2005). A mindfulness-based intervention to improve quality of life among individuals who sustained traumatic brain injuries: One-year follow-up. *Journal of Cognitive Rehabilitation, 23*, 8–13.

Berges, I. M., Kuo, Y. F., Markides, K. S., & Ottenbacher, K. (2007). Attendance at religious services and physical functioning after stroke among older Mexican Americans. *Experimental Aging Research, 33*(1), 1–11.

Buchwald, D., Beals, J., & Manson, S. M. (2000). Use of traditional health practices among Native Americans in a primary care setting. *Medical Care, 38*, 1191–1199.

Bush, A., & NiaNia, W. (2012). Voice hearing and pseudoseizures in a Maori teenager: An example of mate Maori and Maori traditional healing. *Australasian Psychiatry, 20*, 348–351. doi:10.1177/1039856212456090

Campbell, J., Yoon, D. P., & Johnstone, B. (2010). Determining relationships between physical health and spiritual experience, religious practices, and congregational support in a heterogeneous medical sample. *Journal of Religion and Health, 49*, 3–17.

Cohen, D., Yoon, D. P., & Johnstone, B. (2009). Differentiating the impact of spiritual experiences, religious practices, and congregational support on the mental health of individuals with heterogeneous medical disorders. *International Journal for the Psychology of Religion, 19*, 121–138.

Colantonio, A., Kasl, S. V., & Ostfeld, A. M. (1992). Depressive symptoms and other psychosocial factors as predictors of stroke in the elderly. *American Journal of Epidemiology, 136*, 884–894.

Colantonio, A., Kasl, S. V., Ostfeld, A. M., & Berkman, L. F. (1993). Psychosocial predictors of stroke outcomes in an elderly population. *Journal of Gerontology, 48*, S261–S268.

Farah, J., & McColl, M. A. (2008). Exploring prayer as a spiritual modality. *Canadian Journal of Occupational Therapy, 75*(1), 5–13.

Fitchett, G., Rybarczyk, B. D., DeMarco, G. A., & Nicholas, J. J. (1999). The role of religion in medical rehabilitation outcomes: A longitudinal study. *Rehabilitation Psychology, 44*, 333.

Frank, J., & Frank, J. (1993). *Persuasion and healing: A comparative study of psychotherapy* (3rd ed.). Baltimore, MD: The Johns Hopkins University Press.

Franklin, K. L., Yoon, D. P., Acuff, M., & Johnstone, B. (2008). Relationships among religiousness, spirituality, and health for individuals with spinal cord injury. *Topics in Spinal Cord Injury Rehabilitation, 14*, 76–81.

Giaquinto, S., Spiridigliozzi, C., & Caracciolo, B. (2007). Can faith protect from emotional distress after stroke? *Stroke, 38*, 993–997.

Gisi, T. M., & D'Amato, R. C. (2000). What factors should be considered in rehabilitation: Are anger, social desirability, and forgiveness related in adults with traumatic brain injuries? *International Journal of Neuroscience, 105*(1–4), 121–133.

Gurley, D., Novins, D. K., Jones, M. C., Beals, J., Shore, J. H., & Manson, S. M. (2001). Comparative use of biomedical services and traditional healing by American Indian veterans. *Psychiatric Services, 52*(1), 68–74.

Hummer, R. A., Rogers, R. G., Nam, C. B., & Ellison, C. G. (1999). Religious involvement and U.S. adult mortality. *Demography, 36*, 273–285.

Hunter, L. M., Logan, J., Goulet, J., & Barton, S. (2006). Aboriginal healing: Regaining balance and culture. *Journal of Transcultural Nursing, 17*(1), 13–22. doi:10.1177/1043659605278937

Johnstone, B., Bayan, S., Gutierrez, L., Lardizabal, D., Lanigar, K., Yoon, D. P., & Judd, K. (2015). Neuropsychological correlates of forgiveness. *Religion, Brain, and Behavior, 5*(1), 24–35.

Johnstone, B., Franklin, K. L., Yoon, D. P., Burris, J., & Shigaki, C. L. (2008). Relationships among religiousness, spirituality, and health for individuals surviving a stroke. *Journal of Clinical Psychology in Medical Settings, 15*, 308–313.

Johnstone, B., & Glass, B. A. (2008). Evaluation of a neuropsychological model of spirituality in persons with traumatic brain injury. *Zygon, 43*, 861–874.

Johnstone, B., Glass, B. A., & Oliver, R. E. (2007). Religion and disability: Clinical, research and training considerations for rehabilitation professionals. *Disability & Rehabilitation, 29*, 1153–1163.

Johnstone, B., & Yoon, D. P. (2009). Relationships between the Brief Multidimensional Measure of Religiousness/Spirituality and health outcomes for a heterogeneous rehabilitation population. *Rehabilitation Psychology, 54*, 422–431.

Johnstone, B., Yoon, D. P., Cohen, D., Schopp, L. H., McCormack, G., & Smith, M. (2012). Relationships among spirituality, religious practices, personality factors, and health for five different faith traditions. *Journal of Religion and Health, 51,* 1017–1041. doi:10.1007/s10943-012-96158

Johnstone, B., Yoon, D. P., Rupright, J., & Reid-Arndt, S. (2009). Relationships among spiritual beliefs, religious practices, congregational support, and health for individuals with traumatic brain injury. *Brain Injury, 23,* 411–419.

Keightley, M. L., Ratnayake, R., Minore, B., Katt, M., Cameron, A., White, R., . . . Colantonio, A. (2009). Rehabilitation challenges for Aboriginal clients recovering from brain injury: A qualitative study engaging health care practitioners. *Brain Injury, 23,* 250–261.

Kerferi, J., & Riemer-Ross, M. (2007). The spiritual realm of rehabilitation counseling. In P. Leung, C. R. Flowers, W. B. Talley, & P. R. Sanderson (Eds.), *Multicultural issues in rehabilitation and allied health* (pp. 267–280). Linn Creek, MO: Aspen Professional Services.

Kim, J., Heinemann, A. W., Bode, R. K., Sliwa, J., & King, R. B. (2000). Spirituality, quality of life, and functional recovery after medical rehabilitation. *Rehabilitation Psychology, 45,* 365.

Koenig, H. G. (2008). *Medicine, religion, and health: Where science and spirituality meet.* Goshen, IN: Templeton Foundation Press.

Koenig, H. G., Al Zaben, F., & Khalifa, D. A. (2012). Religion, spirituality, and mental health in the West and the Middle East. *Asian Journal of Pyschiatry, 5,* 180–182.

Koenig, J., King, D., & Carson, V. B. (2012). *Handbook of religion and health* (2nd ed.). New York, NY: Oxford University Press.

Koffman, J., Morgan, M., Edmonds, P., Speck, P., & Higginson, I. J. (2008). "I know he controls cancer": The meanings of religion among Black Caribbean and White British patients with advanced cancer. *Social Science & Medicine, 67,* 780–789. doi:10.1016/j.socscimed.2008.05.004

Kosman, B. A., & Keysar, A. (2009). American Religious Identification Survey (ARIS 2008): Summary report. Retrieved from http://commons.trincoll.edu/aris/files/2011/08/ARIS_Report_2008.pdf

Krause, N., & Hayward, R. D. (2013). Trust-based prayer expectancies and health among older Mexican Americans. *Journal of Religious Health.* Advance online publication. doi:10.1007/s10943-013-9786-y

Lomay, V. T., & Hinkebein, J. H. (2006). Cultural considerations when providing rehabilitation services to American Indians. *Rehabilitation Psychology, 51*(1), 36–42. doi:10.1037/0090-5550.51.1.36

Mahalik, J. L., Johnstone, B., Glass, B. A., & Yoon, D. P. (2007). Spirituality, psychological coping, and community integration for persons with traumatic brain injury. *Journal of Religion, Disability, and Health, 11*(3), 65–77.

Matheis, E. N., Tulsky, D. S., & Matheis, R. J. (2006). The relation between spirituality and quality of life among individuals with spinal cord injury. *Rehabilitation Psychology, 51*(3), 265–271.

McColl, M. A., Bickenbach, J., Johnston, J., Nishihama, S., Schumaer, M., Smith, K., . . . Yealland, B. (2000). Spiritual issues associated with traumatic-onset disability. *Disability and Rehabilitation, 22*, 555–564.

McCullough, M. E., Larson, D. B., & Koenig, H. G. (2001). *Handbook of religion and health*. New York, NY: Oxford University Press.

McMillan, T., Robertson, I. H., Brock, D., & Chorlton, L. (2002). Brief mindfulness training for attentional problems after traumatic brain injury: A randomised control treatment trial. *Neuropsychological Rehabilitation, 12*(2), 117–125.

Miller, W. R., & Thoresen, C. E. (2003). Spirituality, religion, and health: An emerging research field. *American Psychologist, 58*(1), 24.

Neimeier, J., & Arango-Lasprilla, J. C. (2007). Toward improved rehabilitation services for ethnically diverse survivors of traumatic brain injury. *Journal of Head Trauma Rehabilitation, 22*(2), 75–84.

Novins, D. K., Beals, J., Moore, L. A., Spicer, P., Manson, S. M. & AI-SUPERPFP Team. (2004). Use of biomedical services and traditional healing options among American Indians: Sociodemographic correlates, spirituality, and ethnic identity. *Medical Care, 42*, 670–679.

Oman, D., Kurata, J. H., Strawbridge, W. J., & Cohen, R. D. (2002). Religious attendance and cause of death over 31 years. *International Journal of Psychiatry in Medicine, 32*(1), 69–89.

Pargament, K. I., Koenig, H. G., Tarakeshwar, N., & Hahn, J. (2004). Religious coping methods as predictors of psychological, physical and spiritual outcomes among medically ill elderly patients: A two-year longitudinal study. *Journal of Health Psychology, 9*, 713–730.

Pew Forum on Religious & Public Life. (2008). *Summary of key findings*. Retrieved from http://religions.pewforum.org/pdf/report-religious-landscape-key-findings.pdf

Pew Forum on Religious & Public Life. (2012). *The global religious landscape: A report on the size and distribution of the world's major religious groups as of 2010*. Retrieved from http:www.//pewforum.org/files/2014/01/global-religion-full.pdf

Rahnama, M., Khoshknab, M. F., Maddah, S. S. B., & Ahmadi, F. (2012). Iranian cancer patients' perception of spirituality: A qualitative content analysis study. *BMC Nursing, 11*, 19.

Rippentrop, E. A., Altmaier, E. M., Chen, J. J., Found, E. M., & Keffala, V. J. (2005). The relationship between religion/spirituality and physical health, mental health, and pain in a chronic pain population. *Pain, 116*, 311–321.

Shatenstein, B., & Ghadirian, P. (1998). Influences on diet, health behaviours and their outcome in select ethnocultural and religious groups. *Nutrition, 14*, 223–230.

Strawbridge, W. J., Shema, S. J., Cohen, R. D., & Kaplan, G. A. (2001). Religious attendance increases survival by improving and maintaining good health behaviors, mental health, and social relationships. *Annals of Behavioral Medicine, 23*, 68–74.

Struthers, R., & Eschiti, V. S. (2005). Being healed by an indigenous traditional healer: Sacred healing stories of Native Americans. Part II. *Complementary Therapies in Clinical Practice, 11*, 78–86.

Struthers, R., Eschiti, V. S., & Patchell, B. (2004). Traditional healing: Part 1. *Complementary Therapies in Nursing & Midwifery, 10*, 141–149. doi:10.1016/j.ctnm.2004.05.001

Wolsko, C., Lardon C., Mohatt, G. V., & Orr, E. (2007). Stress, coping, and well-being among the Yup'ik of the Yukon-Kuskokwim Delta: The role of enculturation and acculturation. *International Journal of Circumpolar Health, 66*(1), 51–61.

World Health Organization. (2000). *General guidelines for methodologies on research and evaluation of traditional medicine.* Retrieved from http://www.who.int/medicinedocs/en/d/Jwhozip42e

CHAPTER TWELVE

ON NEW DIRECTIONS TO ADVANCE THE FIELD OF MULTICULTURAL NEUROREHABILITATION

Jay M. Uomoto

Recovery is a newly achieved state of ordered functioning, that is, responsiveness, hinging on a specifically formed relation between preserved and impaired performances. This new relation operates in the direction of a new individual norm, of new constancy and adequacy.
　　　　　　　　—Kurt Goldstein (1939/1995), *The Organism*, p. 334

Neurorehabilitation has become more of a global phenomenon and is not necessarily limited to industrialized or Westernized societies. Increasing visibility of international perspectives in neurorehabilitation (e.g., Christensen & Uzzell, 2013) and in cross-cultural neuropsychology (e.g., Fletcher-Janzen, Strickland, & Reynolds, 2000; Uzzell, Ponton, & Ardila, 2007) has begun to be disseminated with voices that stretch across different continents. The importance of culture continues to require further focus and depth of research and clinical insights. To understand how various cultures impact the day-to-day execution of neurorehabilitation services, this book examines specific issues from a perspective that Cheung, van de Vijver, and Leong (2011) have posited as an integration of *emic* (culturally unique) concepts into a redefined *etic* (universal) interpretation of neurorehabilitation principles. As noted in the Preface, this is but a start in bettering our understanding and hopefully inculcating cultural perspectives into effective neurorehabilitation practices. The knowledge base is admittedly thin in this topic area. While much has been written about racial and ethnic disparities in neurorehabilitation, less appears in the literature regarding other types of cultural disparities in this arena of health care. Many recommendations have been detailed to overcome such differences (e.g., see American College of Physicians, 2010; Smedley, Stith, & Nelson, 2003), and clearly these insights can be applied to the delivery of neurorehabilitation services. However, as Niemeier, Burnett, and Whitaker (2003) underscore, a call for culturally competent rehabilitative care has much to be desired, where "this new focus [on cultural competence] has not yet led to appreciable changes in actual training and service delivery for today's more ethnically diverse American rehabilitation patient" (p. 1240). In a later article, Niemeier and Arango-Lasprilla (2007) stress the significance of cultural awareness and sensitivity in everyday clinical transactions with patients and their loved ones.

To stimulate further deliberation on the topic of what effective multicultural neurorehabilitation involves, several expansions of the current literature and research are recommended. Clearly, this is not meant to be exhaustive, but merely an attempt at providing a basis to further the discussion and action in the field.

EXPANSION OF THE CONCEPT OF CULTURE

Culture often connotes concepts of race and ethnicity when discussed in the context of health care disparities. Socioeconomic and other demographic variables make up the majority of the balance on discussion regarding culture in health care. However, to advance the field of neurorehabilitation, extending what constitutes the breadth of cultures that impact this field is worth considering. Ardila (2013), in discussing an update of what might be considered significant neuropsychological syndromes that are contemporary and in line with current culture, states, "It can be proposed that it is time to reanalyze most of the neuropsychological syndromes, and eventually, to develop new assessment procedures, more in accordance with the XXI-century living conditions" (p. 761).

Ardila points out that because of new methods of communication, this may spawn new neuropsychological syndromes. For example, with the reliance on keyboarding for multiple methods of verbal information delivery, disorder in these skills may be reflected in a syndrome of memory disturbances for spatial position on the keyboard in the person with brain injury. He goes on to describe how the decline in written arithmetic skills may see the decline of traditional forms of acalculia, but with the ubiquitous use of the pocket calculator may come a rise in a form of "pocket calculator acalculia" (p. 757) for which no neuropsychological test exists. These are just some examples of how modern culture, and even pop culture, can infiltrate everyday neurological functions and therefore requires changes in the way we think about evaluating, and treating rehabilitation deficits in a meaningful way.

Multicultural neurorehabilitation must emphasis "multiple," and do so in a dynamic manner. In other words, at any given time, multiple cultures operate in each interaction and in each therapy delivered in the neurorehabilitation setting. In neurocognitive rehabilitation of those with combat-related blast injuries, for example, one must take into consideration that a younger military cohort is likely to be represented at Veterans Affairs medical centers or military medical facilities. This group may also, for example, be considered more "computer or technology savvy." Whereas paper-and-pencil memory compensatory strategies may be appropriate for some, neurocognitive training may need to focus on the optimal use of smartphones and other mobile devices that provide apps that serve compensatory functions. The technology field is evolving so rapidly that even these features may soon be outdated. The point is that culture spans an array of dimensions, and one cannot limit one's conceptualization of culture in neurorehabilitation to racial or ethnic variables. What this all means is that when one considers the concept of culture in improving neurorehabilitation services, it should be anticipated that these improvements are likely to be dynamic, setting-specific, and ever-changing.

EXPANDING NEUROSCIENCE RESEARCH TO REFLECT THE INFLUENCE OF CULTURE

Recently, there has been increased interest and research into the newly developing field of *cultural neuroscience*. Considered a new field of inquiry, at its core is a cross-pollination of cross-cultural psychology and the neuroscience of culture (Rule, Freeman, & Ambady, 2013). *Culture and Brain*, a journal that began publication in 2013, is evidence of the scientific interest in, and even the legitimacy of, the field of cultural neuroscience. Differences in culture are echoed in changes of neural activity. Neuronal plasticity is thought to covary with variations in cultural environments. Cultural neuroscience is an emerging field whose research paradigm, according to Chiao, Cheon, Pornpattananangkul, Mrazek, and Blizinsky (2009), investigates the interactions among situation, ontogeny, and phylogeny, and thus is interested in the relationships among culture, mind, brain, and genes. They provide the example of their research, showing how "cultural values of individualism and collectivism modulate neural responses during self-processing" (p. 7). They further show how these cultural values influence the neural processing of affect and emotion.

In a functional neuroimaging (fMRI) investigation in cultural neuroscience, Immordino-Yang (2013) reported on her study comparing Chinese participants living in Beijing and Americans living in Los Angeles in their narrative responses to scenarios meant to elicit feelings of compassion and admiration. Whereas American participants reported embodied sensations when describing their reactions to the scenario, Chinese participants focused on the analysis of the situation. These reactions corresponded to fMRI findings of activation of lateral parietal somatosensory and frontal motor cortex brain regions in the American participants, which largely were absent in the Chinese participants. Differential recruitment of brain regions appears to vary among individuals from different cultures. In conclusion, Immordino-Yang observes, "The challenge will be to develop bridges that align neurobiological measures with psychocultural ones" (p. 45). In its infancy as a research tradition in the neurosciences, discovering the interactions of culture and brain functioning is key to understanding culture's influence on brain dysfunction.

By implication, the influence of culture on disturbed neural processing and the consequent phenomenology of neurological disorder can potentially be discovered. As we learn more about what facilitates recovery from brain dysfunction and actionable means by which to invoke neuroplasticity, it is likely that there will not be a "one-size-fits-all" methodology (i.e., singular etic solutions) in neurorehabilitation. Rather, neurorehabilitation may need to incorporate notions of cultural differences in the way processes of neuroplasticity are engaged via the specific types and methods of therapy. We are clearly not yet at the point where we can define such specific therapy.

EXPANDING CONSIDERATIONS OF CULTURE IN AN ECOLOGICAL SYSTEMS MODEL

Several models are available by which to conceptualize the influence of culture in human functioning. The most persuasive model is one that mirrors a dynamic, ecological system. A major figure in human developmental research was Urie Bronfenbrenner (1979/1981), whose famous work *The Ecology of Human Development* articulated an ecological systems view of human existence and development. Foundational to Bronfenbrenner's (1994) ecological perspective on development is his first proposition that "throughout the life course, human development takes place through processes of progressively more complex reciprocal interaction between an active, evolving biopsychological human organism and the persons, objects, and symbols in its immediate environment" (p. 38). Although a comprehensive discussion of Bronfenbrenner's model is beyond the scope of this chapter, the essential tiers of interacting levels in his ecological systems theory is relevant to our consideration of multicultural neurorehabilitation (Table 12.1).

Table 12.1 *Bronfenbrenner's Interacting Ecological Systems*

Ecological System	Description	Multicultural Neurorehabilitation Examples
Microsystem	Immediate social environment of the individual; interpersonal relations and social roles are of prominence; everyday activities within a specific setting	Impact of the immediate family system and inclusion in the neurorehabilitation setting; role expectations based on culture; rituals, beliefs, and cultural practices that may be integrated into care; cultural specific syndromes with correlative interpersonal behaviors and physical manifestations adds to conceptualization of care delivery; engagement in rehabilitation therapies may require special attention to cultural variables; peer group interactions, cross-generational cultural differences in the experience of disability by the individual

(*continued*)

Table 12.1 *Bronfenbrenner's Interacting Ecological Systems (continued)*

Ecological System	Description	Multicultural Neurorehabilitation Examples
Mesosystem	Connections that occur between two or more settings in which the individual participates	Transfer of gains from the neurorehabilitation setting to the home and community—potential challenges to carry over remedial and compensatory strategies to a different cultural environment at home and with the community
Exosystem	Connection between two or more settings in which the individual does not participate in one setting; that other setting influences the setting in which the individual does participate	Return to work or school environments, in which no accommodations are made for language translation in the person whose secondary language (English) may have been compromised secondary to severe brain injury, although such service was available in the neurorehabilitation unit and not problematic at home with bilingual parents. Parents' cultural community shuns the family secondary to stigma of having a child with a severe disability
Macrosystem	Overarching culture and subcultures, belief systems, bodies of knowledge that are embedded in the above systems; cultural meanings that structure the everyday life of the person	Western culture of individualism may conflict with collectivist worldviews that may create a disconnect in the patient's understanding of the sequelae and prognosis for a brain injury (microsystem), cause friction between a traditional family from a particular culture and treatment team interactions (mesosystem), impact support of the family by the immediate community of the person with brain injury after discharge from the hospital
Chronosystem	Impact of prior life events; life transitions; environment changes over time	A person is born and raised in a rural environment, marginal performances in school with truancy, is impacted by the September 11, 2001 terrorist attacks, enlists in the military, is influenced by military culture, with promotions to higher military ranks, commits to a career in the military

At the *microsystem* level, neurorehabilitation activities are seen as an interaction between staff and the treatment environment, and the particular cultural practices that are manifest on the rehabilitation unit or program. Much of what has been discussed in this book has considered the cultural dimension at a microsystem level in neurorehabilitation. In terms of the interactive nature of culture in the neurorehabilitation environment, Bronfenbrenner (1989) reminds us of the importance of not only intraindividual characteristics of the person, but he also proposed a tripartite model of interaction involving the "person-process-context" (p. 35). In this model, intraindividual characteristics interact with process variables, all placed within a specific environmental context. In neurorehabilitation this interaction could be conceptualized as follows:

1. The individual characteristics of a neurological disorder (e.g., traumatic brain injury) experienced by a particular *person* with that person's own makeup influenced by multiple cultures (e.g., race, ethnicity, gender, age, experience of disablement, sexual orientation) interacts with
2. The *process* of engaging in neurorehabilitation (e.g., rehabilitation therapies, patient–family–provider interpersonal interactions, rehabilitation team functioning), which also interacts with
3. The *context* within which neurorehabilitation services are delivered (e.g., intensive care unit, acute and postacute neurorehabilitation, type of hospital organization and hospital culture, third-party insurance determined length of stay).

At the *mesosystem* level, two or more specific environmental settings are the topics of consideration. The connection between the neurorehabilitation environment (and its unique culture of service delivery) and the home and community environment is important. The person with a brain injury resides in both environments, albeit at different times. From a multicultural perspective, generalizing and maintaining gains in the neurorehabilitation setting are paramount to carry over to the home, and they impact one's participation in the community. The *exosystem* refers to two or more settings, where the individual does not participate in at least one of them. However, that setting may still have a significant influence on the individual's functioning in the other setting. There can be indirect impact on the person with an acquired disability due to a neurological disorder if the larger cultural community's norms and mores do not permit acceptance of that individual, even if the acceptance involves health care interactions and recovering at home.

Macrosystems in Bronfenbrenner's model refer to larger, all-encompassing systems in which micro-, meso-, and exosystems are immersed. Bronfenbrenner (1994) refers to this level as "a given culture or subculture, with particular reference to the belief systems, bodies of knowledge, material resources, customs, lifestyles, opportunity structures, hazards, and life course options that are embedded in each of these broader systems" (p. 40). Some of the chapters in this book discuss common cultural themes that serve as an overarching macrosystem for the individual with a brain injury.

More recent to Bronfenbrenner's model is the inclusion of the *chronosystem*, which he describes as encompassing "change or consistency over time, not only in the characteristics of the person but also of the environment in which that person lives" (p. 40). Persons with brain injuries present to the neurorehabiliation setting with their own social-historical developmental history. This is similar to Luria's (1976) early research findings and conceptualization of cognitive development being a product of social-historical influence. Key events and cultural settings in that person's life (e.g., a person grows up in a predominantly politically conservative community with close connections to evangelical social groups, then moves to a highly culturally diverse urban setting for college) provide the backdrop to a further changed life secondary to brain injury.

Bronfenbrenner's insistence on an ecological perspective in analyzing questions of development is apropos for clinical rehabilitation service delivery models in combination with his tiered model of human development. It is befitting for this discussion relative to multicultural neurorehabilitation. To expand the consideration of culture in neurorehabilitation, the interaction between person–process–context variables and not singularly the intraindividual cultural characteristics of the person with neurological disorder needs to be the basis of conceptualizing effective neurorehabilitation services.

EXPANDING THE SCOPE AND DEPTH OF
CULTURAL COMPETENCY TRAINING

Common to many health care systems are staff training requirements at the onboarding phase of employment and mandatory in-service and continuing education offerings that focus on cultural competency. Indeed, psychology licensure requirements in many states include compulsory coursework or continuing education in diversity and culture. These efforts highlight the significance of cultural diversity knowledge in health care provision. However, few training efforts at the medical center or hospital organization level are focused on cultural competencies that are tailored to the treatment setting, type of treatment delivered, and context in which treatment occurs. For example, it is mostly incumbent upon the health care provider to obtain knowledge regarding diversity issues in a specific population (e.g., stroke or traumatic brain injury), with specific cultural characteristics (e.g., socioeconomic, regional or geographic culture), within a specific neurorehabilitation setting (e.g., postacute outpatient rehabilitation, residential neurobehavioral rehabilitation). In regard to neurorehabilitation, cultural competency training for rehabilitation staff should go beyond the mandatory online training that "checks the box" and fulfills an employee's requirement for diversity training per year. Cordoning off cultural diversity training as a standalone activity and as a general employee requirement can minimize its importance and in fact may be too general in its content to sufficiently prepare staff to engage in culturally sensitive and aware clinical practice.

Knowledge of cultural diversity is clearly important. Understanding the interplay between one's own behavior as a clinician and interactions with those of diverse cultural backgrounds is also critical. Lequerica and Krch (2014) note the following in this regard:

> Because one's own worldview impacts the way we see the world and interpret behavior, it is important to understand one's own ethnocentrism when dealing with a diverse population of patients with brain injury. . . . Taking into account cultural and contextual factors is an important step in developing culturally competent rehabilitation practices. (p. 645)

This aspect of cultural competency involves a process of ongoing self-evaluation and in vivo experience and supervision, and it requires constant vigilance to adjusting one's approach and responses depending on the particular clinical situation. Tervalon and Murray-Garcia (1998) refer to this as a process of maintaining "cultural humility," where being aware of the power differential that occurs in patient–provider interactions is critical.

It is still unclear exactly what cultural competence training should consist of. It is even less clear what should be involved in culturally competent neurorehabilitation care. It would be impossible for formal training to cover the multitude of cultural presentations that play a role in neurorehabilitation service delivery. However, some common themes and a working definition of cultural competence are good starting points. Many definitions of cultural competence exist. Sue (1998) said, "Cultural competence (along with the broader concept of multiculturalism) is the belief that people should not only appreciate and recognize other cultural groups but also be able to effectively work with them" (p. 440). Hence, one's knowledge is not required to be so vast as to be aware of all the nuances of each culture encountered, but effective service delivery (however outcome may be measured) is a marker of culturally competent treatment. Whaley and Davis (2007) understand cultural competency as including problem-solving skills that acknowledge cultural heritage and adaptation as dynamic factors in shaping human behavior. They also emphasize the element of internalization of cultural dynamics in one's clinical problem-solving practices. Such internalization is likely a competency that occurs over time and with experience, where mentoring and supervision are key aspects to build these problem-solving skills.

These skills cannot be easily taught, and most likely training of cultural competencies in the neurorehabilitation setting should involve a multimodal methodology (didactic, interactive, in vivo supervision) and be implemented in a developmental manner—from the classroom, to practice in the clinic, to competencies as a trainer/supervisor for some, and to a train-the-trainer model to extend expertise in multicultural neurorehabilitation. Much in the same way that cultural formulation is included as part of current psychiatric diagnostic nosology in the *Diagnostic and Statistical Manual of Mental Disorders*, 5th Edition (American Psychiatric Association, 2013), discussion of cultural formulation could be integrated into case conferences and interdisciplinary neurorehabilitation team discussions on patient care. Cultural competency training may need to be neurorehabilitation-setting specific. For example, one setting may have a higher proportion of Native American and Latino/Latina patients and families, whereas another setting may see more of those who are from a rural and older cohort, or where there are military service members and veterans who live closer to the neurorehabilitation facility. Other types of cultural training might cut across cohorts, such as training in religious and spirituality issues that might arise in the neurorehabilitation setting.

EXPANDING THE NOTION OF RECOVERY OF FUNCTION

In Luria's (1963) classic book *Restoration of Function After Brain Injury*, he discussed the specific mechanisms of recovery that form the basis of his approach to neuropsychological rehabilitation. He acknowledged that with brain tissue destruction come damaged brain functions that are irreversible. He also makes the case, based on research available at that time, for a "second component" of brain dysfunction that he states "under certain conditions, may be reversible" (p. 1). There may be spontaneous recovery of temporarily suppressed brain function, and similarly he talks of the influences on "mediator metabolism" (p. 9) and the idea of facilitating synaptic conduction via what was implicated to be neuropharmacological solutions. Luria also discussed the importance of restoring brain function by what he called an adjustment of the "mental orientation" (p. 24), citing examples of how this was evident in certain prolonged postconcussion syndromes. In this situation, he discussed the implications of psychological mechanisms of the inhibition of function. The rest of his book is devoted to his theory of the reorganization of the functional systems as a general framework to restore brain function. This appears to represent a large portion of his life's work in neuropsychological rehabilitation.

Much of the work in neurorehabilitation, especially in the acute phase of recovery after neurological injury, is spent in the restoration of function, as well as ways to compensate for functional impairments. This represents the neurorehabilitation specialist's core job. In advancing the field of multicultural neurorehabilitation, the restoration of function and developing compensatory strategies for dysfunction are crucial, but they may not be sufficient in themselves because of the cultural context of the patient's situation (e.g., Bronfenbrenner's model). These ideas may in fact apply to neurorehabiliation in general but are seen here as critical when examining the enterprise of neurorehabilitation from a cultural perspective.

EXPANSION OF QUALITY OF LIFE PARAMETERS

It is common in acute and postacute neurorehabilitation for the rehabilitation team, usually in coordination with the patient and family, to determine outcome goals that in turn set the agenda for rehabilitation therapies. It would be interesting to see how much variation truly exists when comparing interdisciplinary goals across neurorehabilitation settings. In many settings, interdisciplinary goals appear to be linked to the functional pathology presented by the patient, and with possibly lower priority assigned to goals that align with the patient's life circumstances. A patient's life circumstances are nested within a rich social-historical developmental background, with converging cultural elements. Yet, rehabilitation goals may appear somewhat generic across patient populations. Paternalism in defining goals *for* the patient may be a subtle, and sometimes not so subtle, process in neurorehabilitation. Although Luria was focused on the restoration of brain function, as we should be, neurorehabilitation may also require an examination of what quality-of-life goals may be relevant for a particular patient, depending on his or her cultural background. Negotiating goals for what might be achievable and what might not be logistically (e.g., due to length of stay limitations) or physiologically possible (e.g. full restoration of anterograde memory in a patient with severe anoxic brain injury) is essential for effective and relevant neurorehabilitative care.

Case Vignette: A patient (who did not have a brain injury) was a park ranger whose job involved traveling to remote areas of the state he lived in. He often had to struggle through mud and snow in adverse weather conditions. He presented with what was formerly called a "hysterical gait" disorder; no physiological pathology could be found to account for his complete inability to walk. He had recently experienced a trauma and a minor lower extremity injury, to which he presented with a catastrophic psychological response, fearing that he would no longer be able to work and provide for his family.

The physician team leader, who was very familiar with hysterical gait disorder, organized the team to gradually increase this patient's walking ability in a systematic and graded behavioral manner. He also brought in a rehabilitation psychologist to work on individual and couples therapy with the patient. The physical therapist felt the patient made appropriate gains (he was able to walk inside the parallel bars) and was planning on an imminent discharge from treatment. The physician, somewhat alarmed, instructed the physical therapist and occupational therapist to take the patient out to a muddy area near the treatment facility and have him walk with snowshoes—an example of ecologically valid treatment. This latter tactic proved to be significantly therapeutic, because the patient's demeanor, cognitive view of the future, and stated quality of life improved markedly. Many cultural aspects come to mind when reviewing what might account for his conception of quality of life: being the family breadwinner and his concept of masculinity as evidenced by his ability to financially provide for his family, his upbringing in a rural environment and the social expectations of the physical independence that comes along with that social history, and his life career and identity as a park ranger. The particular trauma likely had psychological significance based at least in part on his social-historical heritage (in Bronfenbrenner's typology, the *chronosystem*) and cultural identity. If his rehabilitation had ended as soon as he could walk in the parallel bars, the risk of future disability could have been very high.

THE CONCEPT OF HEALTH–QUALITY OF LIFE

The World Health Organization (WHO) and specifically the World Health Organization Quality of Life (WHOQOL) Group (see Power, Bullinger, Harper, & WHOQOL Group, 1999) developed a comprehensive measure to assess universal (etic) aspects of the concept of quality of life. Their work led to the development of the WHOQOL-100, a measure that assesses 24 facets of quality of life, represented under the four larger categories of physical, psychological, social relationship, and environment domains. The measure was developed in 15 international locations, representing 14 separate countries (two cities in India were in the development sample), totaling 4,802 participants. The four higher-order domains all correlated highly with an overall dimension of quality of life. The authors of the WHOQOL-100 purport the measure to be appropriate across multiple cultures to measure health–quality of life. The concept of the measure may provide common ground that could be applied in neurorehabilitation settings to gauge and help determine culturally relevant rehabilitation goals. The caveat, of course, is that this is an international measure and perhaps should not be dogmatically applied without local analysis of cultural nuances that may need to be considered in the individual case (emic aspect).

AN EXISTENTIAL-CULTURAL VIEW OF CHANGED IDENTITY

Suffering is a universal phenomenon. It is an experience that is closely allied to the perception of quality of life and immersed within the totality of the existence of the patient with a neurological disorder. As Cassell (2004) so aptly states in his book *The Nature of Suffering and the Goals of Medicine*, "Doctors do not treat diseases, they treat patients" (p. 19). He goes on to talk about suffering as a highly individualized and personal experience, only known in its fullest extent by the person who is suffering. Suffering can also be attached to any aspect of personhood. In his view, Cassell defines suffering as what occurs when "an impending destruction of the person is perceived; it continues until the threat of disintegration has passed or until the integrity of the person can be restored" (p. 32).

In the context of multicultural neurorehabilitation, it is therefore important to understand what suffering means to that individual and ensure that the health care provider's view of suffering is from an *insider's* point of view. The individual's cultural heritage and the "leading edge" aspects of culture that may be relevant in the situation must be taken into account when ascertaining that patient's suffering. It may be that the suffering is due to a loss of identity in the patient's ethnic cultural community. The stigma of having a brain injury while living in a small rural community may account for the suffering. A person may be suffering because his or her socioeconomic status (e.g., wage-earning potential) is threatened by the onset of a neurological disorder. A threat can occur even within the family when a brain injury changes a person's social role and responsibilities where these are held in high esteem in a particular culture. For example, once the author met with an Asian father to conduct psychoeducation and provide support and advice on how to care for his son who had been diagnosed with schizophrenia. The father, clearly shaken by the news, stated, "My son is garbage, just garbage." One could easily frown upon this father for being uncaring, yet in this Asian father, there was perceived loss of his first son and loss of his son's position in the family. The father likely experienced this situation as a significant level of suffering—a perceived threat to his position as the patriarch, seeing himself as having failed in that role in some manner. In certain cultures, one could easily see how a change in identity can occur not just in the individual with brain injury but also within the extended social network. Comprehending the experience of suffering in the patient, family, and social network, in all of its cultural dimensions and nuances, is a clearly difficult clinical task, and even a challenging human task. In defining what the term *experience* means in the context of cross-cultural concepts of suffering, Kleinman and Kleinman (1991) stated the following:

> Experience may . . . be thought of as the intersubjective medium of social transactions in local moral words. It is the outcome of cultural categories and social structures interacting with psychophysiological processes such that a mediating world is constituted. (p. 277)

Rebuilding self-identity is a universal goal in neurorehabilitation, and the way this is achieved may require cultural interpretations of human behavior and a cultural view of the individual experience of suffering. It is not enough to assume that improvement of function is sufficient to the task of the relief of suffering and the facilitation of quality of life from the patient's perspective. Goldstein (1939/1995) said it well when speaking of changed self-identity after brain injury:

> Every recovery with residual defect entails some loss in "essential nature." There is no real substitution. (p. 334)

REFERENCES

American College of Physicians. (2010). *Racial and ethnic disparities in health care, updated 2010.* Philadelphia, PA: American College of Physicians.

American Psychiatric Association. (2013). *Diagnostic and statistical manual of mental disorders* (5th ed.). Washington, DC: American Psychiatric Association.

Ardila, A. (2013). A new neuropsychology for the XXI century. *Archives of Clinical Neuropsychology, 28,* 751–762.

Bronfenbrenner, U. (1979/1981). *The ecology of human development: Experiments by nature and design.* Cambridge, MA: Harvard University Press.

Bronfenbrenner, U. (1989). Interacting systems in human development. Research paradigms: Present and future. In N. Bolger, A. Caspi, G. Downey, &

M. Moorehouse (Eds.), *Persons in context: Developmental processes* (pp. 25–49). Cambridge, MA: Cambridge University Press.

Bronfenbrenner, U. (1994). Ecological models of human development. In *International encyclopedia of education*, vol. 3 (2nd ed.). Oxford, UK: Pergammon/Elsevier Science. (Reprinted from *Readings on the development of children*, pp. 37–43, by M. Gauvain, & M. Cole, Eds., 2nd ed., 1993, New York: Freeman.)

Cassell, E. J. (2004). *The nature of suffering and the goals of medicine* (2nd ed.). New York, NY: Oxford University Press.

Cheung, F. M., van de Vijver, F. J. R., & Leong, F. T. L. (2011). Toward a new approach to the study of personality in culture. *American Psychologist, 66*, 593–603.

Chiao, J. Y., Cheon, B. K., Pornpattananangkul, N., Mrazek, A. J., & Blizinsky, K. D. (2013). Cultural neuroscience: Progress and promise. *Psychological Inquiry, 24*, 1–19.

Christensen, A.-L., & Uzzell, B. P. (Eds.). (2000). *International handbook of neuropsychological rehabilitation*. New York, NY: Springer Publishing.

Fletcher-Janzen, E., Strickland, T. L., & Reynolds, C. R. (Eds.). (2000). *Handbook of cross-cultural neuropsychology*. New York, NY: Kluwer Academic/Plenum Publishers.

Goldstein, K. (1939/1995). *The organism: A holistic approach to derived biology from pathological data in man*. New York, NY: Zone Books.

Immordino-Yang, M. H. (2013). Studying the effects of culture by integrating neuroscientific with ethnographic approaches. *Psychological Inquiry, 24*, 42–46.

Kleinman, A., & Kleinman, J. (1991). Suffering and its professional transformation: Toward an ethnography of interpersonal experience. *Culture, Medicine, and Psychiatry, 15*, 275–301.

Lequerica, A., & Krch, D. (2014). Issues of cultural diversity in acquired brain injury (ABI) rehabilitation. *NeuroRehabilitation, 34*, 645–653.

Luria, A. R. (1963). *Restoration of function after brain injury*. New York, NY: The Macmillan Company.

Niemeier, J. P., & Arango-Lasprilla, C. (2007). Toward improved rehabilitation services for ethnically diverse survivors of traumatic brain injury. *Journal of Head Trauma Rehabilitation, 22*, 75–84.

Niemeier, J. P., Burnett, D. M., & Whitaker, D. A. (2003). Cultural competence in the multidisciplinary rehabilitation setting: Are we falling short of meeting needs? *Archives of Physical Medicine and Rehabilitation, 84*, 1240–1245.

Power, M., Bullinger, M., Harper, A., & World Health Organization Quality of Life Group. (1999). The World Health Organization WHOQOL-100: Tests of the universality of quality of life in 15 different cultural groups worldwide. *Health Psychology, 18*, 495–505.

Rule, N. O., Freeman, J. B., & Ambady, N. (2013). Culture in social neuroscience: A review. *Social Neuroscience, 8*, 3–10.

Smedley, B. D., Stith, A. Y., Nelson, A. R., Committee on Understanding and Eliminating Racial and Ethnic Disparities in Health Care. (2003). *Unequal treatment: Confronting racial and ethnic disparities in health care.* Washington, DC: National Academy of Sciences, National Academies Press.

Sue, S. (1998). In search of cultural competence in psychotherapy and counseling. *American Psychologist, 53,* 440–448.

Tervalon, M., & Murray-Garcia, J. (1998). Cultural humility versus cultural competence: A critical distinction in defining physician training outcomes in multicultural education. *Journal of Health Care for the Poor and Underserved, 9,* 117–125.

Uzzell, B. P., Ponton, M., & Ardila, A. (Eds.). (2007). *International handbook of cross-cultural neuropsychology.* Mahwah, NJ: Lawrence Erlbaum Associates, Inc.

Whaley, A. L., & Davis, K. E. (2007). Cultural competence and evidence-based practice in mental health services: A complementary perspective. *American Psychologist, 62,* 563–574.

AFTERWORD

It is only fitting to end this book by citing the work of Dr. Tony Wong, to whose memory and legacy this volume was dedicated. I had the distinct honor of working with him on a prior book chapter (Uomoto & Wong, 2000) that addressed the issue of multicultural aspects of brain injury rehabilitation. He examined the aftereffects of brain injury in a cultural context by delineating different levels of analysis and the corresponding attention that should be paid to multicultural specificity in patient services and family and support services. One quickly sees that as one examines the patient from a biopsychosocial standpoint: Beyond the physiological level of analysis, culture plays a moderate to critical role in case conceptualization and therefore in defining appropriate rehabilitation services. As noted earlier in this chapter, perhaps what is changing is that even at that physiological level, culture and its social-historical significance also must be considered.

In the meantime, his work and clinical pearls of wisdom remain timeless and practical. In one of his last written works (Wong, 2011), Dr. Wong wrote about the neuropsychology of Chinese Americans. At the end of that book chapter, as was characteristic of his other writings, he provided recommendations for the practicing clinician. Considerations of the socioeconomic status and history, as well as the primary language and dialect of the patient, were emphasized. The influence of culture on neuropsychological testing (and by implication for the goals of this book), neurorehabilitation care of the patient, was emphasized. Finally, sensitivity to the worldview of the patient was seen as critical. These recommendations by Dr. Wong, and at the end of this chapter and book, remain relevant and continue to be clinically influential for advancing the field of multicultural neurorehabilitation.

REFERENCES

Uomoto, J. M., & Wong, T. M. (2000). Multicultural perspectives on the neuropsychology of brain injury assessment and rehabilitation. In E. Fletcher-Janzen, T. L. Strickland, & C. R. Reynolds (Eds.), *Handbook of cross-cultural neuropsychology* (pp. 169–184). New York, NY: Kluwer Academic/Plenum Publishers.

Wong, T. M. (2011). Neuropsychology of Chinese Americans. In D. E. M. Fujii (Ed.), *The neuropsychology of Asian Americans* (pp. 29–46). New York, NY: Taylor & Francis.

INDEX